A Practical Approach to Regional Anesthesia

Fourth Edition

MICHAEL F. MULROY, MD
Faculty Anesthesiologist
Virginia Mason Medical Center
Seattle, Washington

CHRISTOPHER M. BERNARDS, MD
Faculty Anestheiologist
Virginia Mason Medical Center
Seattle, Washington

SUSAN B. MCDONALD, MD
Faculty Anestheiologist
Virginia Mason Medical Center
Seattle, Washington

FRANCIS V. SALINAS, MD
Faculty Anesthesiologist
Virginia Mason Medical Center
Seattle, Washington

Wolters Kluwer | Lippincott Williams & Wilkins
Health

Philadelphia • Baltimore • New York • London
Buenos Aires • Hong Kong • Sydney • Tokyo

Acquisitions Editor: Brian Brown
Developmental Editor: Nicole Dernoski
Managing Editor: Grace Caputo
Marketing Manager: Angela Panetta/Lisa Parry
Project Manager: Paula C. Williams
Designer: Doug Smock
Production Services: Laserwords Private Limited, Chennai, India

Fourth Edition

351 West Camden Street
Baltimore, MD 21201

530 Walnut Street
Philadelphia, PA 19106

Printed in China

9 8 7 6 5 4 3 2 1

Library of Congress Cataloging-in-Publication Data
A practical approach to regional anesthesia / Michael F. Mulroy . . . [et al.].—4th ed.
p. ; cm.
Rev. ed. of: Regional anesthesia / Michael F. Mulroy. 3rd ed. c2002.
Includes bibliographical references and index.
ISBN 978-0-7817-6854-2
1. Conduction anesthesia—Handbooks, manuals, etc. I. Mulroy, Michael F. II. Mulroy, Michael F. Regional anesthesia.
[DNLM: 1. Anesthesia, Conduction—Handbooks. WO 231 P8953 2008]
RD84.M85 2008
617.9′64—dc22

2008003349

❖

To my parents who made everything possible and to Nathan and Elizabeth who make it all worthwhile.

CMB

I would like to thank my wife Joanne and children, Alex, Brandon, and Cameryn for their love and support. I would be remiss if I did not also express my heartfelt gratitude to Dr. Mike Mulroy who has been my teacher, mentor and role-model, colleague, and most of all a great friend.

FVS

To my parents, my husband, and to all my mentors and colleagues at Virginia Mason, especially Dr. Mulroy, for all their encouragement and support.

SBM

To my family for their patience, but especially to all those colleagues, residents and faculty, at Virginia Mason who have created and nourished the tradition of regional anesthesia and its teaching for so many years.

MFM

Contents

Contributor

Kathleen L. Larkin, MD
Acting Assistant Professor
Department of Anesthesiology
Children's Hospital and Regional Medical Center
Seattle, Washington

Preface

A Practical Approach to Regional Anesthesia is in fact the fourth iteration of *Regional Anesthesia: An Illustrated Procedural Guide,* which was conceived to build on the foundation created in the anesthesiology department of the Virginia Mason Medical Center by Daniel C. Moore, MD, the author of the second major text of regional anesthesia in North America. Dr. Moore's book remained a valued resource for many decades after its original publication in 1953. The *Regional Anesthesia* manuals have attempted to continue the tradition that he and the Department of Anesthesia at Virginia Mason established and that continues to this day.

The early practitioners in the department could have had no idea of how extensive the use of regional anesthesia would become, nor of how their vision of superior perioperative pain relief would have been confirmed by many studies and expanded by recent developments in pharmacology and equipment. Long-acting local anesthetics, especially when used in combination with opioids for neuraxial analgesia and in peripheral nerve infusions, clearly provide superior pain relief in the immediate and extended postoperative period. The application of these techniques has been enhanced and expanded by the continuing development of new and improved needles, catheters, and nerve localization devices.

The use of regional techniques is a heritage worth preserving and expanding. Unfortunately, many practitioners are not exposed to extensive training in regional techniques during their residencies and are reluctant to attempt these advantageous methods in private practice because of insecurities about success and the pressures of time and productivity in the modern medical environment. Fortunately for all of us, multiple educational resources, such as the American Society of Regional Anesthesia and Pain Medicine, and many centers of regional anesthesia expertise have emerged in North America. Moreover, useful atlases and exhaustive texts on the subject are also now available. Nevertheless, there continues to be a demand and a use for a straightforward manual such as this one. This book attempts to focus on the practical considerations for choosing and applying regional anesthesia, and emphasizes the clinical application of these techniques in an efficient and effective manner.

A Practical Approach to Regional Anesthesia does not aspire to be a definitive reference source. We have not included every contribution to the art and science of regional anesthesia, and we apologize to those authors and researchers who have added to our knowledge but whose specific contributions are not acknowledged by name. Nor does this handbook pretend to be a definitive atlas of anatomy. There are many such textbooks available, and readers are certainly encouraged to use them. This book *does* aspire, however, to be a useful and practical manual, and we hope that it will add to your understanding, dexterity, and comfort with the regional anesthetic techniques that offer patients so many advantages.

Changes in format and content are apparent in this fourth edition. With the expanding body of knowledge in regional anesthesia, the need for multiple authors became inevitable. This has no doubt led both to some repetition between chapters and to some differences in the style of presentation. Nevertheless, we have attempted to provide a consistent and balanced approach throughout. To improve readability and speed access to information, the text has been presented in an outline format. And to enhance the usefulness of the illustrations, the number of figures has increased, with the addition of many new and revised images, and nearly all have been reproduced in full color.

Most importantly, the content has been adjusted to reflect current practices. The chapters on obstetric anesthesia and management of chronic pain have been deleted since these areas have expanded so extensively that they require separate textual approaches, of which several such are available. Those deletions enabled the inclusion of substantially expanded coverage of recent developments in nerve localization, especially the use of ultrasound. While this new technique is not yet simple or economical enough to replace all other techniques, it appears to have significant advantages in nerve localization and potentially in safety that certainly merit the attention we have given it. We hope that the readers find it equally useful and advantageous in their practices.

While the textual material is primarily the responsibility of the four authors, we must recognize our other contributors, especially our colleagues at the Virginia Mason Medical Center, who continue to stimulate and support each of us in our practice of regional anesthesia. Many of the ideas for techniques and applications have come from this group and certainly will continue to evolve with their input in the future. This includes our surgical colleagues and our residents, who are constantly stimulating us to improve our techniques, standardize our procedures, and share them in an educational format. We thank them all. We especially thank Dr. Kathleen Larkin from the Children's Hospital Medical Center in Seattle for her kind revision of the chapter on pediatric regional anesthesia. And, of course, the book would have not made it to press without the constant editorial management of Grace Caputo of Dovetail Content Solutions and the oversight of Brian Brown at Lippincott Williams & Wilkins and we also are indebted again to Jennifer Smith for her skillful and insightful updating of the artwork. But we owe by far the most gratitude to our patient and accepting families, who have supported the long hours of additional work that made this text possible.

We hope you will find *A Practical Approach to Regional Anesthesia* to be a useful and relied-on manual in your anesthesia practice, and that it will encourage you to continually improve upon these techniques and to apply them even more widely to our perioperative patients to provide them the greatest advantages in analgesia and anesthesia.

Michael F. Mulroy, MD

Preface to Previous Edition

THIS IS A PRACTICAL MANUAL of regional anesthesia for both students and practitioners. It is a "how to" guide for common regional techniques to be used and referred to in the operating room. It provides information to justify the reasons and purposes of the techniques. It also provides the pharmacologic and physiologic data to support the choices of drugs and doses and to avoid common complications. The manual presents commonly performed techniques for all regions of the body, while discussing their application in the subspecialty areas of pediatrics, obstetrics, and pain management. In a practical manual of this breadth, however, encyclopedic depth is not the goal. For definitive texts on any of the subjects discussed, the reader should consult standard texts and original reports listed in the references at the end of each chapter.

Familiarity with the first five chapters of the manual supplements the procedural chapters that follow. Discussions of premedication, equipment, and common complications are presented in this introductory section, but are referred to only briefly in subsequent chapters. The discussions of specific techniques are organized into chapters on axial blockade and techniques involving the upper and lower extremities, head, and trunk. In addition to detailed step-by-step description of block techniques, each chapter reviews relevant anatomy, drug considerations, and specific complications. The final chapters deal with the application of regional techniques in the subspecialty areas of pediatrics, obstetrics, and acute and chronic pain management. Greater detail is available in subspecialty texts, but the practitioner who is called on only occasionally to provide pain management or pediatric regional anesthesia will find helpful guidelines in these final chapters. These chapters will be particularly useful to the novice.

The manual is designed to be used as a practical guide where anesthesia is performed. Successful regional anesthesia, however, requires more than the use of a simple map at the time of the procedure. The reader, especially the novice, is encouraged to review the anatomy in more detailed standard anatomy texts and atlases before approaching the patient. Three-dimensional visualization and appreciation of anatomy is essential for successful regional anesthesia, and review of the landmarks on a skeleton or a live model is helpful. Knowledge of the drugs to be used and their potential complications is also essential before approaching the patient.

The techniques described here are those generally used at the Virginia Mason Medical Center. Where scientific data are available to substantiate a preference for a specific approach or technique, they are included in the references. Much of regional anesthesia, however, remains an art. Personal experience and preference still dictate many of the approaches described. There is substantial variation, even within our department, in the performance of common techniques. All of the individual variations cannot be included, but it would be unfortunate if medicine of any kind were practiced by the use of a "cookbook" formula accepted by all. The art of regional anesthesia is dynamic, as reflected in the new drugs, equipment, and techniques included in this new edition and there is no doubt that further changes lie ahead.

This manual would not have been possible without the contributions and support of the entire Anesthesia Department of the Virginia Mason Clinic. The final product reflects the contributions of each staff member (though not necessarily expressing opinions that everyone will agree with!). The resident staff and the graduates have also made invaluable suggestions regarding content and clarity over the years; as always, we learn as much from our students as they learn from us. Specific appreciation goes to Linda Jo Rice, MD, for her contribution on the application of regional techniques to the pediatric population, which we do not serve at Virginia Mason, and to James Helman, MD, for his expertise in approaching the management of chronic pain. I thank Iris Nichols for her patient efforts in providing the original illustrations that support the text, and Jennifer Smith for her additions and modifications in the art for this edition. Finally, Craig Percy deserves the credit for nurturing this third edition. It is hoped that these efforts have produced a manual that will help the novice and graduate alike in improving their regional anesthesia skills.

Michael F. Mulroy, MD

1 Local Anesthetics

Christopher M. Bernards

I. History

Local anesthetics are compounds that produce reversible block of nerve action potentials. A number of compounds with local anesthetic activity occur in nature including cocaine and eugenol derived from plants, saxitoxin derived from algae (dinoflagellates), and tetrodotoxin derived from several fish species in the family *tetraodontiformes* (although it is actually a *Pseudoalteromonas* bacterium that produces the toxin within the fish). Although undoubtedly used for centuries by native peoples, the first reported medicinal use of a drug as a local anesthetic occurred in 1884 when German medical intern Carl Koller reported (by proxy) the use of cocaine he had received from Sigmund Freud to anesthetize the eye by topical application.

Because of the potential toxicity of cocaine, chemists began trying to synthesize a substitute for cocaine in the early 1890s. This effort resulted in the synthesis of procaine by Einhorn et al. in 1905. All local anesthetics currently available for regional anesthesia are effectively variations of procaine.

II. Chemistry

A. Structure. All local anesthetics used for nerve block consist of a hydrophobic aromatic ring connected to a tertiary amine group by a hydrocarbon chain (Figure 1.1). Hydrocarbon chain length varies between 6 and 9 angstroms; longer or shorter chains result in ineffective drugs. Benzocaine, which is used only for topical anesthesia, lacks the tertiary amine group and does not have a hydrogen that is exchangeable at physiologic pH ($pK_a = 3.5$).

B. Ester versus amide. Local anesthetics are divided into esters and amides depending on whether the hydrocarbon chain is joined to the benzene-derived moiety by an ester or an amide linkage (Figure 1.1). The type of linkage is important in determining how drugs are metabolized (see Chapter 2 [Section VII]).

C. Chirality. Many local anesthetics have at least one asymmetric carbon atom and therefore exist as two or more enantiomers. Most are used clinically as racemic mixtures containing both enantiomers. Exceptions are ropivacaine and levobupivacaine, which are supplied as single enantiomers because the clinically used enantiomer is more potent and less toxic than the racemate.

III. Physicochemical properties

A. Acid–base. Because the tertiary amine group can bind a proton to become a positively charged quaternary amine (Figure 1.1), all local anesthetics (except benzocaine) exist as a weak acid–base pair in solution. The ability to generate a positive charge is critical to sodium channel blockade (see Section IV.E).

1. pK_a (Table 1.1). In solution, local anesthetics exist in both the uncharged form (base) and positively charged form (conjugate acid). The percentage of each species present in a particular solution or tissue depends on the pH of the solution/tissue and can be calculated from the Henderson-Hasselbalch equation:

$pK_a = pH - \log [base]/[acid]$

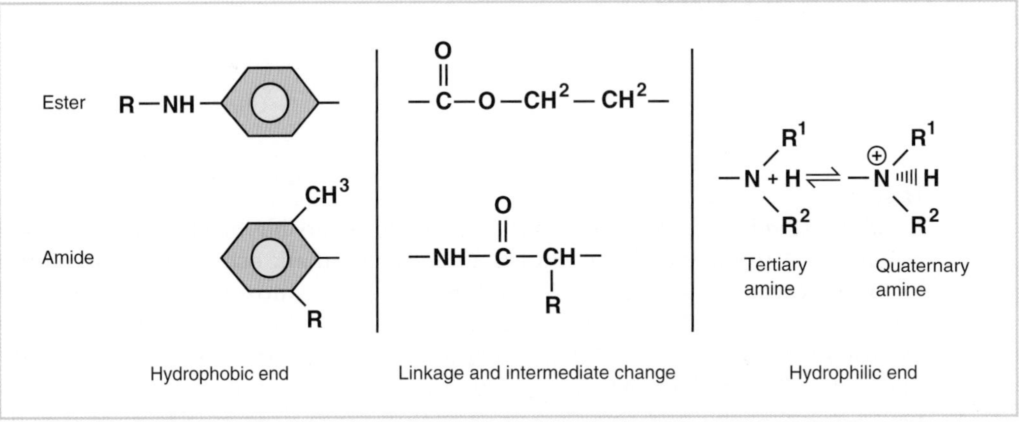

Figure 1.1. Typical structures of local ester and amine anesthetic molecules.

where
pH is the solution or tissue pH and
pK_a is the pH at which half the local anesthetic molecules are in the base form and half in the acid form.

The value for pK_a is unique for any local anesthetic and is a measure of the tendency for the molecule to accept a proton when in the base form or to donate a proton when in the acid form. Most local anesthetics have a pK_a between 7.5 and 9.0.

Because local anesthetics are supplied as unbuffered acidic solutions (pH = 3.5–5.0), there are approximately 1,000 to 100,000 times more molecules in the charged form than the uncharged form (which helps to keep the local anesthetic in solution). Because extracellular tissue pH is approximately 7.4, the proportion of molecules in the charged form decreases by a factor of somewhere between 500 and 10,000 when injected into tissue. For example, because mepivacaine has a pK_a of 7.6, there would be 1,000 times as many molecules in the protonated form (weak acid) than in the uncharged form in a commercially supplied solution at pH 4.6. Once injected into tissue with a pH of 7.4, many of the charged mepivacaine molecules would "donate" their protons so that only approximately 1.6 times as many will be charged as uncharged. As discussed in Section IV.E, it is critical to local anesthetic action that they are capable of transitioning between the charged and uncharged forms.

B. **Hydrophobicity** (Table 1.1). Local anesthetics vary in the degree to which they dissolve in aqueous (hydrophilic) versus lipid (hydrophobic) environments. Differences in hydrophobicity are primarily the result of differences in the types of chemical groups bound to the tertiary amine (Figure 1.1). The charged form of any individual local anesthetic is more hydrophilic than is the corresponding uncharged form. Hydrophobic character is often, and inaccurately, referred to as *lipid solubility*. Greater hydrophobicity correlates with greater local anesthetic potency and duration of action (see Section V.A and Chapter 2).

1. Hydrophobicity is determined by adding the local anesthetic to a vessel containing two immiscible liquids—an aqueous buffer and a hydrophobic "lipid." Lipids are usually chosen in an effort to mimic the hydrophobic character of cellular lipid membranes; octanol, olive oil, and n-heptane are

Table 1.1 Physicochemical properties of local anesthetics

Drug (brand name)	Type (year introduced)	Chemical structure	Relative *in vitro* potency Rat sciatic nerve	pK_a	Partition coefficient[a]	Plasma protein binding
Cocaine	Ester	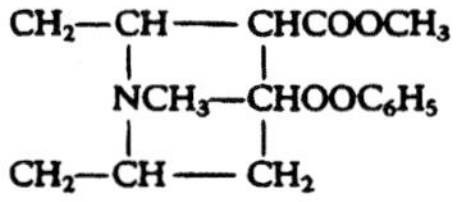 CH_2—CH—CHCOOCH_3 NCH_3—CHOOC_6H_5 CH_2—CH—CH_2	—	8.6	—	92
Procaine (Novocaine)	Ester (1905)	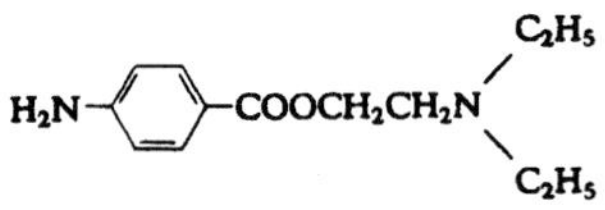 H_2N–[ring]–COOCH_2CH_2N(C_2H_5)(C_2H_5)	1	8.9	1.7	5.8
Benzocaine	Ester (1900)	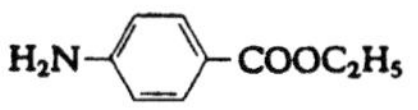 H_2N–[ring]–COOC_2H_5	—	3.5	81	—
Tetracaine (Pontocaine)	Ester (1930)	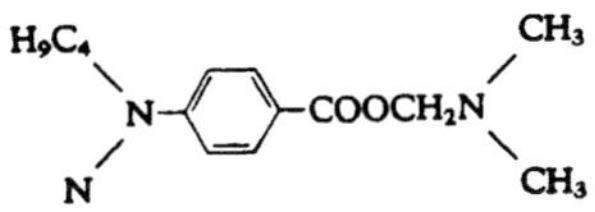 H_9C_4, N–N–[ring]–COOCH_2N(CH_3)(CH_3)	8	8.5	221	75.6
2-Chloroprocaine (Nesacaine)	Ester (1952)	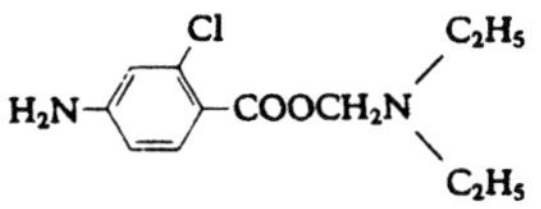 H_2N–[ring(Cl)]–COOCH_2N(C_2H_5)(C_2H_5)	1	8.7	9.0	NA
Lidocaine (Xylocaine)	Amide (1944)	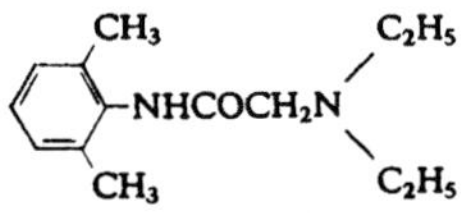 [ring(CH_3)(CH_3)]–NHCOCH_2N(C_2H_5)(C_2H_5)	2	7.72	2.4	64.3
Mepivacaine (Carbocaine, Polocaine)	Amide (1957)	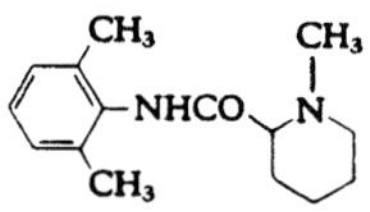 [ring(CH_3)(CH_3)]–NHCO–[piperidine N–CH_3]	2	7.6	21	77.5
Prilocaine (Citanest)	Amide (1960)	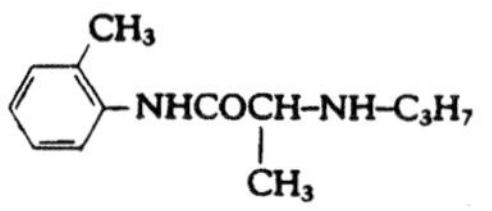 [ring(CH_3)]–NHCOCH(CH_3)–NH–C_3H_7	2	7.7	25	55
Ropivacaine (Naropin)	Amide (1995)	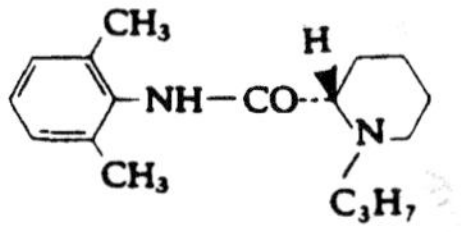 [ring(CH_3)(CH_3)]–NH–CO–[H, piperidine N–C_3H_7]	4	8.1	115	95
Bupivacaine (Marcaine, Sensorcaine) Levobupivacaine (Chirocaine)	Amide (1963)	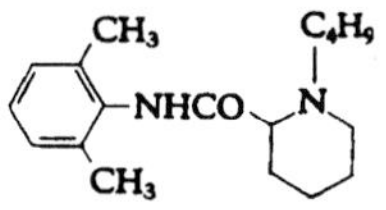 [ring(CH_3)(CH_3)]–NHCO–[piperidine N–C_4H_9]	8	8.1	346	95.6
Etidocaine (Duranest)	Amide (1972)	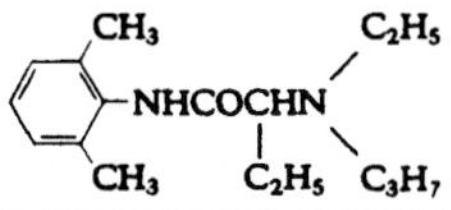 [ring(CH_3)(CH_3)]–NHCOCH(C_2H_5)N(C_2H_5)(C_3H_7)	8	7.74	800	94

[a]Octanol: buffer pH 7.4.

(Adapted from Covino BG, Vasallo HG. *Local anesthetic: mechanism of action and clinical use*. New York: Grune & Stratton, 1976; deJong RH. *Local anesthetics*. St. Louis: Mosby–Year Book, 1993; Cousing MJ, Bridenbaugh PO. Neural blockade and management of pain, Philadelphia: Lippincott Williams & Wilkins, 1998.)

commonly used lipids. The local anesthetic is added to the vessel and the vessel is agitated to "mix" the two liquids. The solution is allowed to sit and the liquid phases to separate. After separation, the concentration of local anesthetic is measured in the aqueous phase and in the lipid phase. The resultant ratio of the concentrations is the "distribution coefficient," which is often inappropriately simplified as the "lipid solubility."

2. Importantly, the distribution coefficient so determined will vary greatly depending on:
   a. The **pH of the aqueous phase** because this will determine what percentage of the local anesthetic is charged (more hydrophobic) or uncharged (more hydrophilic). A pH of 7.4 is common and the resulting distribution coefficient is termed the *partition coefficient*. The distribution coefficient is commonly measured using the local anesthetic base and an aqueous phase pH significantly above the drug's pK_a, so all of the local anesthetic is effectively uncharged.
   b. The **lipid** used. Different lipids will yield very different distribution coefficients and the values determined in one solvent system cannot be compared with those determined in a different system. Referring to a drug's "lipid solubility" without defining the system in which it was determined is incomplete information.
   c. The **form of the local anesthetic** (i.e., base or salt). Consequently, tables that simply list a local anesthetic's "lipid solubility" without information as to how it was determined are not particularly useful. In Table 1.1, local anesthetic partition coefficients are reported for chloride salts of local anesthetics in octanol and buffer at pH 7.4 (octanol: $buffer_{7.4}$).

C. **Protein binding.** Binding to plasma proteins varies between 5% and 95% (Table 1.1). In general, more hydrophobic drugs have higher protein binding. In fact, properties sometimes attributed to a drug's degree of "protein binding" are probably actually related to their hydrophobicity. Whether plasma protein binding has any relationship to tissue protein binding is unknown and should not be assumed.

1. α_1-Acid glycoprotein and albumin are the primary plasma proteins to which local anesthetics bind. Binding to these proteins is pH dependent and binding decreases during acidosis, because the number of available binding sites decreases in an acidic environment.
2. In plasma, it is the **unbound** or "free" fraction of local anesthetic that is capable of leaving plasma to enter organs like the brain or heart. Consequently, it is the free fraction that is responsible for systemic toxicity.
   a. Patients with low plasma protein concentrations (e.g., malnutrition, cirrhosis, and nephrotic syndrome) are at greater risk of systemic toxicity than are patients with normal plasma protein concentrations and patients with high plasma protein concentrations (e.g., some cancers) are afforded a degree of protection (1).

IV. The sodium channel and nerve conduction

A. **Sodium channel structure** (Figure 1.2). The mammalian sodium channel is a **transmembrane protein** composed of three subunits that form a voltage-sensitive, sodium-selective channel through the neuronal membrane. To date, ten distinct human genes coding for ten structurally different sodium channels have been identified. Different isoforms are expressed in different tissues (e.g., muscle, heart, central nervous system, and peripheral nervous system). It is possible that there are mutations that confer either increased or decreased sensitivity to local anesthetics [in fact, such induced mutations have been produced in experimental systems (2,3)], but to date none have been identified clinically.

B. Conduction. At rest, neurons maintain an electrochemical gradient across their membranes because Na^+/K^+-ATPase (adenosine triphosphatase) pumps three Na^+ ions out of the axoplasm for every two K^+ ions pumped in. Consequently, the axon interior is relatively negative (−50 to −90 mV) and sodium poor compared to the exterior (Figure 1.2). When the nerve is sufficiently "stimulated," sodium channels in a very localized region of the nerve membrane open thereby permitting Na^+ ions to move down their electrochemical gradient into the axon interior and locally "depolarize" the axonal membrane. If the magnitude of the depolarization exceeds "threshold" (i.e., the transmembrane potential decreases sufficiently), then sodium channels in the adjacent membrane are induced to open (this is what is meant by "voltage-sensitive") which in turn depolarizes even more membrane areas and induces even more distant sodium channels to open. In this way, the depolarization spreads down the axonal membrane producing an action potential.

C. Repolarization. After a few milliseconds, the sodium channel is inactivated by a time-dependent conformation change that closes an inactivation gate (Figure 1.2). In the **inactivated state**, the sodium channel cannot conduct Na^+ and cannot be reopened if stimulated (analogous to the cardiac refractory period). Initially, resting membrane potential recovers toward normal by the extracellular movement of K^+ and later by Na^+/K^+ exchange by ATPase. As the resting membrane potential is restored, the sodium channel undergoes additional conformation changes to enter the **closed (resting) state** during which it does not conduct Na^+ ions, but a sufficient stimulus (e.g., depolarization, sensory transduction, neurotransmitter binding) will convert the channel to the **open state**. Importantly, the binding affinity of local anesthetics varies with the state of the sodium channel, being greatest in the inactivated state and least in the resting (closed) state. These state-dependent differences in binding affinity underlie "phasic" or "rate-dependent" block (see Section V.B). Also, differences between local anesthetics in the degree to which they exhibit state-dependent differences in binding affinity underlie the differences in their relative cardiovascular toxicity (see Chapter 3).

D. Local anesthetic binding. There is no "receptor" for local anesthetics; rather there is a "*binding site.*" Directed mutagenesis studies indicate that the local anesthetic binding site is located within the **sodium channel** near its intracellular opening (Figure 1.2) (2). Local anesthetics block action potentials by preventing Na^+ movement through the sodium channel; either by physically blocking Na^+ or by preventing a necessary change in sodium channel conformation that would permit Na^+ to traverse the pore.

1. The local anesthetic **binding site** consists of a **hydrophobic region** to which the hydrophobic portion of the local anesthetic molecule is assumed to interact and a hydrophilic region where the quaternary amine interacts (Figure 1.2). Amino acid substitutions at these sites prevent local anesthetics from being effective.

E. Model of local anesthetic action. *In vitro* experiments using giant squid axon have shown that permanently charged quaternary amine local anesthetics have relatively weak local anesthetic activity when applied outside the nerve

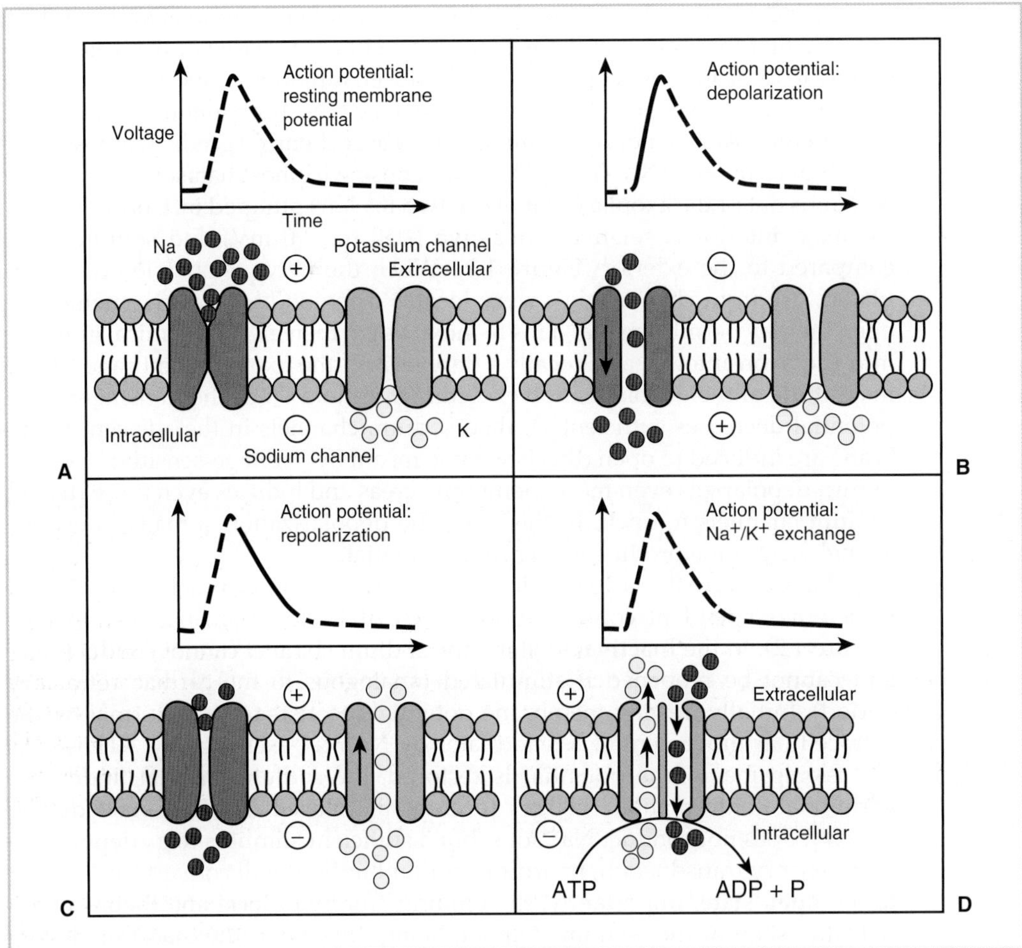

Figure 1.2. Sodium and potassium channel function and ion movements during nerve depolarization. **A:** At rest, the sodium channel is in the closed confirmation and there is a relative excess of sodium ions (*solid circles*) in the extracellular space and a relative excess of potassium ions in the intracellular space (*open circles*). Because there are approximately three positively charged sodium ions in the extracellular space for every two charged sodium–potassium ions in the intracellular space, the intracellular space is negative (−50 to −90 mV) relative to the extracellular space. **B:** Following a sufficient stimulus, the voltage-gated sodium channel confirmation changes to the open configuration, and sodium ions flow down their electrochemical gradient into the interior of the neuron, resulting in depolarization. **C:** At the peak of the action potential, the sodium channel conformation changes spontaneously to the inactivated state, which prevents further sodium entry and is refractory to reopening in response to a stimulus. Simultaneously, the voltage-gated potassium channels open, and potassium flows down its concentration gradient to render the neuron interior negative relative to the exterior (repolarization). **D:** The sodium–potassium pump (Na^+/K^+ adenosine triphosphatase [ATPase]) exchanges three intracellular sodium molecules for every two extracellular potassium molecules, thereby restoring the resting membrane potential and moving the sodium channel to the closed confirmation. ADP, adenosine diphosphate; ATP, adenosine diphosphate; P, phosphate. (Adapted from Baras K, Clitten S. Clinical Anesthesia, 3rd edition.)

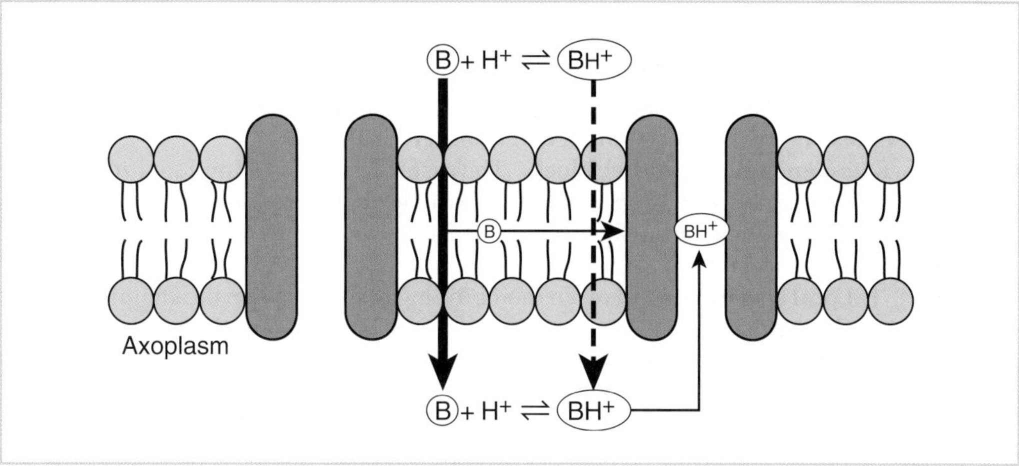

Figure 1.3. Model of local anesthetic interaction with the sodium channel. In the extracellular fluid, the local anesthetic molecule is in re-equilibrium as both a neutral tertiary amine base (*B*) and a positively charged quaternary amine (BH^+). The uncharged tertiary form of the local anesthetic crosses the cell membrane much more readily than does the charged quaternary form, but the uncharged form does cross to some extent. The same equilibrium between the uncharged tertiary amine and the charged quaternary amine exists within the interior of the nerve as well, although the lower pH within the neuron will tend to favor the quaternary form more than in the extracellular fluid. Only the charged quaternary form is capable of interacting with the local anesthetic binding site *within* the sodium channel, and it can reach that site only from inside the neuron. Uncharged local anesthetics (e.g., benzocaine) are thought to interact with sodium channels at a separate site that may be reached from within the axonal membrane. Alternatively, uncharged local anesthetics may alter sodium channel function by altering the properties of the axonal membrane and therefore the interaction of the sodium channel with the membrane.

membrane, but are quite potent when inserted directly into the nerve cytoplasm. Conversely, uncharged tertiary amine local anesthetics applied intraneurally are not very effective local anesthetics. These observations lead to the following model for tertiary amine local anesthetics (Figure 1.3).

1. Local anesthetics must cross the axonal plasma membrane to reach their binding site.
2. The **uncharged**, more hydrophobic, tertiary amine form of the local anesthetic more readily crosses the axonal membrane.
3. The **charged** quaternary form of the local anesthetic is responsible for sodium channel blockade.
4. **Exceptions.** There are several exceptions to this model.
   a. **Benzocaine,** which lacks an amine group and thus is permanently uncharged, still blocks sodium channels. Benzocaine may have a different binding site and may reach it directly from the plasma membrane instead of the axoplasm (Figure 1.3).
   b. Permanently charged **quaternary amine** local anesthetics (e.g., tonicaine) do produce slow onset but long-lasting sodium channel blockade *in vivo* (4,5).

V. ***In vitro*** **pharmacodynamic characteristics**

A. **Potency.** Local anesthetic potency is commonly defined as the **minimal local anesthetic concentration** required to produce neural blockade. *In vitro*, using isolated nerves, potency correlates very well with hydrophobicity. *In vivo*, the correlation, although still present, is less robust. Also, minimal blocking concentrations *in vitro* are an order of magnitude or more lower than required *in vivo* because of uptake, non-specific tissue binding tissue diffusion barriers, and so on that are encountered *in vivo* (see Chapter 2).

B. **Rate-dependent (phasic) block.** The faster a nerve is stimulated *in vitro*, the lower the concentration of local anesthetic that is required to block it. This phenomenon is variously termed *use-dependent, rate-dependent*, or *phasic* block. It occurs because:

1. Local anesthetics can reach their binding site only when the channel is open. Consequently, a resting nerve cannot be blocked and the more frequently a nerve is stimulated the more time channels will be open to admit local anesthetic.
2. The affinity of the local anesthetic for its binding site is greatest in the inactivated state and least in the resting state (Figure 1.2). During the interval the channel moves from the inactivated to the resting state, the local anesthetic can move away from the binding site so that subsequent depolarization finds the channel unblocked. As firing rate increases, the channels spend less time in the resting state and therefore there is less time for local anesthetics to move away from the binding site. In effect, sodium channel blockade is the result of the balance between local anesthetic binding in the inactivated state and local anesthetic dissociation in the resting state.

Phasic block occurs to a greater degree with more potent (hydrophobic) local anesthetics because the magnitude of the differences in their binding affinity between the open/inactivated states and the resting state is greater than for more hydrophilic drugs. Although readily demonstrated *in vitro*, it is unclear to what extent rate-dependent block occurs in neurons *in vivo*. However, rate-dependent block of cardiac sodium channels *in vivo* is an important reason that hydrophobic local anesthetics are more cardiotoxic than are hydrophilic local anesthetics (see Chapter 3).

C. **Length of nerve exposed and local anesthetic block.** *In vitro*, the greater the length of nerve exposed to local anesthetic, the lower the concentration of local anesthetic necessary to produce blockade (6). This effect peaks at exposure lengths of 2.5 to 3 mm; as exposure length increases beyond 3 mm the minimal blocking concentration does not decrease further.

1. **Myelinated axons.** Myelin consists of Schwann cell plasma membranes wrapped around axons (Figure 1.2). There are gaps, called *nodes of Ranvier*, at fixed intervals between the myelinated areas. Myelination results in much **faster conduction** velocities because the axonal membrane needs only to be depolarized at the node. In effect, depolarization "jumps" from node to node in a process called *saltatory conduction*.
   a. Local anesthetics can gain access to the axonal membrane of myelinated axons only at the nodes of Ranvier. *In vitro*, the sodium channels in approximately three consecutive nodes (0.4–4 mm) need to be blocked by local anesthetic for axonal conduction to fail. The large variability in length stems from the fact that larger-diameter axons have larger "internodal" distances than do smaller diameter axons. Whether the same number of nodes needs to be blocked *in vivo* is unknown.
2. **Unmyelinated axons.** As with myelinated axons, the concentration of local anesthetic required to block conduction of unmyelinated axons

Table 1.2 Axon classification[a]

Fiber type	Size (μ)	Function	Local anesthetic sensitivity (*in vitro*)	Illustrations
A alpha	12–20	Somatic motor, proprioception	++	
beta	5–12	Touch, pressure	++	
gamma	3–6	Motor to muscle spindles	+++	
delta	2–5	Pain, temperature, touch	+++	
B	<3	Autonomic (preganglionic)	++	
C	0.3–1.4	Pain, reflex responses Autonomic (postganglionic)	+	

[a]Human axons are classified by size, presence or absence of myelin, and function. *In vitro,* small unmyelinated axons are most resistant to local anesthetic blockade, whereas large myelinated axons are the most sensitive. *In vivo*, however, the sensitivity to local anesthetic block is different for reasons that are not fully understood (see Chapter 2). '+' indicates the relative sensitivity to local anesthetic block.

decreases with increasing length of nerve exposed to the local anesthetic.

D. Axon type, axon size, and local anesthetic blockade. Human axons are classified with respect to their structure (myelinated, unmyelinated), size (i.e., diameter), and function (Table 1.2). The characteristics of local anesthetic blockade vary among different axon types but the role that size, myelination, or function play in axonal blockade is not entirely clear.

1. Under equilibrium conditions *in vitro*, unmyelinated axons (C fibers) are the most resistant to local anesthetic blockade, followed by large (A_α, A_β) and small (B) myelinated axons (7–9). Intermediate-sized myelinated axons (A_δ, A_γ) are the easiest axons to block *in vitro*. The mechanism responsible for this differential sensitivity is not precisely known, but it is clearly not related to nerve size or to myelination *per se*.

VI. Summary

The chemistry and molecular pharmacology of local anesthetics described in this chapter underlie the clinical pharmacology described in the following chapters. Familiarity with the principles described here will make it easier to understand the clinical pharmacology of individual local anesthetics when used for specific blocks. However, bear in mind that the clinical arena involves numerous factors (e.g., uptake, distribution, and metabolism) not present in the simple systems used to investigate chemistry and pharmacology at the cellular level. Therefore, the following chapters are essential for understanding the clinical use of this important class of drugs.

REFERENCES

1 Molitor RE, Lain D, DuPen SL Jr. Home epidural infusions of opiate agonists and bupivacaine – epinephrine. *Am J Hosp Pharm* 1988;45(9):1861–1862.

2 Yarov-Yarovoy V, Brown J, Sharp EM, et al. Molecular determinants of voltage-dependent gating and binding of pore-blocking drugs in transmembrane segment IIIS6 of the Na+ channel alpha subunit. *J Biol Chem* 2001;276(1):20–27.

3 Ragsdale DS, McPhee JC, Scheuer T, et al. Molecular determinants of state-dependent block of Na+ channels by local anesthetics. *Science* 1994;265(5179):1724–1728.

4 Gerner P, Nakamura T, Quan CF, et al. Spinal tonicaine: potency and differential blockade of sensory and motor functions. *Anesthesiology* 2000;92(5):1350–1360.

5 Khan MA, Gerner P, Sudoh Y, et al. Use of a charged lidocaine derivative, tonicaine, for prolonged infiltration anesthesia. *Reg Anesth Pain Med* 2002;27(2):173–179.

6 Raymond SA, Steffensen SC, Gugino LD, et al. The role of length of nerve exposed to local anesthetics in impulse blocking action. *Anesth Analg* 1989;68(5):563–570.

7 Huang JH, Thalhammer JG, Raymond SA, et al. Susceptibility to lidocaine of impulses in different somatosensory afferent fibers of rat sciatic nerve. *J Pharmacol Exp Ther* 1997;282(2):802–811.

8 Wildsmith JA, Gissen AJ, Gregus J, et al. Differential nerve blocking activity of amino-ester local anaesthetics. *Br J Anaesth* 1985;57(6):612–620.

9 Franz DN, Perry RS. Mechanisms for differential block among single myelinated and non-myelinated axons by procaine. *J Physiol* 1974;236(1):193–210.

2 Local Anesthetic Clinical Pharmacology

Christopher M. Bernards

I. Introduction

Much of the information in Chapter 1 described the cellular pharmacology of local anesthetics in isolated nerves studied *in vitro*. Although this information is applicable to the clinical situation in general terms, there are some important differences in local anesthetic pharmacology *in vivo*. For example, *in vitro* the minimal blocking concentration of lidocaine in isolated nerve is 0.07%. In contrast, nerve block *in vivo* requires concentrations between 1.5% and 2%; an approximately 30-fold higher concentration.

Most differences between the *in vitro* and *in vivo* pharmacology of local anesthetics can be attributed to differences in pharmacokinetics. Unlike the *in vitro* situation, *in vivo*, there are numerous competing sites for local anesthetic to end up other than within the nerve (Figure 2.1). For example, drug may be cleared into plasma or lymphatics, may be sequestered in muscle or fat, may nonspecifically bind to connective tissue, and so on.

II. Factors determining block onset

A. Injection site. Arguably the most important factor determining the speed at which a block sets up is the proximity of the injection site to the targeted nerve(s). The closer the local anesthetic is placed to the nerve(s), the less time required for drug to diffuse from the injection site to the target.

1. Neuronal barriers. Even if local anesthetic is placed immediately adjacent to the nerve, multiple tissue barriers (i.e., **epineurium, perineurium, endoneurium,** fat) must still be crossed before the drug reaches the axons (Figure 2.2). What physicochemical properties of local anesthetics govern and how rapidly this occurs is not known. Also, it is not known whether partitioning of hydrophobic drugs into neuronal fat serves as a drug reservoir and, therefore, prolongs the block or serves as a drug sink that decreases local anesthetic access to axons.

B. Dose, volume, and concentration. Although results vary somewhat with the type of block and the local anesthetic used, in general, it is the total local anesthetic dose, and not the volume or concentration that determines the onset rate, depth, and duration of nerve block (1).

C. Local anesthetic choice. Local anesthetics must move through the aqueous extracellular fluid space to get from their injection site to the targeted nerve. *En route,* hydrophobic local anesthetics are more likely to partition from the hydrophilic extracellular fluid space and into surrounding tissues or to bind nonspecifically to hydrophobic sites on connective tissue than are more hydrophilic drugs (Figure 2.1). This likely explains the slower onset of hydrophobic local anesthetics despite their inherently greater potency.

III. Factors determining duration

Block duration is largely a function of drug clearance rate.

A. Dose. Larger doses of local anesthetic produce **longer-duration** block than do smaller doses because it takes longer to clear enough drug from the

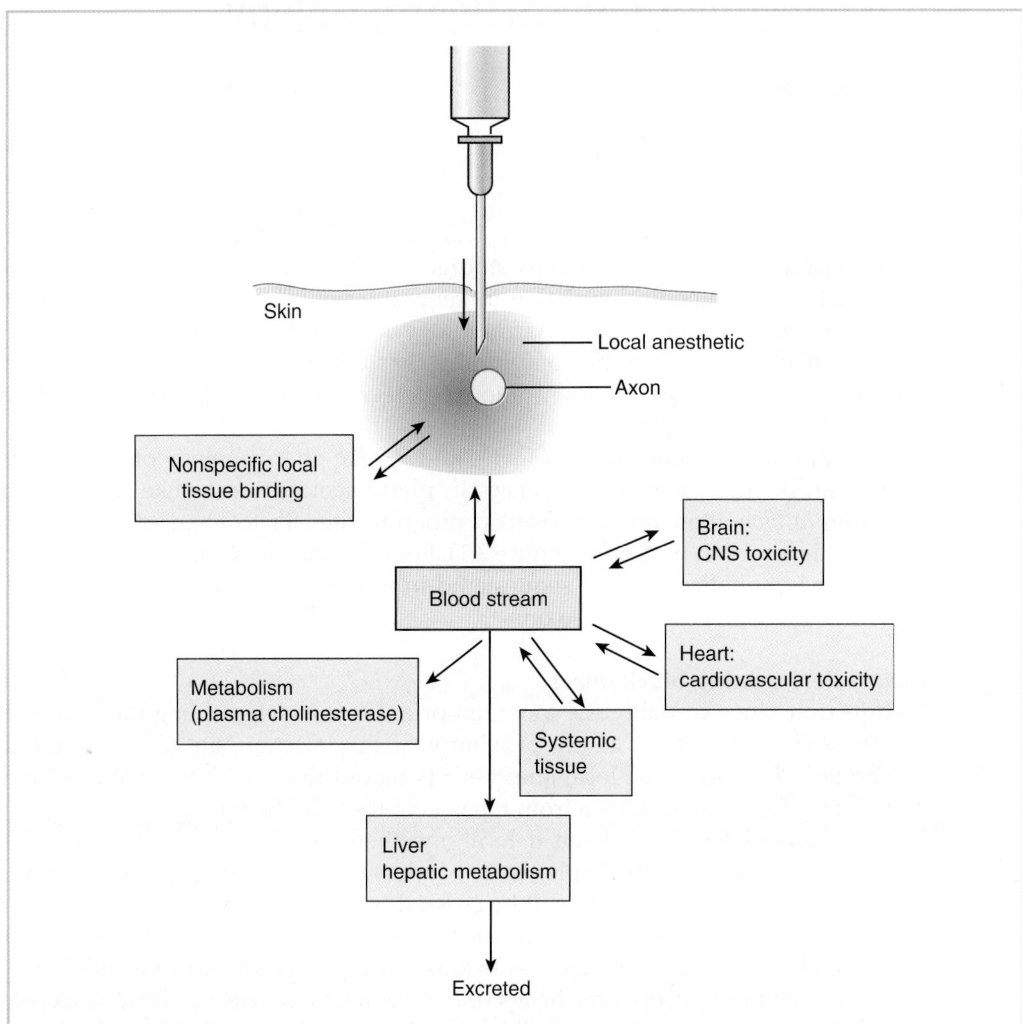

Figure 2.1. Disposition of sites for local anesthetics following peripheral nerve blocks. Nonspecific binding to extraneuronal tissues (e.g., tissue proteins, fat) and uptake into the blood stream limit the amount of drug available to produce neural blockade, and thereby affects the likelihood of adequate neural blockade. Placing the drug closer to the nerve decreases the impact of drug loss due to tissue and blood. Following uptake into the vascular system, some drugs are metabolized by plasma cholinesterases (e.g., chloroprocaine) or are delivered to the liver for metabolism (or both). Uptake into blood also plays a vital role in producing central nervous system (CNS) of cardiovascular toxicity.

nerve/surrounding tissues for the concentration to fall below the minimum necessary for blockade.

B. **Local anesthetic choice.** In general, hydrophobic local anesthetics are cleared more slowly from an injection site than are hydrophilic drugs for the reasons noted earlier. In addition, hydrophobic drugs are intrinsically more potent than hydrophilic local anesthetics. Consequently, hydrophobic local anesthetics produce longer-duration blocks than do more hydrophilic drugs.

1. **Vascular effects.** Local anesthetics have a complex and variable effect on local blood vessels and consequently on their own clearance. In general,

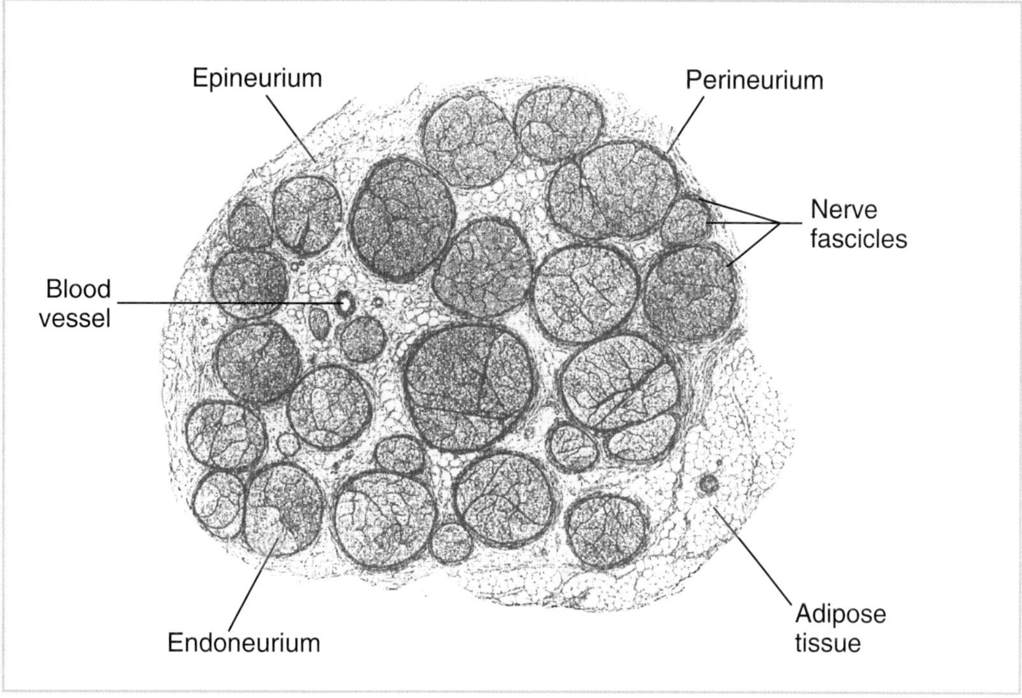

Figure 2.2. Drawing of a human peripheral nerve in cross section. Axons are gathered into fascicles, which contain dozens to a hundred or more axons. Each individual axon in the fascicle is surrounded by loose connective tissue (endoneurium). Each fascicle is surrounded by perineurium, and the collections of fascicles that make up the individual nerve are surrounded by epineurium. Perineurium and epineurium are more substantial barriers than is the endoneurium.

at high concentrations local anesthetics tend to produce **vasodilatation**, thereby increasing local blood flow and consequently their own clearance. As local anesthetic concentration falls, either as a function of distance from the injection site or because of clearance, **vasoconstriction** occurs thereby reducing clearance and prolonging duration (see specific drugs given in the subsequent text for individual differences).

IV. Adjuncts

Multiple "adjuncts" are added to local anesthetics to alter their onset or duration. The most common follow:

A. Vasoconstrictors

1. Epinephrine added to a local anesthetic decreases local blood flow and, consequently drug clearance, thereby, prolonging block duration (2) and decreases local anesthetic peak plasma concentration following spinal, epidural, and peripheral nerve blocks. Lower peak plasma concentration decreases the risk of central nervous system (CNS) toxicity from systemic absorption and increases the local anesthetic dose that can be used safely. Importantly, epinephrine does not provide protection from the toxic effects of accidental intravascular local anesthetic injection (3).
   a. The effect of epinephrine is generally greater for **shorter acting**, more hydrophilic drugs.

b. Most commonly, epinephrine is added to local anesthetics at a concentration of 5 μg/mL. There is insufficient data available to determine whether this is the optimal concentration for all local anesthetics and blocks.

c. The addition of epinephrine to 2-chloroprocaine for spinal anesthesia has been shown to produce "flu-like" symptoms (malaise, myalgias, arthralgia, anorexia) for unknown reasons (4). These symptoms do not occur when using plain 2-chloroprocaine for spinal anesthesia or when adding epinephrine to other local anesthetics for spinal anesthesia. Consequently, epinephrine should not be added to 2-chloroprocaine for spinal anesthesia. Fentanyl (20 μg) is an alternative that effectively prolongs spinal 2-chloroprocaine sensory block (5).

2. Phenylephrine has also been added to local anesthetics for spinal anesthesia. The dose is usually 1 to 2 mg (potency of 1 mg phenylephrine is equivalent to 0.1 mg epinephrine). However systemic absorption and subsequent hemodynamic effects when used in epidural or peripheral solutions limits its use. The dose is usually 1 to 2 mg (potency of 1 mg phenylephrine is equivalent to 0.1 mg epinephrine).

B. Clonidine

1. α_2-Adrenergic agonists are analgesic drugs in their own right and have been shown to inhibit both C-fibers and A-fibers (6) and to modestly inhibit local anesthetic clearance (7). When added to local anesthetics, clonidine prolongs sensory block during peripheral, central neuraxial, and intravenous regional anesthesia to a degree comparable to that produced by epinephrine. However, unlike epinephrine, clonidine does not prolong motor block. Interestingly, clonidine is as effective at prolonging spinal block when administered orally as when added to the intrathecal local anesthetic (8).

2. The use of clonidine is limited by side effects, primarily sedation, hypotension, and bradycardia. These side effects result from the fact that presynaptic α_2 adrenergic receptors inhibit norepinephrine release from noradrenergic neurons in the CNS.

C. Bicarbonate. Sodium bicarbonate (1 mEq/mL) is sometimes added to local anesthetics to increase speed of onset. However, studies are conflicting as to whether bicarbonate is effective in this regard. In general, bicarbonate does not speed the onset of hydrophobic local anesthetics (e.g., bupivacaine, etidocaine) and a positive effect with hydrophilic drugs has been demonstrated more often with epidural block than with peripheral nerve block. Even in those studies that have demonstrated a faster onset by adding bicarbonate, the effect is small and is of questionable clinical significance in most instances (i.e., it may take more time to locate and add the bicarbonate than is gained in faster onset). If bicarbonate is added to local anesthetics, care must be taken not to add too much (i.e., render the solution too alkaline) lest the local anesthetic precipitate. The most common recommendation is to add 1 mEq of bicarbonate to each 10 mL of lidocaine or mepivacaine, and one-tenth that amount to bupivacaine, if at all.

D. Hyaluronidase. This enzyme breaks down hyaluronic acid, which is an important component of connective tissue. It is added to local anesthetics in an effort to breakdown connective tissue in the extracellular matrix and thereby increase drug dispersion through tissue. It is of questionable clinical benefit and has been virtually abandoned for regional anesthesia except for peribulbar blocks. In peribulbar anesthesia the use of hyaluronidase is associated with a faster onset of motor block (9), but it has also been implicated in case reports of allergic reaction and injury to extraocular muscles.

E. **Opioids**

1. When added to short-duration local anesthetics used for **spinal anesthesia**, short-acting opioids (e.g., fentanyl, sufentanil) **prolong and intensify sensory block** without prolonging motor block or time to void (10), which is particularly advantageous for ambulatory spinal anesthesia. However, itching can be a problem (11). When added to local anesthetics for **peripheral nerve block**, fentanyl has also been shown to prolong sensory block, but at the expense of significantly slowing onset in some studies (12).
2. Systemic opioid effects/side effects cannot be ignored when they are added to local anesthetics. For example, when added to **epidural** local anesthetic infusions, fentanyl augments analgesia by systemic uptake and redistribution to brainstem, with all of the attendant risks of systemically administered opioids (13). Similarly, when added to **intrathecal** local anesthetics, the peak plasma concentration of sufentanil occurs between 20 and 30 minutes and is greater than what is necessary for postoperative analgesia (14). This explains the many reports of "early" respiratory depression in mothers (15) and fetal heart rate abnormalities in infants (16) when sufentanil is added to intrathecal local anesthetics for labor analgesia or cesarean (C)-section.

V. Differential block

Clinically, differential block refers to the observation that some nerve functions are blocked before others. This is probably a different phenomenon that occurs *in vitro* wherein different classes of nerve fibers are blocked at different local anesthetic concentrations.

A. In general, **pain, autonomic function, temperature** sensation (especially cold), and **light touch** are blocked **before proprioception, deep pressure, and motor** function.

B. Traditionally, this phenomenon was assumed to result from some nerve types having greater **sensitivity** to local anesthetic block. However, this explanation is at odds with *in vitro* studies showing that C-fibers (sympathetic, pain, temperature) are more resistant to local anesthetic block than Aδ-fibers (motor neurons) (see Chapter 1).

C. The mechanism responsible for differential block *in vivo* is still unknown but may involve the length of nerve exposed to local anesthetic, the position of the individual axons in the nerve bundle, the frequency at which the nerve fires, interference with neuronal firing pattern (which plays a role in the coding of sensory information projected centrally), and so on.

D. Differential blockade is more prominent with some local anesthetics, and is manifest by blockade of sensory propagation with apparent sparing of motor blockade at lower concentrations of drug. This **sensory-motor dissociation** is considered a beneficial effect for postoperative analgesia.

VI. Mantle effect

In addition to differential nerve block causing temporal differences in the sequence that various modalities are blocked, there are also spatial differences in block onset. That is, when blocking nerves that innervate an extremity, it is common to see that the more proximal parts of the extremity (i.e., those closer to the local anesthetic injection site) are blocked before more distal areas. This phenomenon is thought to result from the arrangement of axons within the nerve bundle such that nerves innervating distal parts of the extremity lie at the core of the nerve bundle, whereas those innervating more proximal portions lie in the mantle. Because local anesthetics move centripetally from the exterior of the nerve to the interior, the mantle fibers are blocked first.

VII. **Individual local anesthetics** (Table 2.1)

A. **Cocaine.** Cocaine was the first local anesthetic used medicinally. It was abandoned as a local anesthetic for peripheral and central neuraxial blocks because of neural toxicity and abuse potential.

1. Cocaine is an ester local anesthetic metabolized in the liver to produce active metabolites. The half-life in humans is approximately 45 minutes. In the presence of alcohol, the metabolic pathway is altered to produce cocaethylene, which is more toxic than cocaine.
2. Currently, its "sole" medical use is as a topical local anesthetic (4%) in ear, nose, and throat (ENT) surgery because it produces intense vasoconstriction (thereby reducing bleeding) in addition to sensory block.
3. Maximum cocaine dose is 200 mg and because local anesthetic toxicity is additive, the common practice of performing awake nasal intubation with topical application of cocaine in the nose followed by liberal amounts of lidocaine (4%) or benzocaine spray to the pharynx/trachea increases the risk of systemic toxicity.
4. Cocaine can cause coronary artery spasm and concomitant use of cocaine and phenylephrine in nasal septoplasty has been associated with acute myocardial infarction in a 23-year-old patient without cardiac risk factors (17).

B. **Benzocaine.** Benzocaine was the first synthetic local anesthetic (although procaine was the first synthetic local anesthetic used clinically for nerve block).

1. It is an ester and a secondary amine with a pK_a of 3.5. Consequently, it exists only in the uncharged form at physiological pH and is poorly soluble in aqueous solutions.
2. Because it is sparingly soluble in water, benzocaine is used exclusively as a topical spray, lozenge, or troche for mucous membranes or as a cutaneous cream/gel for dermal hypesthesia.
3. Although most local anesthetics have been implicated in causing methemoglobinemia, benzocaine appears to be particularly high risk in this regard. Adding to the inherent risk of methemaglobinemia is the fact that it is relatively easy to administer an excessive dose because of the difficulty in quantifying the amount of drug administered when it is applied as a spray or cream.

C. **Procaine.** Procaine is an ester and was the first synthetic local anesthetic used clinically.

1. Procaine is rapidly metabolized in plasma by **cholinesterase** and has an elimination half-life less than 8 minutes. Consequently, the risk of systemic toxicity is low.
2. Procaine is used primarily for subcutaneous **infiltration** (0.25%–1.0%). It is ineffective topically and is unreliable for epidural block. It is a poor choice for peripheral nerve block because of its slow onset and short duration.
3. Procaine is used for **spinal** anesthesia (50–100 mg). When compared to lidocaine, it produces a slightly shorter block and has a high failure rate

Table 2.1 Local anesthetic drug clinical doses

Drug (brand name)	Topical	Spinal	Epidural[f]		Peripheral nerve block	Intravenous regional	Maximum recommended doses			
							Plain		With epinephrine	
			Surgical	Obstetric			Total	mg/kg	Total	mg/kg
Cocaine	4%	NA	NA	—	NA	NA	200	1.5	—	—
Benzocaine	5%–20%	NA	NA	—	NA	NA	—	—	—	—
Short duration										
Procaine (Novocaine)	NA	10%	NI	NI	1%	NI	500	—	—	—
2-Chloroprocaine (nesacaine)	NI	NA	2%–3%	2%–3%	1%–2%	NI	800	11	1,000	14
Intermediate duration Lidocaine (Xylocaine)	4%	5%	1.5%	1.5%	0.5%	0.5%	300	4.5	500	7
Mepivacaine (Carbocaine, Polocaine)	NA	NA	2% 1% 1.5% 2%	2%[a] NI	1% 1%	NA	400	—	550	[e]
Prilocaine (Citanest)	NA	NA	2%–3%	NI	1%	0.5%	—	—	500	—
Long duration										
Ropivacaine (Naropin)	NA	0.5%[b]	0.75%, 1%[c]	0.2%	0.5%	NA	250	—	250	3
Bupivacaine (Marcaine, Sensorcaine)	NA	0.5% 0.75%	0.5% 0.75%[c]	0.125%[d] 0.25% 0.5%[a]	0.25% 0.5%	0.25%[b]	175	—	225	3
Levobupivacaine (Chirocaine)										
Etidocaine (Duranest)	NA	NA	1% 1.5%	NI	1%	NI	300	4	400	6
Tetracaine (Pontocaine)	1%–2%	1%	NA	NA	NA	NA				

Drugs are grouped in general duration of action. Concentrations listed are those recommended for particular application.
NA, not available; NI, not indicated; PDR, Physicians' Desk Reference.
[a]Produces motor blockade suitable for cesarean delivery.
[b]Not approved for this use.
[c]For single injection only; lower concentrations should be used for follow-up injections of catheters.
[d]Not prepared commercially; must be diluted at time of use.
[e]Specific dose for epinephrine-containing solution not identified; this is largest described dose.
[f]Preservative free solutions only.

(i.e., inadequate sensory block) but a significantly lower incidence of transient neurologic symptoms (TNS) (18). The commercial 10% solution should be diluted to 5% in dextrose, water, saline, or cerebrospinal fluid (CSF).

4. As with all synthetic ester local anesthetics, procaine is metabolized to para-aminobenzoic acid (PABA), which is a molecule frequently associated with **allergic reactions**.

D. **Tetracaine.** Tetracaine is the longest acting ester local anesthetic and before the advent of amide local anesthetics it was the preferred drug for long-lasting blocks.

1. As with procaine, slow onset when used for epidural or peripheral nerve block led to the abandonment of tetracaine for these uses when alternative amides were developed.
   a. At one time, tetracaine was mixed with faster-onset local anesthetics (e.g., chloroprocaine) a failed effort to speed its onset while preserving its long duration (see Section VIII).
2. Tetracaine is metabolized (hydrolysis) more slowly than procaine (although it is still faster than the amide local anesthetics) are metabolized; consequently, **risk of systemic toxicity is greater**.
3. Tetracaine is used primarily for **spinal anesthesia** for which it is available as a 1% solution and as a powder (''niphanoid crystals'') that can be diluted with CSF, water, saline, or dextrose.
   a. Tetracaine plus phenylephrine (5 mg) or epinephrine (0.2 mg) produces the longest-lasting spinal block (4–6 hours).
4. Tetracaine is very effective on **mucosal membranes** (commercially available in combination with benzocaine for this purpose) and is used for topical **ophthalmologic anesthesia**.

E. **2-Chloroprocaine.** 2-Chloroprocaine, a derivative of procaine, was the last ester local anesthetic introduced into clinical practice.

1. Unlike procaine, 2-chloroprocaine has a **rapid onset of action,** and at concentrations of 2% to 3% is an effective drug for epidural, spinal, and peripheral nerve blocks. Because it has a duration of action between 30 and 60 minutes, it is suitable for **short outpatient procedures**.
2. 2-Chloroprocaine is hydrolyzed in plasma even more rapidly than procaine and has a half-life less then 1 minute. Therefore, the **risk of systemic toxicity is lower** than for any other local anesthetic.
   a. The low risk of toxicity to mother and newborn plus its rapid onset makes chloroprocaine an attractive drug for epidural anesthesia for **C-section**.
3. **Formulations.** Chloroprocaine is available commercially as a **preservative-free solution** and as solution containing sodium bisulfite as an antioxidant (1). Because of concern regarding potential neurotoxicity, only the preservative-free solution should be used for central neuraxial block.
4. Use of 2-chloroprocaine for **spinal anesthesia is controversial** and is discussed in detail in Chapter 6. In brief, intrathecal 2% chloroprocaine, at a dose of 40 mg, produces good quality spinal anesthesia with a faster recovery and a lower incidence of TNS than lidocaine (19).
5. Interestingly, use of 2-chloroprocaine for epidural anesthesia has been shown to reduce the subsequent analgesic duration of epidural morphine, fentanyl, and clonidine. The mechanism is unknown.

F. **Lidocaine.** Lidocaine was the **first amide** local anesthetic introduced into clinical practice and it rapidly replaced the esters because of its longer duration and better quality block than procaine, its lower toxicity than tetracaine, and a much lower risk of allergy. It is the "archetypal" amide local anesthetic against which all others amides are compared.

1. Lidocaine is effective for **peripheral nerve block** (1% and 1.5%), **epidural** anesthesia (2%), **spinal** anesthesia (0.2%–5%), **intravenous regional anesthesia** (0.5%), and **mucosal** anesthesia (4%).
2. Lidocaine produces moderate **vasodilatation.**
3. Lidocaine is the local anesthetic most likely to cause **TNS** and while all local anesthetics can cause spinal cord injury, lidocaine may well be one of the most dangerous agents in this regard (20).
4. Although very rare, lidocaine allergy has been reported (21).

G. **Mepivacaine.** Mepivacaine is a cyclic tertiary amine like ropivacaine and bupivacaine, but clinically it is **similar to lidocaine**. It differs chemically from bupivacaine and ropivacaine in that it has a methyl group as a substituent on the tertiary nitrogen.

1. Mepivacaine is useful for **infiltration, epidural, spinal,** and **peripheral** nerve blocks. It is not very effective topically.
2. Mepivacaine has a mild **vasoconstricting** effect, which may explain its approximately 25% longer duration than lidocaine.
3. Mepivacaine is poorly metabolized in the fetus and neonate and is probably not a good choice for epidural anesthesia/analgesia in obstetrics (22).

H. **Prilocaine.** Prilocaine is clinically similar to lidocaine and although not commercially available for regional anesthesia in the United States, it is used in other countries.

1. Prilocaine has a large volume of distribution and is the **most rapidly metabolized** amide local anesthetic. These pharmacokinetic properties have led some to consider it an ideal drug for **intravenous regional anesthesia**.
2. Prilocaine is used in local anesthetic **creams** for cutaneous anesthesia.
3. Prilocaine's unique metabolite, o-toluidine, causes **methemoglobinemia**, which has limited the clinical acceptance of prilocaine.

I. **Bupivacaine.** Bupivacaine was the first **long-acting amide** local anesthetic. It has a butyl group on the tertiary nitrogen where mepivacaine has a methyl group. This substituent makes bupivacaine significantly more hydrophobic than mepivacaine (and lidocaine), slower in onset but of much longer duration.

1. Bupivacaine is used for **infiltration** (0.25%), **spinal** (0.5% and 0.75%), **epidural** (0.5% and 0.75%), and **peripheral nerve blocks** (0.375%–0.5%). It is less desirable for intravenous regional anesthesia because of its cardiovascular toxicity. Peripheral nerve blocks with bupivacaine often provide sensory block for 4 to 12 hours and on occasion 24 hours. This has made it a useful agent for outpatient regional anesthesia of the extremities when prolonged analgesia is desirable. When instilled intraperitoneally, bupivacaine provides effective analgesia following laparoscopic surgery (23).
2. In the **epidural** space, dilute concentrations of bupivacaine (0.1% or less) provide good sensory analgesia with little or no motor block. This has made it a popular choice for both postoperative and labor epidural analgesia.
3. Bupivacaine, like other hydrophobic amides, has a **lower therapeutic index** with respect to **cardiovascular toxicity** than lidocaine. High plasma concentrations required for cardiovascular toxicity are usually associated with intravascular injection. Because bupivacaine is more slowly absorbed into plasma than lidocaine, it produces peak plasma concentrations that are

approximately 40% lower (mg/mL per 100 mg administered). Consequently, bupivacaine is less likely to cause systemic toxicity than lidocaine *if intravascular injection is avoided.*

4. Reports of **cardiac arrest** following intravascular bupivacaine administration during attempted epidural anesthesia using 0.75% bupivacaine in pregnant women led the U.S. Food and Drug Administration (FDA) to warn against the use of this concentration for obstetric epidural anesthesia.

J. Levobupivacaine. Bupivacaine exists as two **enantiomers**, (R) and (S). Commercial bupivacaine is a racemic mixture of both enantiomers, whereas levobupivacaine is the pure (S)-enantiomer. It is not available in the United States at this time.

1. Levobupivacaine is approximately **equivalent to the racemic mixture** (i.e., bupivacaine) with respect to its use in regional anesthesia.
2. Human volunteer and animal studies indicate that the CNS and **cardiovascular toxicity of levobupivacaine is less than that of bupivacaine** (24,25). From a practical point of view, this means that patients can be expected to tolerate a somewhat larger dose of levobupivacaine before experiencing cardiovascular collapse. However, levobupivacaine is still quite cardiotoxic if a sufficient dose is administered intravenously and care must be taken to prevent intravascular injection (e.g., test dose, incremental injection). Quoting Mather and Chang, levobupivacaine "... may be viewed as 'safer', but must not be viewed as 'safe'" (25).

K. Ropivacaine. Ropivacaine is part of the homologous series that includes bupivacaine and mepivacaine. Ropivacaine has an isopropyl group bound to the tertiary nitrogen in place of mepivacaine's methyl group and bupivacaine's butyl group. Like levobupivacaine, it is supplied commercially as a single enantiomer. It is available as 0.2%, 0.5%, 0.75%, and 1% solutions.

1. The **potency** of ropivacaine is suggested to be clinically equivalent to that of bupivacaine. However, that is probably an overly simplistic view. In truth, the relative potency of these two drugs differs depending on the system being studied. For example, Casati et al. demonstrated that the ED50 dose for femoral nerve block was the same for bupivacaine and ropivacaine. In contrast, both Polley et al. and Capogna et al. demonstrated ropivacaine was **40% less potent** than bupivacaine when used in dilute solutions for epidural analgesia in labor (26,27). Similarly, Camorica et al. demonstrated that ropivacaine was approximately 35% less potent than bupivacaine when administered intrathecally for labor analgesia (28). In addition, studies comparing the two drugs for peripheral nerve block generally find that equivalent doses produce similar onset and quality of block, but bupivacaine has a significantly longer duration. Therefore, ropivacaine is probably not equipotent with bupivacaine on a milligram per milligram basis, at least not in all clinical situations. This should be kept in mind when comparing the drugs with respect to "motor-sparring" effects and cardiotoxicity.
2. Ropivacaine is clearly **less cardiotoxic** than bupivacaine on a milligram per milligram basis. However, when comparing equipotent doses the difference in toxicity is less clear. Therefore, as with levobupivacaine, ropivacaine should not be considered a "safe" local anesthetic whether it is "safer" than bupivacaine or not.

3. As with cardiovascular toxicity, myotoxicity of ropivacaine is less than that of bupivacaine on a milligram per milligram basis. It is unclear if myotoxicity is less when comparing equipotent doses.
4. Ropivacaine produces **vasoconstriction** at concentrations used clinically for nerve block. This likely explains why epinephrine has little effect on the duration of ropivacaine epidural or peripheral nerve block (29,30).

L. **Etidocaine.** Etidocaine is a derivative of lidocaine with an additional ethyl group on the intermediate chain and a longer aliphatic group on the tertiary amine. These chemical differences make etidocaine a very hydrophobic local anesthetic. It is commercially available outside the United States as 1%, 1.5%, or 2% solutions.

1. Etidocaine's **onset is similar to lidocaine but its duration is comparable to bupivacaine**.
2. Etidocaine's clinical potency is similar to that of mepivacaine with 1.5% solutions commonly used in the epidural space and 1% solutions used for peripheral nerve block.
3. Etidocaine is the only local anesthetic that blocks transmission in the **spinal cord** dorsal column during spinal anesthesia. It is tempting to attribute this to its greater lipid solubility resulting in more extensive partitioning into the myelin of sheaths of dorsal column neurons.
4. Etidocaine fell out of favor clinically because of its tendency to produce **motor block that outlasted sensory block** (lack of "sensory-motor dissociation").

M. **Articaine.** Articaine is a structurally interesting local anesthetic that has a 5-membered thiophene ring instead of a benzene ring as the "hydrophobic tail." It is classified as an amide because the thiophene ring is connected to the intermediate chain by an amide linkage, but it also has an ester side chain attached to the thiophene ring.

1. Articaine (4%) is used "exclusively" as a dental local anesthetic and has become the second most commonly used local anesthetic for dentistry in the United States since its introduction in 2000. Its popularity stems from its **rapid onset**, long duration, and lack of ester-related allergy risk.

VIII. Local anesthetic mixtures

Before the advent of modern amide local anesthetics, it was common to mix a **rapid-onset but short-acting** ester (e.g., procaine) with a **slow-onset but long-acting** drug (e.g., tetracaine). The goal was to produce a solution with both a rapid onset and a long duration. Mixing local anesthetics for this purpose is still practiced, particularly by surgeons. However, it is of questionable value at best. First, local anesthetic toxicity is additive, therefore the total dose of each local anesthetic must be reduced by half when they are mixed. Consequently, the total number of "fast-onset" and "long-acting" local anesthetic molecules present at the injection site will be half of what it would be if the drugs were used singly. Therefore, onset will be slower than usually results from the "rapid-onset" drug and will be shorter than that produced by the "long-acting" drug. For example, mixing chloroprocaine and bupivacaine will produce a mixture with onset and duration characteristics comparable to lidocaine. Consequently, mixing local anesthetics is a practice that should probably be relegated to historical interest.

IX. Depo local anesthetic preparations

The potential benefit of long-acting local anesthetic blocks without the need for catheters and pumps has driven an effort to produce depot-like preparations of currently available local anesthetics.

A. Animal models have shown the ability of multiple preparations, including gels, liposomes, polymer microspheres, and oil–water emulsions to produce long-duration local anesthetic blocks. To date, none of these preparations have come to market for parenteral use in humans. When they do, their benefit and their liability may well be the same. Specifically, unlike a catheter technique, local anesthetic administration cannot be "turned off" with a depo preparation; if the patient (or the physician) does not like the block they will simply have to "wait it out"—perhaps for days. Also, if the preparation produces toxicity, for example allergy, there will be no way to remove it quickly.

B. There are commercially available depo-preparations in the form of local anesthetic patches and creams intended for cutaneous anesthesia before dermatologic procedures or to treat cutaneous pain (e.g., "shingles"). These are reasonably effective but not without risk. Several cases of methemaglobinemia and CNS toxicity have been attributed to local anesthetic creams applied to children (31,32).

X. Summary

Local anesthetics differ from one another in terms of their onset, duration, relative sensory versus motor block, metabolism, and so on. In addition to their inherent properties, various adjuncts can be added to local anesthetics to change their clinical profile to meet the requirements of individual clinical situations. Awareness of these facts will allow clinicians to make rational local anesthetic/adjuvant selections to provide safe and effective regional anesthesia for their patients.

REFERENCES

1 Pippa P, Cuomo P, Panchetti A, et al. High volume and low concentration of anaesthetic solution in the perivascular interscalene sheath determines quality of block and incidence of complications. *Eur J Anaesthesiol* 2006;23:855–860.

2 Bernards CM, Kopacz DJ. Effect of epinephrine on lidocaine clearance *in vivo*: a microdialysis study in humans. *Anesthesiology* 1999;91:962–968.

3 Bernards CM, Carpenter RL, Kenter ME, et al. Effect of epinephrine on central nervous system and cardiovascular system toxicity of bupivacaine in pigs. *Anesthesiology* 1989;71:711–717.

4 Smith KN, Kopacz DJ, McDonald SB. Spinal 2-chloroprocaine: a dose-ranging study and the effect of added epinephrine. *Anesth Analg* 2004;98:81–88.

5 Vath JS, Kopacz DJ. Spinal 2-chloroprocaine: the effect of added fentanyl. *Anesth Analg* 2004;98:89–94.

6 Butterworth JF, Strichartz GR. The alpha 2-adrenergic agonists clonidine and guanfacine produce tonic and phasic block of conduction in rat sciatic nerve fibers. *Anesth Analg* 1993;76:295–301.

7 Kopacz DJ, Bernards CM. Effect of clonidine on lidocaine clearance *in vivo*: a microdialysis study in humans. *Anesthesiology* 2001;95:1371–1376.

8 Ota K, Namiki A, Iwasaki H, et al. Dose-related prolongation of tetracaine spinal anesthesia by oral clonidine in humans. *Anesth Analg* 1994;79:1121–1125.

9 Mantovani C, Bryant AE, Nicholson G. Efficacy of varying concentrations of hyaluronidase in peribulbar anaesthesia. *Br J Anaesth* 2001;86:876–878.

10 Liu S, Chiu AA, Carpenter RL, et al. Fentanyl prolongs lidocaine spinal anesthesia without prolonging recovery. *Anesth Analg* 1995;80:730–734.

11 Mulroy MF, Larkin KL, Siddiqui A. Intrathecal fentanyl-induced pruritus is more severe in combination with procaine than with lidocaine or bupivacaine. *Reg Anesth Pain Med* 2001;26:252–256.

12 Nishikawa K, Kanaya N, Nakayama M, et al. Fentanyl improves analgesia but prolongs the onset of axillary brachial plexus block by peripheral mechanism. *Anesth Analg* 2000;91:384–387.
13 Ginosar Y, Riley ET, Angst MS. The site of action of epidural fentanyl in humans: the difference between infusion and bolus administration. *Anesth Analg* 2003;97:1428–1438.
14 Lu JK, Schafer PG, Gardner TL, et al. The dose-response pharmacology of intrathecal sufentanil in female volunteers. *Anesth Analg* 1997;85:372–379.
15 Fournier R, Gamulin Z, Van Gessel E. Respiratory depression after 5 micrograms of intrathecal sufentanil. *Anesth Analg* 1998;87:1377–1378.
16 Van de Velde M, Teunkens A, Hanssens M, et al. Intrathecal sufentanil and fetal heart rate abnormalities: a double-blind, double placebo-controlled trial comparing two forms of combined spinal epidural analgesia with epidural analgesia in labor. *Anesth Analg* 2004;98:1153–1159.
17 Ashchi M, Wiedemann HP, James KB. Cardiac complication from use of cocaine and phenylephrine in nasal septoplasty. *Arch Otolaryngol Head Neck Surg* 1995;121:681–684.
18 Le Truong HH, Girard M, Drolet P, et al. Spinal anesthesia: a comparison of procaine and lidocaine. *Can J Anaesth* 2001;48:470–473.
19 Kouri ME, Kopacz DJ. Spinal 2-chloroprocaine: a comparison with lidocaine in volunteers. *Anesth Analg* 2004;98:75–80.
20 Hodgson PS, Neal JM, Pollock JE, et al. The neurotoxicity of drugs given intrathecally (spinal). *Anesth Analg* 1999;88(4):797–809.
21 Duque S, Fernandez L. Delayed-type hypersensitivity to amide local anesthetics. *Allergol Immunopathol (Madr)* 2004;32:233–234.
22 Meffin P, Long GJ, Thomas J. Clearance and metabolism of mepivacaine in the human neonate. *Clin Pharmacol Ther* 1973;14:218–225.
23 Alkhamesi NA, Peck DH, Lomax D, et al. Intraperitoneal aerosolization of bupivacaine reduces postoperative pain in laparoscopic surgery: a randomized prospective controlled double-blinded clinical trial. *Surg Endosc* 2007;21:602–606.
24 Gristwood RW. Cardiac and CNS toxicity of levobupivacaine: strengths of evidence for advantage over bupivacaine. *Drug Saf* 2002;25:153–163.
25 Mather LE, Chang DH. Cardiotoxicity with modern local anaesthetics: is there a safer choice? *Drugs* 2001;61:333–342.
26 Capogna G, Celleno D, Fusco P, et al. Relative potencies of bupivacaine and ropivacaine for analgesia in labour. *Br J Anaesth* 1999;82:371–373.
27 Polley LS, Columb MO, Naughton NN, et al. Relative analgesic potencies of ropivacaine and bupivacaine for epidural analgesia in labor: implications for therapeutic indexes. *Anesthesiology* 1999;90:944–950.
28 Camorcia M, Capogna G, Columb MO. Minimum local analgesic doses of ropivacaine, levobupivacaine, and bupivacaine for intrathecal labor analgesia. *Anesthesiology* 2005;102:646–650.
29 Cederholm I, Anskar S, Bengtsson M. Sensory, motor, and sympathetic block during epidural analgesia with 0.5% and 0.75% ropivacaine with and without epinephrine. *Reg Anesth* 1994;19:18–33.
30 Weber A, Fournier R, Van Gessel E, et al. Epinephrine does not prolong the analgesia of 20 mL ropivacaine 0.5% or 0.2% in a femoral three-in-one block. *Anesth Analg* 2001;93:1327–1331.
31 Raso SM, Fernandez JB, Beobide EA, et al. Methemoglobinemia and CNS toxicity after topical application of EMLA to a 4-year-old girl with molluscum contagiosum. *Pediatr Dermatol* 2006;23:592–593.
32 Rincon E, Baker RL, Iglesias AJ, et al. CNS toxicity after topical application of EMLA cream on a toddler with molluscum contagiosum. *Pediatr Emerg Care* 2000;16:252–254.

3 Complications of Regional Anesthesia

Christopher M. Bernards

I. Introduction

A. Injuries of any kind to patients as a result of regional anesthesia are uncommon; permanent, devastating injuries are quite rare. In fact, the low frequency of injury makes it difficult to study regional anesthesia–related complications because it is hard to accrue enough patients to achieve sufficient statistical power to draw reliable conclusions about incidence, risk factors, demographics, and so on. Most large studies rely on either retrospective chart reviews or voluntary reporting of complications to a central database. These methods often suffer from reporting bias (clinicians may choose not to report their serious complications or they may dismiss minor complications as too trivial to merit reporting) and they generally lack the accuracy, detail, or follow-up necessary to fully characterize cause, risk factors, recovery, and so on. Even large prospective studies often fail to ask the right questions or to follow patients long enough to identify late developing problems. For example, Philips et al.'s prospective study of 10,440 patients undergoing lidocaine spinal anesthesia did not detect what we now recognize as transient neurologic symptoms (TNSs) (1).

B. Animal studies provide some insight into mechanisms and risk factors for injury in regional anesthesia, because they permit investigators to actually create an injury instead of waiting for it to occur "randomly" in clinical practice. Of course, animals are hot humans and care must be taken when extrapolating quantitative data between species. However, qualitative relationships are very likely valid, for example, the observation that risk of causing neural injury in animal models increases as the dose and concentration of local anesthetic is increased.

C. With these caveats in mind, the most recent large clinical study of regional anesthesia–related complications was conducted in France using a voluntary reporting model (2). The authors collected data on 158,083 blocks of all kinds from 487 anesthesiologists. They reported the incidence of serious complications (e.g., seizure, central or peripheral neural injury, death) to be 3.5/10,000 blocks. The risk of death was reported to be 1/400,000 regional blocks; all but one of which occurred during spinal anesthesia. Therefore, in the aggregate, the available evidence would suggest that regional anesthesia is no more likely to be associated with complications than is general anesthesia.

II. Local tissue injury

A. Nerve injury. All local anesthetics are neurotoxic and capable of producing permanent neurologic injury if the dose/concentration is high enough. That said, temporary or permanent injury to neural tissue caused by local anesthetics (as opposed to needle trauma) is a rare complication of regional anesthesia. Multiple risk factors have been identified and include:

1. Local anesthetic **dose/concentration**. In animal models, the risk of neurotoxicity increases with increasing local anesthetic dose and concentration (3–5). See Chapter 2, Table 2.1, for recommended local anesthetic doses/concentrations.

2. **Epinephrine.** Adding epinephrine to local anesthetics increases the risk of neuronal injury in animal models of spinal and peripheral nerve block (5,6). Whether this is the result of a pharmacokinetic effect of epinephrine (i.e., reduced local anesthetic clearance and therefore greater exposure of the nerve to local anesthetic) or direct toxicity is unclear.
3. **Microspinal catheters.** Use of very small diameter (''microspinal'') catheters for continuous spinal anesthesia has been associated with spinal cord injury (cauda equina syndrome) (7). Injury is presumed to result because the very slow injection speeds achievable with these catheters results in limited mixing of the local anesthetic with cerebrospinal fluid (CSF); consequently, spinal tissue can be exposed to very high local anesthetic concentrations, especially if using hyperbaric or hypobaric solutions that pool in a dependant area of the subarachnoid space (8). These catheters were banned in the United States by the U.S. Food and Drug Administration (FDA) in 1992 but continue to be used in other parts of the world.
   a. Importantly, spinal cord injury can occur even when intrathecal catheters are not used. Therefore, for reasons of safety, it is best **not to ''redo''** a spinal block that is ''patchy'' because the patchiness of the block may signify that local anesthetic distribution is restricted within the subarachnoid space of that individual for reasons unknown. Repeating the block would potentially result in very high local anesthetic concentrations and neurologic injury.
4. **Skin prep solutions. Betadine, chlorhexidine, alcohol,** and other agents used to decontaminate the skin before regional anesthesia procedures are all neurotoxic. Care must be taken to avoid contaminating local anesthetics with any of these solutions. Most commercial ''kits'' used for regional anesthesia include a removable tray into which the antiseptic solution is poured before loading onto sponges. These trays should be **removed from the kit** and placed away from the remainder of the kit *before* the antiseptic solution is poured in to it. This practice will reduce the risk of splashing these neurotoxic solutions onto regional anesthesia needles or into local anesthetic solutions. Similarly, packets containing swabs preloaded with antiseptic should be opened away from the regional anesthesia tray to prevent contamination.
5. **Preexisting neurologic disease.** It has long been taught/assumed that patients with preexisting neurologic conditions (e.g., **multiple sclerosis [MS], peripheral neuropathy, amyotrophic lateral sclerosis [ALS]**, etc.) were at increased risk of neurologic injury from regional anesthesia techniques. This concern was based, at least in part, on the *''double-crush''* concept, that is, that a second injury to a nerve at a different site may result in a greater injury than could be explained by a simple additive effect. Also, the natural history of many of these diseases is that they have a waxing–waning course and are worsened by stress. Consequently, clinicians feared that they would be blamed for causing injury when, in fact, disease progression unrelated to the anesthetic was the real ''culprit.'' The only large study (n =139) of regional anesthesia in patients with preexisting neurologic conditions was a retrospective review of patients with central nervous system (CNS) disorders (e.g., post polio syndrome, ALS, MS, and spinal cord injury) undergoing epidural or spinal anesthesia (9). The authors found no evidence of new neurologic injury or disease progression.

Although this is a retrospective study with all of the attendant limitations of such a study design, it does suggest that the "conventional wisdom" regarding the use of regional anesthesia in patients with preexisting neurologic lesions needs further investigation.

B. Transient neurologic syndrome. TNS refers to **temporary pain or dysesthesia in the legs or buttocks** following spinal anesthesia. It generally **resolves in 2 to 7 days** without sequelae (10). Although all local anesthetics can cause TNS, the risk is an order of magnitude greater with lidocaine than with any other local anesthetic, and is most likely with knee arthroscopy or procedures involving the lithotomy position. The mechanism is unknown, although it is assumed, but not proved, to be neurologic in origin. It occurs with low concentrations and even low doses of lidocaine, and has led some clinicians to seek alternative drugs despite the absence of permanent injury.

1. The severity of TNS pain is not trivial for some patients; 65% report verbal analog scale (VAS) pain scores in the moderate to severe range (VAS = 4–10). Neither is it always short lived with 27% reporting symptoms lasting 3 to 7 days (11).

C. Myotoxicity. All local anesthetics produce dose-dependent myotoxicity in all individuals, although bupivacaine appears to be the most myotoxic local anesthetic (12). The mechanism is not entirely clear, but disruption of mitochondrial function has been demonstrated (13). Edema, necrosis, apoptosis, and inflammatory cell infiltrate are observed in biopsy specimens (12). Animal studies of long-term (1–4 weeks) local anesthetic infusion for femoral nerve block demonstrate calcific myonecrosis and scar formation (14). This has only very rarely been identified as a cause of clinically identifiable injury in humans; primarily in retrobulbar blocks causing extraocular muscle dysfunction and consequent diplopia (15,16). Complete recovery is the norm.

D. Neurotrauma. Historically, **needle trauma** and **intraneural injection** were thought to be important causes of neurologic injury, and they may be. However, recent observations using ultrasonography have shown that both nerve impalement by block needles and intraneural injection occur without producing significant neural injury (17). Animal studies have also shown that intentional intraneural injection does not necessarily result in permanent injury **if injection pressures are low** (less than 12 psi), but does produce severe injury if pressures are high (18). Spearing peripheral nerves with block needles and injecting local anesthetics intraneurally are inherently distasteful and should be avoided. However, they may not be the high-risk events once thought. In searching for ways to reduce the already low incidence of nerve injury during regional anesthesia, it may behoove us to identify additional potential risk factors. Two aspects of nerve localization have been considered to prevent neurotrauma:

1. **Nerve stimulators, paresthesias, and neurotrauma.** Nerve stimulators were introduced as an alternative to using paresthesias to localize peripheral nerves. The assumption was that the magnitude of the current necessary to elicit a motor response was correlated with the proximity of the needle tip to the nerve and by inference that use of the nerve stimulator would reduce the risk of nerve injury from needle to nerve contact. However, two studies over the last several years have demonstrated that the correlation between needle-nerve proximity and the current necessary to elicit a motor response is poor (19,20). Using ultrasonography, Perlas et al. demonstrated

that nerve stimulation failed to produce a motor response at less than 0.5 mA in 25% of patients even when the needle tip was in contact with the nerve (20). In these patients, currents as high as 1.0 mA were required to elicit a motor response while the needle was in contact with the nerve. Even more surprising was the fact that this same study found that needle contact with a peripheral nerve failed to produce a paresthesia 62% of the time. Therefore, one wonders how often a block needle pierces a nerve during attempted localization using either a paresthesia or a nerve stimulator as an endpoint. **Neither nerve stimulators nor paresthesias** appear to be reliable predictors of the proximity of a needle to a peripheral nerve.

2. **Ultrasonography and neurotrauma.** It is tempting to assume that use of ultrasonography to visualize the targeted nerve during needle placement and drug injection will decrease the risk of trauma-related nerve injury. However, further study is necessary to determine whether or not this assumption is valid.

III. Systemic toxicity

Systemic toxicity is manifest primarily in the CNS and the cardiovascular system, although allergy can also produce systemic reactions. CNS and cardiovascular toxicity are dependant on local anesthetic peak plasma concentration; systemic allergic reactions are not.

A. Relevant pharmacokinetics

1. Most cases of CNS toxicity, and probably all cases of serious cardiovascular toxicity, result from **unintended intravascular injection**.
2. Peak local anesthetic plasma concentration varies approximately **linearly with dose**, that is, if you double the dose of local anesthetic administered to an individual you will double their peak local anesthetic plasma concentration.
3. Peak plasma concentration **does not depend on body weight** in adults (Figure 3.1). Basing maximum local anesthetic dose on the weight of adult patients has no scientific foundation and is, therefore, medically inappropriate (except in the pediatric population). However, using doses greater than the mg/kg maximum recommended by the manufacturer does pose a medicolegal risk.
4. The **timing and magnitude** of peak local anesthetic plasma concentration also varies with the **type of block** performed, probably because of differences in the local vascularity and the surface area for drug absorption (Table 3.1). Given that peak plasma concentrations vary with the type of block performed (Figure 3.2), it is inappropriate (from a systemic toxicity viewpoint) to apply the same maximum dose recommendations to all blocks (21). However, using larger maximum doses than recommended by the manufacturer does carry a medicolegal risk.
5. It is the **free (not protein bound) fraction** of local anesthetic that is responsible for systemic toxicity because only unbound drug can exit plasma to enter tissues.
   a. **Acidosis** (respiratory or metabolic) displaces local anesthetics from their plasma protein binding sites and therefore increases the risk of toxicity (22).
6. **Epinephrine** delays absorption and decreases the peak concentration of most local anesthetics during most types of blocks by counteracting local

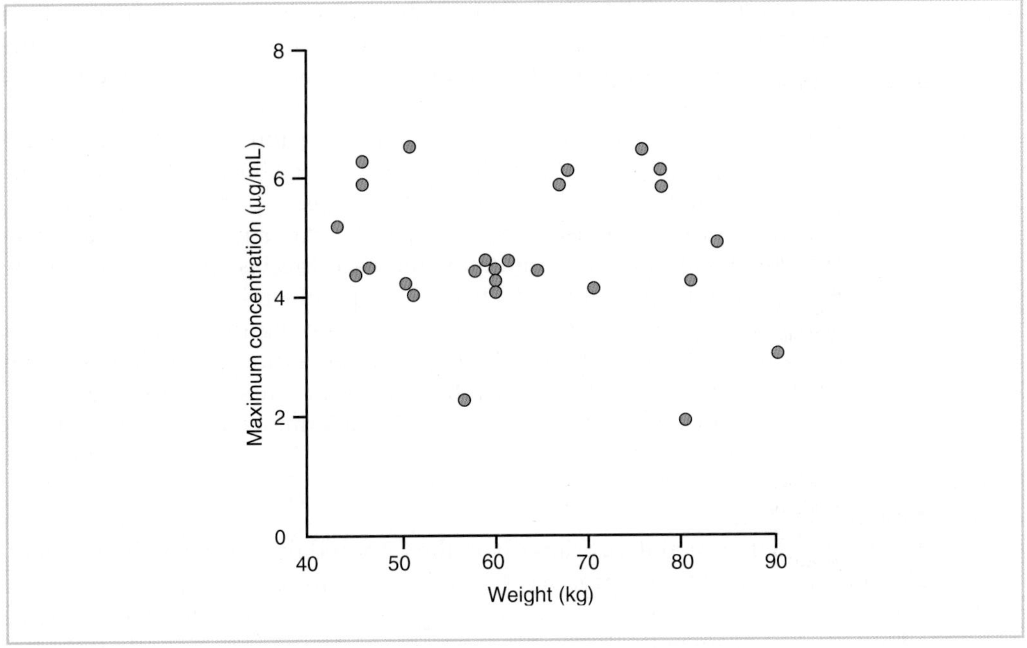

Figure 3.1. Lack of correlation between patient weight and peak plasma concentration after epidural administration of 400 mg of lignocaine. This same lack of a relationship between patient weight and peak plasma concentration has been demonstrated for multiple local anesthetics and different types of block. (Redrawn from Braid DP, Scott DB. Dosage of lignocaine in epidural block in relation to toxicity. *Br J Anaesth* 1966;38:596.)

anesthetic–mediated vasodilatation. The magnitude of the effect is greater with shorter-acting, more hydrophilic drugs.

7. Among **esters, chloroprocaine** and **procaine** are **least likely** to cause systemic toxic reactions because of their relatively rapid metabolism by plasma cholinesterase. Among amides, **prilocaine** is least likely to cause systemic toxicity because of its relatively extensive redistribution (large volume of distribution) and relatively rapid hepatic metabolism.
8. Because of their much slower absorption, hydrophobic drugs like bupivacaine and etidocaine are less likely to cause systemic toxicity than lidocaine *if intravascular injection is avoided.*
9. **Toxicity is additive** when multiple local anesthetics are used, that is, mixing two different local anesthetics does not reduce the risk of toxicity.
10. Often, one local anesthetic **enantiomer** is less toxic than the other. For example, the levorotary isomer of bupivacaine is less toxic than the dextrorotary isomer.

B. CNS toxicity

1. If local anesthetic plasma concentrations rise slowly enough (e.g., absorption from tissues), patients progress through a **reproducible series of CNS signs and symptoms** (23) (Figure 3.3). With a rapid increase in plasma concentrations (e.g., intravascular injection), seizures may be the first manifestation.
2. The **therapeutic to CNS toxicity ratio is the same** for all local anesthetics, that is, there is no difference in their propensity to cause seizures.

Table 3.1 Typical C_{max} after regional anesthetics with commonly used local anesthetics

Local anesthetic	Technique	Dose (mg)	C_{max} (μg/mL)	T_{max} (min)	Toxic plasma concentration (μg/mL)
Bupivacaine	Brachial plexus	150	1.0	20	3
	Celiac plexus	100	1.50	17	
	Epidural	150	1.26	20	
	Intercostal	140	0.90	30	
	Lumbar sympathetic	52.5	0.49	24	
	Sciatic/femoral	400	1.89	15	
L-bupivacaine	Epidural	75	0.36	50	4
	Brachial plexus	250	1.2	55	
Lidocaine	Brachial plexus	400	4.00	25	5
	Epidural	400	4.27	20	
	Intercostal	400	6.8	15	
Mepivacaine	Brachial plexus	500	3.68	24	5
	Epidural	500	4.95	16	
	Intercostal	500	8.06	9	
	Sciatic/femoral	500	3.59	31	
Ropivacaine	Brachial plexus	190	1.3	53	4
	Epidural	150	1.07	40	
	Intercostal	140	1.10	21	

C_{max}, peak plasma concentration; T_{max}, time until C_{max}.

(Data from: Liu SS. Local anesthetics and analgesia. In: Ashburn MA, Rice LJ, eds. *The management of pain*. New York: Churchill Livingstone, 1997:141–170; Berrisford RG, Sabanathan S, Mearns AJ, et al. Plasma concentrations of bupivacaine and its enantiomers during continuous extrapleural intercostal nerve block. *Br J Anaesth* 1993;70:201; Kopacz DJ, Helman JD, Nussbaum CE, et al. A comparison of epidural levobupivacaine 0.5% with or without epinephrine for lumbar spine surgery. *Anesth Analg* 2001;93:755; Crews JC, Weller RS, Moss J. Levobupivacaine for axillary brachial plexus block: a pharmacokinetic and clinical comparison in patients with normal renal function or renal disease. *Anesth Analg* 2002;95:219.)

3. Sedative-hypnotic (e.g., **benzodiazepine, propofol, and barbiturate**) premedication raises seizure threshold (24) and probably prevents many seizures that would otherwise occur in patients not receiving sedative/hypnotic premedication.
4. **Treatment.** Treatment consists primarily of **airway management** to prevent hypoxia and cardiovascular support, if necessary, until plasma concentrations fall below the seizure threshold. Importantly, the **hypercarbia and acidosis** produced by seizures displaces local anesthetics from plasma protein binding sites, thereby increasing the free plasma concentration and potentially worsening toxicity (e.g., prolonged seizures, cardiovascular toxicity). Consequently, there is potential value in stopping the tonic/clonic convulsion. Seizures can be rapidly terminated with a sedative hypnotic (e.g., benzodiazepine, barbiturate) or the motor component (which is the source of the hypercarbia and metabolic acidosis) with a muscle relaxant (succinylcholine is most rapid).

C. **Cardiovascular toxicity**

1. The very high local anesthetic plasma concentrations necessary to cause significant cardiovascular toxicity can probably only be reached by **intravascular injection**.

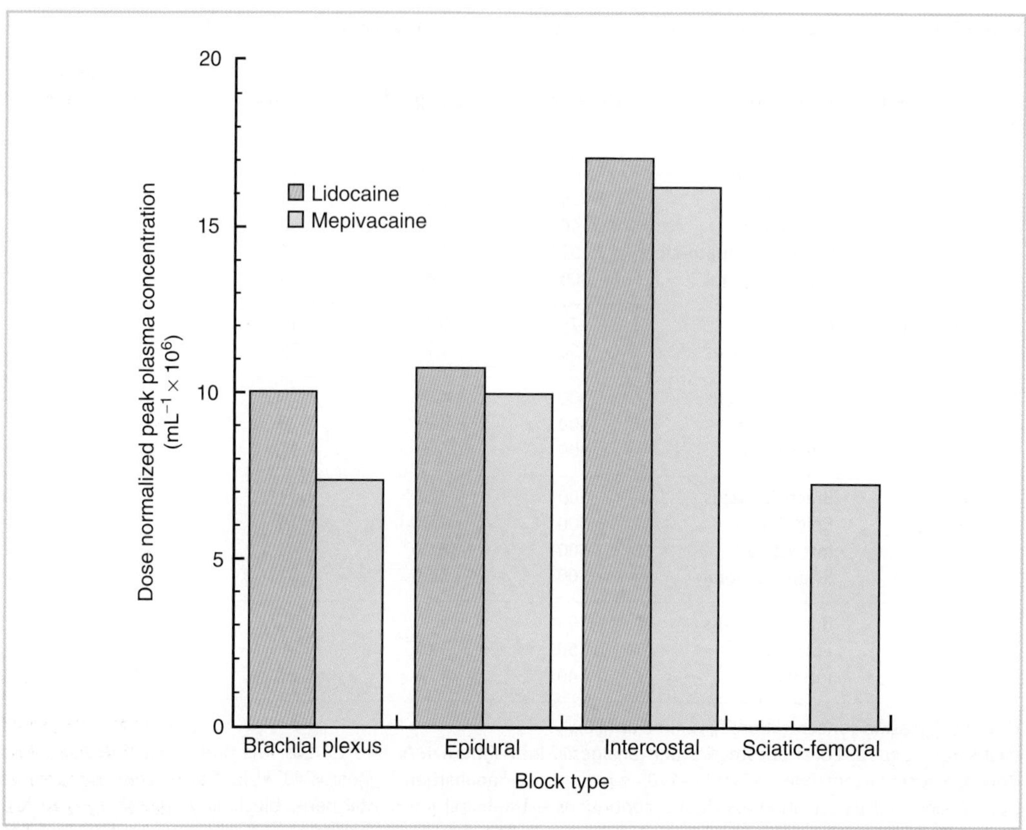

Figure 3.2. Dose-normalized peak plasma concentrations of lidocaine and mepivacaine following different types of nerve block. Highest concentrations occur following intercostal blocks.

2. The **therapeutic/cardiotoxic ratio is lower for hydrophobic local anesthetics** (e.g., etidocaine, bupivacaine) than for more hydrophilic drugs.
   a. The difference in relative myocardial toxicity between hydrophilic and hydrophobic local anesthetics is, at least in part, the result of **rate-dependent block**. That is, between myocardial contractions local anesthetics can diffuse away from their binding sites in myocardial sodium channels so that when the next depolarization occurs the sodium channel can conduct Na^+ normally. Because hydrophilic local anesthetics require less time to dissociate from the sodium channel binding site, it is more likely that myocardial sodium channels will function normally at physiological heart rates (HRs) when exposed to hydrophilic local anesthetic than to hydrophobic ones (Figure 3.4).
3. Cardiovascular toxicity is manifest as either malignant dysrhythmias, including **ventricular fibrillation**, and/or **pulseless electrical activity** (PEA) (24–26).
4. **Treatment**
   a. **Dysrhythmis** should *not* be treated with **lidocaine** or any other local anesthetic. **Amiodarone** has not been extensively studied but is probably the best choice for treatment of serious local anesthetic–induced dysrhythmias.

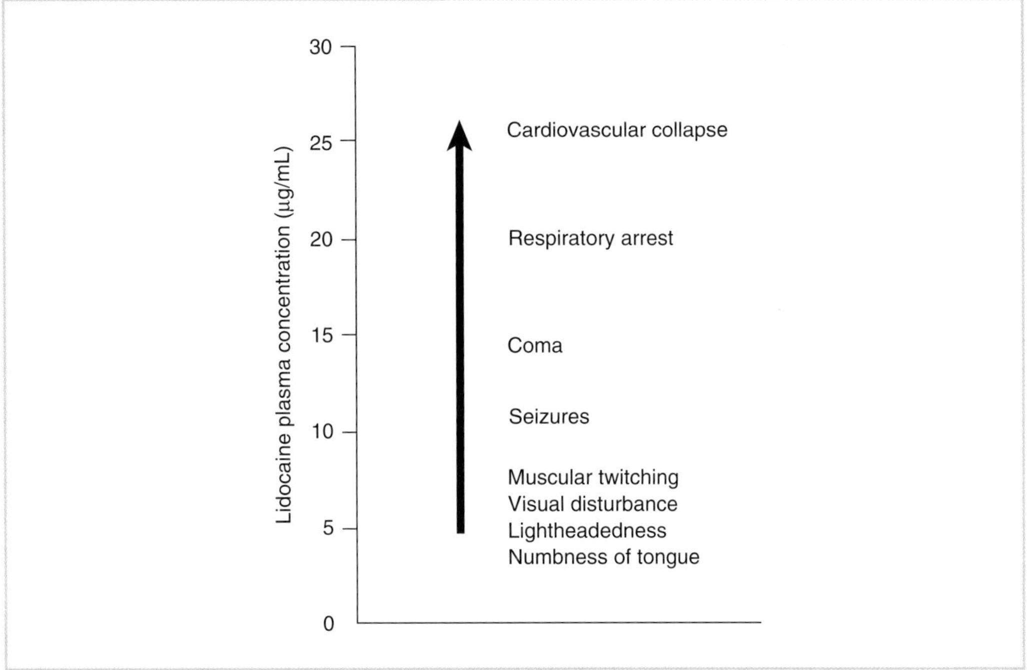

Figure 3.3. The signs and symptoms of local anesthetic toxicity progress through a fairly stereotypical sequence regardless of local anesthetic used, as long as plasma concentrations rises relatively slowly. A very rapid increase in plasma concentration may result in "skipping" of some signs and symptoms. Premedication, especially with sedative hypnotics, may modify the sequence (e.g., deay seizures) or obscure the patient's ability to report symptoms.

b. Animal studies demonstrate that standard **advanced cardiac life support (ACLS) protocols are inadequate** to treat local anesthetic–induced PEA. Much **larger and more frequent dosing with epinephrine** is required (24–27). Calcium should also be considered to help counteract the profound vasodilatation and impaired contractility produced by the very high local anesthetic plasma concentrations associated with cardiovascular toxicity. Bicarbonate may be useful in the setting of metabolic acidosis because it will help prevent displacement of local anesthetic from plasma protein binding sites.

c. **Intralipid.** Animal studies (28,29) and limited human experience (30) demonstrate that intralipid is an effective treatment for local anesthetic–induced cardiovascular toxicity. *In vitro* studies in isolated hearts suggest that intralipid changes the hydrophobic character of blood so that hydrophobic local anesthetics partition from the myocardium back into the plasma (31).

   (1) **Dose.** 1 mL/kg bolus of 20% intralipid followed by 0.25 mL/kg/min infusion. Bolus may be repeated twice. Maximum total dose not to exceed 8 mL/kg.

   (2) Just as dantrolene is kept on hand to treat rare cases of malignant hyperthermia, current evidence suggests that it is reasonable to keep a bottle of intralipid on hand to treat local anesthetic–mediated cardiovascular toxicity.

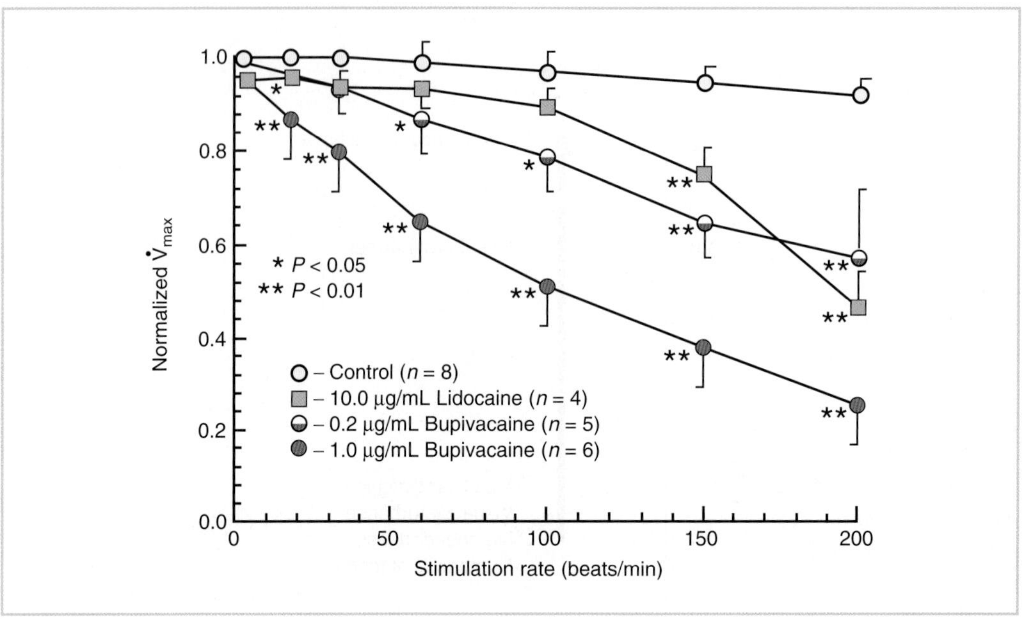

Figure 3.4. Heart rate–dependent effects of lidocaine and bupivacaine on velocity of the cardiac action potential (V_{max}). Bupivacaine progressively decreases V_{max} at heart rates above 10 beats/min due to accumulation of sodium channel block, whereas lidocaine does not decrease V_{max} until heart rate exceeds 150 beats/min. (Adapted with permission from Clarkson CW, Hondegham LM. Mechanisms for bupivacaine depression of cardiac conduction: fast block of sodium channels during the action potential with slow recovery from block during diastole. *Anesthesiology* 1985:62:396.)

5. **Preventing systemic toxicity**
   a. Use the **smallest local anesthetic dose** possible.
   b. Inject local anesthetics **slowly** and **incrementally** so that intravascular injection can be recognized before a toxic or fatal dose is administered.
   c. **Test dose.** Use of a test dose to identify intravascular injection is arguably the single most important step to prevent CNS and cardiovascular toxicity (32). Multiple types of test dose have been evaluated, including:
      (1) Drugs intended to produce a subjective CNS effect when accidentally administered intravenously, for example, **local anesthetics, opioids**. This approach works well in nonsedated subjects trained in what to expect, but midazolam premedication makes local anesthetic symptoms unreliable (32).
      (2) Cardioactive drugs (e.g., **epinephrine, norepinephrine**) are added to local anesthetics because they produce objective cardiovascular effects (increased HR and/or blood pressure) when injected intravascularly (33). The recommended test dose is 3 mL of a local anesthetic solution containing 15 µg epinephrine (1:200,000 = 5 µg/mL). Guinard et al. have shown that a HR increase of 20 beats/min occurring within 2 minutes of administering this test dose is a 100% sensitive and 100% specific indicator of intravascular injection in young adults (34). Therefore, the 15-µg epinephrine test dose is an excellent indicator of intravascular injection *if* the following caveats are kept in mind (Table 3.2):

Table 3.2 Hemodynamic responses to epinephrine test doses in different populations

Study population	Epinephrine dose (μg)	Maximal change in HR BPM (range)	Maximal change in SBP mm Hg (range)
Adult surgical patients 35			
21–40 yr	15	39 (21–53)	28 (1–43)
41–60 yr	15	29 (20–45)	28 (20–53)
61–80 yr	15	31 (9–52)	33 (18–66)
Anesthetized adult patients 36			
0.5 MAC	15	20 (12–35)	36 (16–54)
1.0 MAC	15	10 (1–18)	22 (6–44)
0.5 MAC	30	31 (18–42)	40 (25–60)
1.0 MAC	30	20 (5–50)	39 (15–66)
Acutely β-blocked adult volunteers 34			
Control	15	37 (29–46)	26 (18–33)
β-blockade	15	−28 (−23–33)	35 (24–46)

HR, heart rate; BPM, beats per minute; SBP, systolic blood pressure; MAC, minimum alveolar concentration.

(a) The magnitude of the HR increase is reduced as **patients age**, particularly after the age of 40 (32). In fact, some elderly patients may not demonstrate an HR increase in response to 15-μg epinephrine. Blood pressure response is not significantly altered by age.

(b) The **HR response is reduced**, if not eliminated, in subjects who are acutely **β-blocked** (34). In this group, systolic blood pressure response (α_1-adrenergic effect) is a better indicator of intravascular injection (Table 3.2).

(i) The effect of chronic β-adrenergic blockade on the hemodynamic response to an epinephrine-containing test dose is not known.

(ii) The effect of an epinephrine-containing test dose in patients taking β-blockers plus a vasodilating antihypertensive (e.g., angiotensin-converting enzyme [ACE inhibitor], angiotensin-II receptor blocker) is unknown.

(c) The HR and blood pressure response is reduced in **anesthetized patients** (32). As with acutely β-blocked subjects, systolic blood pressure is a better indicator of intravascular injection of an epinephrine-containing test dose than is HR increase in anesthetized patients (Table 3.2).

(3) **T-wave changes.** Reductions in T-wave amplitude (25% or 0.1 mV) have also been shown to be a reliable indicator of intravascular injection of an epinephrine-containing test dose (37). The shortcoming of this approach is that it is **often difficult to adequately quantify** T-wave changes "on-the-fly" using available electrocardiogram (ECG) monitors.

(4) **Air.** Air injected while listening for "mill-wheel" murmur over right atrium/ventricle has been shown to be an effective indicator of intravascular injection (32). This test is perhaps most useful in **labor** because contractions may produce hemodynamic changes that mimic an epinephrine-containing test dose.

IV. Allergy

The risk of allergic reaction to ester-type local anesthetics is low and to amide local anesthetics is extremely low (38). Many cases of local anesthetic "allergy" probably result from patients mistakenly attributing a side effect to an allergic reaction, for example, intravascular injection, epinephrine-induced tachyarrhythmias, vasovagal reactions, and so on.

A. Esters. Most allergic reactions to ester local anesthetics are probably reactions to their common metabolite, **para-aminobenzoic acid** (PABA). This explains why there is allergic cross-reactivity between different ester local anesthetics. Patients with a known allergy to PABA (common in cosmetics and sunscreens) should probably not receive ester local anesthetics.

B. Amides. Documented amide allergy is extremely rare. Allergic cross-reactivity between esters and amides probably does not occur.

C. Diagnosis. If an allergic reaction is suspected, blood can be drawn for measurement of plasma esterase, which is generally increased in the event of a "true" allergic reaction. Skin testing can be performed to prospectively identify patients with local anesthetic allergy (39).

V. Non–local anesthetic-mediated toxicity

Unintentional injection of toxic chemicals is an ever-present danger given the proximity of chemicals for skin prep (e.g., Betadine, chlorhexidine) and local anesthetics for nerve block. Similarly, other toxins in the operating room (OR) environment have accidentally been injected (e.g., formaldehyde for preserving biopsy specimens) causing injury and death. Another danger is the use of peripheral, epidural, or intrathecal catheters for continuous drug infusion. Everything you can imagine (propofol, thiopental, intralipid, antibiotics, muscle relaxants, etc.) has accidentally been injected through these catheters in the OR or on the surgical ward by persons mistaking the catheter for intravenous tubing; sometimes causing serious injury.

A. To reduce these risks:

1. Clearly **label** the catheter at the catheter's connector.
2. Use tubing that does not resemble intravenous tubing and that lacks in-line access ports when connecting epidural or peripheral nerve catheters to infusion pumps.
3. Do not connect stopcocks to the catheter.
4. Continually educate nurses who are responsible for administering drugs in the hospital wards.

VI. Bleeding complications

At least some bleeding is probably a universal occurrence during peripheral and central neuraxial blocks. Bleeding that produces a hematoma during peripheral nerve blocks may make landmarks difficult to palpate but is generally not serious. However, epidural or intrathecal hematomas can cause devastating neurologic injury. The increased use of prophylaxis for thromboembolism in the perioperative period has increased this risk. The American Society of Regional Anesthesia and Pain Medicine has reviewed the risks attendant to performance of regional blocks in the anticoagulated patient and published guidelines (40) that are also posted on their website (www.asra.com), which should be considered the most current source of recommendations in this area.

A. **Coagulopathy.** Whether iatrogenic (e.g., **heparin, Coumadin, platelet inhibitors**, etc.), self-induced (e.g., ginkgo, garlic, and ginseng), or the result of a disease process, coagulopathy is probably the biggest risk factor for serious bleeding complications. Regional anesthesia, especially epidural and spinal anesthesia, should probably be avoided in fully anticoagulated patients unless there is a clear benefit that outweighs the added risk.

1. **Nonsteroidal anti-inflammatory drugs (NSAIDS).** In the absence of other coagulation defects, aspirin and other NSAIDS do not appear to significantly increase hematoma risk.
2. Low-dose **unfractionated heparin**. "Minidose" or thromboprophylactic subcutaneous heparin does not appear to increase the risk of epidural hematoma in twice-daily dosing.
3. Case reports suggest that epidural catheter **removal** may be as great a risk for epidural hematoma as catheter placement in the anticoagulated patient (41). Therefore, clinicians need to consider the possibility of intraoperative or postoperative anticoagulation before placing an epidural catheter.
   a. It appears safe to place an epidural catheter in a patient who will subsequently be fully anticoagulated with heparin (e.g., cardiac or vascular surgery), under the following conditions (40):
      (1) At least **1 hour elapses** between catheter placement and anticoagulation.
      (2) Care is taken to time catheter removal so that it is done when the patient's coagulation status has normalized.
      (3) Surgery is cancelled if a **free aspiration of blood** occurs. "Traumatic block" has been implicated as increasing the risk of hematoma, but it should be noted that the original recommendation for cancellation of surgery was applied to only 4 patients in the original series of 4,011 cases (42).
      (4) Patients are not taking any other anticoagulant drugs, for example, NSAIDS.

B. **Epidural/intrathecal hematoma.** A rare but potentially devastating complication. Incidence estimated at less than 1:150,000 central neuraxial blocks.

1. **Risk factors.** In addition to anticoagulation, multiple attempts and/or traumatic (bloody) needle insertion is a feature of approximately 50% of reported cases.
2. **Presentation.** Most often presents as **motor weakness** and/or sensory loss, which can make it difficult to distinguish from block associated with continuous postoperative epidural analgesia. **Back pain is not a universal presentation**. Presentation is often more than 24 hours after block performed. Any onset of unexpected weakness is an indication for **immediate neurologic evaluation and diagnostic imaging** (magnetic resonance imaging [MRI] preferred, computed axial tomography [CT] scan acceptable), because urgent intervention is necessary.
3. **Treatment.** A few cases of successful conservative (nonoperative) treatment have been reported (43); however, expeditious (**less than 8 hours** from symptom onset) **surgical evacuation** of the hematoma is the treatment of choice. The rate and extent of recovery depends on how rapidly the hematoma is evacuated.

VII. **Infection**

Infection is **uncommon**. Risk factors include immunocompromise, indwelling catheters, duration of indwelling catheter, and lack of perioperative antibiotics. Although not specifically studied, performing blocks through **infected tissues** probably increases the risk of further infectious complications and should be avoided.

A. **Peripheral nerve blocks.** The risk of infection caused by "single-shot" peripheral nerve blocks placed using appropriate aseptic technique is extremely low. The risk of infection or colonization increases when **indwelling catheters** are used. Still, although catheters are frequently colonized (approximately 70%; primarily *Staphylococcus epidermidis*), clinical evidence of infection is uncommon (less than 3%).

B. **Central neuraxial blocks.** The risk of infection from "single-shot" spinal and epidural anesthesia is low, although probably higher than for peripheral nerve blocks. Incidence of meningitis following spinal anesthesia is estimated at less than 1:40,000 and the risk of abscess following epidural anesthesia is estimated at less than 1:10,000 (2).

1. **Risk factors**

a. As with peripheral nerve catheters, epidural catheters increase the risk of epidural abscess.

b. Animal data suggest that untreated **bacteremia** increases the risk of meningitis following lumbar puncture. When appropriate antibiotic treatment was given, lumbar puncture did not increase the risk of meningitis in the setting of bacteremia (44). It is unknown if this is true in humans.

c. **Chorioamnionitis.** Studies to date suggest that chorioamnionitis in the peripartum period does not result in increased risk of infectious complications during regional anesthesia for labor analgesia.

C. **Signs/symptoms of infection.** Local **tenderness**, **erythema**, fever, and **leukocytosis** are to be expected with peripheral infections. Meningitis typically presents with fever, headache, photophobia, meningismus, and later altered mental status. Epidural abscess often presents with back and/or radicular pain, which may be indolent. Onset of sensory/motor changes may progress rapidly to paralysis.

D. **Treatment.** Peripheral catheter-related infections generally respond to catheter removal and appropriate antibiotic therapy as determined by culture. Epidural abscess and meningitis are medical emergencies with high morbidity/mortality and aggressive medical and/or surgical intervention is warranted.

REFERENCES

1 Phillips OC, Ebner H, Nelson AT, et al. Neurologic complications following spinal anesthesia with lidocaine: a prospective review of 10,440 cases. *Anesthesiology* 1969;30:284–289.

2 Auroy Y, Benhamou D, Bargues L, et al. Major complications of regional anesthesia in France: the SOS Regional Anesthesia Hotline Service. *Anesthesiology* 2002;97:1274–1280.

3 Muguruma T, Sakura S, Saito Y. Epidural lidocaine induces dose-dependent neurologic injury in rats. *Anesth Analg* 2006;103:876–881.

4 Sakura S, Bollen AW, Ciriales R, et al. Local anesthetic neurotoxicity does not result from blockade of voltage-gated sodium channels. *Anesth Analg* 1995;81:338–346.

5 Selander D, Brattsand R, Lundborg G, et al. Local anesthetics: importance of mode of application, concentration and adrenaline for the appearance of nerve lesions. An experimental study of axonal degeneration and barrier damage after intrafascicular injection or topical application of bupivacaine (Marcain). *Acta Anaesthesiol Scand* 1979;23:127–136.

6 Hashimoto K, Hampl KF, Nakamura Y, et al. Epinephrine increases the neurotoxic potential of intrathecally administered lidocaine in the rat. *Anesthesiology* 2001;94:876–881.

7 Rigler ML, Drasner K, Krejcie TC, et al. Cauda equina syndrome after continuous spinal anesthesia. *Anesth Analg* 1991;72:275–281.

8 Ross BK, Coda B, Heath CH. Local anesthetic distribution in a spinal model: a possible mechanism of neurologic injury after continuous spinal anesthesia. *Reg Anesth* 1992;17:69–77.

9 Hebl JR, Horlocker TT, Schroeder DR. Neuraxial anesthesia and analgesia in patients with preexisting central nervous system disorders. *Anesth Analg* 2006;103:223–228.

10 Pollock JE. Transient neurologic symptoms: etiology, risk factors, and management. *Reg Anesth Pain Med* 2002;27:581–586.

11 Freedman JM, Li DK, Drasner K, et al. Transient neurologic symptoms after spinal anesthesia: an epidemiologic study of 1,863 patients. *Anesthesiology* 1998;89:633–641.

12 Zink W, Seif C, Bohl JR, et al. The acute myotoxic effects of bupivacaine and ropivacaine after continuous peripheral nerve blockades. *Anesth Analg* 2003;97:1173–1179.

13 Irwin W, Fontaine E, Agnolucci L, et al. Bupivacaine myotoxicity is mediated by mitochondria. *J Biol Chem* 2002;277:12221–12227.

14 Zink W, Bohl JR, Hacke N, et al. The long term myotoxic effects of bupivacaine and ropivacaine after continuous peripheral nerve blocks. *Anesth Analg* 2005;101:548–554.

15 Porter JD, Edney DP, McMahon EJ, et al. Extraocular myotoxicity of the retrobulbar anesthetic bupivacaine hydrochloride. *Invest Ophthalmol Vis Sci* 1988;29:163–174.

16 Rao VA, Kawatra VK. Ocular myotoxic effects of local anesthetics. *Can J Ophthalmol* 1988;23:171–173.

17 Bigeleisen PE. Nerve puncture and apparent intraneural injection during ultrasound-guided axillary block does not invariably result in neurologic injury. *Anesthesiology* 2006;105:779–783.

18 Kapur E, Vuckovic I, Dilberovic F, et al. Neurologic and histologic outcome after intraneural injections of lidocaine in canine sciatic nerves. *Acta Anaesthesiol Scand* 2007;51:101–107.

19 Choyce A, Chan VW, Middleton WJ, et al. What is the relationship between paresthesia and nerve stimulation for axillary brachial plexus block? *Reg Anesth Pain Med* 2001;26:100–104.

20 Perlas A, Niazi A, McCartney C, et al. The sensitivity of motor response to nerve stimulation and paresthesia for nerve localization as evaluated by ultrasound. *Reg Anesth Pain Med* 2006;31:445–450.

21 Rosenberg PH, Veering BT, Urmey WF. Maximum recommended doses of local anesthetics: a multifactorial concept. *Reg Anesth Pain Med* 2004;29:564–575.

22 Burney RG, DiFazio CA, Foster JA. Effects of pH on protein binding of lidocaine. *Anesth Analg* 1978;57:478–480.

23 Scott DB, Lee A, Fagan D, et al. Acute toxicity of ropivacaine compared with that of bupivacaine. *Anesth Analg* 1989;69:563–569.

24 Bernards CM, Carpenter RL, Rupp SM, et al. Effect of midazolam and diazepam premedication on central nervous system and cardiovascular toxicity of bupivacaine in pigs. *Anesthesiology* 1989;70:318–323.

25 Bernards CM, Carpenter RL, Kenter ME, et al. Effect of epinephrine on central nervous system and cardiovascular system toxicity of bupivacaine in pigs. *Anesthesiology* 1989;71:711–717.

26 Kasten GW, Martin ST. Comparison of resuscitation of sheep and dogs after bupivacaine-induced cardiovascular collapse. *Anesth Analg* 1986;65:1029–1032.

27 Chadwick HS. Toxicity and resuscitation in lidocaine- or bupivacaine-infused cats. *Anesthesiology* 1985;63:385–390.

28 Weinberg G, Ripper R, Feinstein DL, et al. Lipid emulsion infusion rescues dogs from bupivacaine-induced cardiac toxicity. *Reg Anesth Pain Med* 2003;28:198–202.

29 Weinberg GL, VadeBoncouer T, Ramaraju GA, et al. Pretreatment or resuscitation with a lipid infusion shifts the dose-response to bupivacaine-induced asystole in rats. *Anesthesiology* 1998;88:1071–1075.

30 Rosenblatt MA, Abel M, Fischer GW, et al. Successful use of a 20% lipid emulsion to resuscitate a patient after a presumed bupivacaine-related cardiac arrest. *Anesthesiology* 2006;105:217–218.

31 Weinberg GL, Ripper R, Murphy P, et al. Lipid infusion accelerates removal of bupivacaine and recovery from bupivacaine toxicity in the isolated rat heart. *Reg Anesth Pain Med* 2006;31:296–303.

32 Mulroy MF, Norris MC, Liu SS. Safety steps for epidural injection of local anesthetics: review of the literature and recommendations. *Anesth Analg* 1997;85:1346–1356.

33 Moore DC, Batra MS. The components of an effective test dose prior to epidural block. *Anesthesiology* 1981;55:693–696.

34 Guinard JP, Mulroy MF, Carpenter RL, et al. Test doses: optimal epinephrine content with and without acute beta-adrenergic blockade. *Anesthesiology* 1990;73:386–392.

35 Guinard JP, Mulroy MF, Carpenter RL. Aging reduces the reliability of epidural epinephrie test doses. *Reg Anesth* 1995;20:193.

36 Liu SS, Carpenter RL. Hemodynamic response to intravascular injection of epinephrine-containing epidural test doses in adults during regional anesthesia. *Anesthesiology* 1996;84:81.

37 Tanaka M, Goyagi T, Kimura T, et al. The efficacy of hemodynamic and T wave criteria for detecting intravascular injection of epinephrine test doses in anesthetized adults: a dose-response study. *Anesth Analg* 2000;91:1196–1202.

38 Amsler E, Flahault A, Mathelier-Fusade P, et al. Evaluation of re-challenge in patients with suspected lidocaine allergy. *Dermatology* 2004;208:109–111.

39 Hein UR, Chantraine-Hess S, Worm M, et al. Evaluation of systemic provocation tests in patients with suspected allergic and pseudoallergic drug reactions. *Acta Derm Venereol* 1999;79:139–142.

40 Horlocker TT, Wedel DJ, Benzon H, et al. Regional anesthesia in the anticoagulated patient: defining the risks (the second ASRA Consensus Conference on Neuraxial Anesthesia and Anticoagulation). *Reg Anesth Pain Med* 2003;28:172–197.

41 Yin B, Barratt SM, Power I, et al. Epidural haematoma after removal of an epidural catheter in a patient receiving high-dose enoxaparin. *Br J Anaesth* 1999;82:288–290.

42 Rao TL, El-Etr AA. Anticoagulation following placement of epidural and subarachnoid catheters: an evaluation of neurologic sequelae. *Anesthesiology* 1981;55:618–620.

43 Groen RJ. Non-operative treatment of spontaneous spinal epidural hematomas: a review of the literature and a comparison with operative cases. *Acta Neurochir (Wien)* 2004;146:103–110.

44 Carp H, Bailey S. The association between meningitis and dural puncture in bacteremic rats. *Anesthesiology* 1992;76:739–742.

4 Premedication and Monitoring

Michael F. Mulroy

Premedication and intraoperative sedation are important components of regional techniques. "Pure" regional anesthesia can be performed without supplementation, especially in ambulatory surgery. Omission of sedation is appropriate in the obstetric suite or the emergency room, where systemic medications must be carefully limited. In the operating room, however, successful regional anesthesia is facilitated by skillful use of adjuvants to produce cooperation and acceptance. This may include sedation and analgesia for the performance of the block, as well as sedation during prolonged surgical procedures.

I. Goals

A. Basically, supplemental medication is given to attain one of three objectives:

1. To **decrease apprehension and increase the degree of cooperation** in the anxious patient
2. To **provide analgesia** to reduce the degree of discomfort associated with the procedure, particularly with insertion of needles or search for paresthesias
3. To **produce amnesia** or lack of awareness of the intraoperative and perioperative events

B. A fourth motive is sometimes mentioned: the hope of raising the **seizure threshold** to local anesthetic drugs. This is not attained with the conventional sedative doses of benzodiazepines or barbiturates, but only with doses sufficient to produce unconsciousness in most patients. This approach is not warranted because it carries its own risk of respiratory and cardiac depression, and such sedation may mask the response to a test dose (1) or the early warning signs that usually precede bupivacaine cardiotoxicity (2).

C. A wide range of sedation can be produced depending on the patient and the situation (Table 4.1). There are different stages in the execution of a regional anesthetic: the performance of the block itself and the intraoperative management. Each stage requires appropriate tailoring of sedation.

1. **Outpatients,** minor procedures. These are usually associated with little anxiety and require little sedation; the use of excessive amounts will negate the advantages of rapid recovery and discharge.
2. The anxious **inpatient.** Major procedures, such as upper abdominal surgery will require sedation and an amnestic agent for insertion of an epidural catheter, as well as intraoperative supplementation with a light general anesthetic.
3. A **teaching** situation. Heavy sedation and an amnestic agent are often appropriate.
4. **Children.** Infants usually require a general anesthetic for the performance of the block itself. Although the use of a general anesthetic to facilitate regional block in children is accepted as reducing the chance of injury, in the adult such a practice may increase the risk of unrecognized nerve injury (3).

Table 4.1 Common sedative medications used to supplement regional anesthetic

Drug (brand name)	Dose range	Applications	Comments
Benzodiazepines			
Midazolam (Versed)	1–5 mg i.v.	Rapid-onset sedation in induction, operating rooms	Amnesia potential
Narcotics			
Fentanyl (Sublimaze)	25–200 μg i.v.	Rapid-onset analgesia in induction and operating rooms	Useful adjunct for painful procedures (needle insertion), potential for respiratory depression
Ketamine (Ketalar)	Bolus of 20–50 mg i.v.	Sedation during blocks	Some analgesic properties, supports respiration and blood pressure; risk of confusion with higher doses
Sedative/hypnotics			
Dexmedetomidine (Precedex)	Bolus followed by infusion (0.7 μg/kg/h)	Intraoperative sedation	Potential bradycardia, hypotension
Propofol (Diprivan)	Boluses of 30–60 mg, infusion of 25–100 μg/kg/min	Rapid sedation for procedures in induction room, good sedation intraoperatively	Pain on injection

i.v., intravenous.

II. Drugs

A. Opioids. The opioid class of drugs produce analgesia and sedation without loss of consciousness. Therefore, they are excellent in enhancing patient cooperation and in reducing the discomfort associated with needle insertion or paresthesias. They also possess the desirable feature of easy reversibility with naloxone. **Respiratory depression** is the main drawback of the opioids, and doses must be individually titrated and the patient monitored appropriately. All of the opioids share the propensity to stimulate the chemoreceptor trigger zone and induce nausea. This is dose related and rarely occurs in the sedative dose range. Some respiratory depression will occur, and pulse oximetry and supplemental oxygen are appropriate.

1. **Fentanyl** is the most popular opioid sedative because of its rapid onset, short but adequate duration, and easy titratability. It is most appropriate for the ambulatory surgery setting, but is also effective for sedation while performing blocks in an inpatient induction area. Increments of 25 to 50 μg give rapid analgesia for 20 to 30 minutes, usually waning as the block is completed. Dosage is a function of patient vitality, not body size; **microgram per kilogram schedules should be avoided.**
2. **Derivatives of fentanyl** are available. Sufentanil is similar, although roughly ten times as potent; suitable dilution is advisable. Alfentanil is similar in effect but shorter in duration and less potent than fentanyl. Although perhaps ideal as an intravenous infusion anesthetic for outpatients, its sedative properties after a bolus injection may be too short to facilitate regional techniques. Remifentanil is even shorter in duration and is suitable

only as an infusion. The expense and need of a pump for these two drugs make bolus fentanyl doses more often the drug of choice.

3. **Morphine and meperidine** are long acting and provide good sedation as well as analgesia, but their **longer duration** and slower onset make them less useful.
4. Several opioids with both **agonist and antagonist** properties are intended to reduce the potential for respiratory depression, but they have not been shown to have significant advantages in efficacy or safety.

B. **Benzodiazepines** are extensively used as premedicants or sedatives. They are effective, centrally acting anxiolytics, and they have the additional potential to produce **amnesia**. These drugs are effective in the treatment of local anesthetic toxicity and are therefore useful to have in induction areas in the event of a toxic reaction. The amnestic property, especially of the longer-acting lorazepam (1- to 2-mg doses), is advantageous for inpatients desiring to be unaware of procedures. Like morphine, it may require 30 to 60 minutes to reach peak effect, and care must be used when titrating intravenous supplemental sedation during this period of increasing blood levels. Prolonged sedation in the recovery room is seen frequently, particularly in the elderly patient. Because of concern about prolonged postoperative effects, there is less use of the long-acting drugs.

1. **Midazolam** is the most popular benzodiazepine, and has essentially replaced diazepam for parenteral use because of its predictable dose response and absence of venous irritation. Midazolam is **rapid and short acting** and produces less respiratory depression than opioids. It is useful for intraoperative sedation once an adequate block has been achieved. It is also useful in producing amnesia for the block itself, although it is **not analgesic** in this situation and profits from opioid supplementation. The amnestic effect can be a disadvantage by producing **unwanted confusion** and **lack of cooperation** in patients if excessive doses are used. Sedation can be long lasting, so the dosage should be kept to a minimum (1–3 mg intravenously, titrated intravenously in 0.5- to 1-mg increments). Its duration of sedation is short with these doses, lasting approximately 30 minutes. The **amnestic effect is unpredictable**, and occurs at doses lower than those required to produce sedation, which may present a problem in outpatients. Intraoperative observations and postoperative instructions may not be remembered by an apparently alert outpatient. Nevertheless, midazolam is an excellent anxiolytic, and the amnestic effect is useful both during performance of blocks and for intraoperative sedation. Larger doses may prolong recovery, and will also increase the potential for respiratory depression when used in conjunction with opioids.
2. **Antagonists.** The availability of the specific antagonist drug flumazenil has increased the safety margin of benzodiazepines, but it is more reasonable to shift to a shorter-acting infusion of propofol or dexmedetomidine if prolonged sedation is necessary.

C. **Propofol** is not only primarily a general anesthetic drug but also an **excellent sedative** in lower doses. Although it (like the benzodiazepines) **does not have analgesic properties**, it is not an antianalgesic like the barbiturates. It also lacks the subhypnotic amnestic properties of the benzodiazepines, but it provides more **rapid recovery and an antiemetic effect** that is beneficial, especially in outpatients.

1. It can be used as a **bolus** for brief deep sedation during performance of some selected blocks (such as retrobulbar block) where consciousness is not necessary.
2. As an **infusion** during surgical procedures, it provides anxiolytic, sedative, and amnestic properties, with the best results in the dose range of 30 to 60 μg/kg/min **(4)**. Its rapid recovery, antiemetic effect, and easy titratability make it ideal for sedation in short outpatient procedures.
3. The **combination** of small doses of midazolam and fentanyl to enhance the performance of a regional block, followed by a propofol infusion for sedation, provides an ideal formula for patient satisfaction and rapid recovery.

D. **Barbiturates** have basically been replaced by these other two classes of drugs because they are not true analgesics or amnestics; they produce these effects only in doses sufficient to produce unconsciousness. At lower doses, they are actually **antianalgesic** and may produce exaggerated responses to pain and decreased cooperation.

E. **Dexmedetomidine** is an α_2 agonist that has been used for sedation in the intensive care unit and for surgical procedures **(5)**. It has the advantage of **avoiding respiratory depression**, but may produce **hemodynamic side effects**, particularly bradycardia and hypotension. It appears to potentiate analgesia and reduce inhalation anesthetic requirements. It is administered as an intravenous bolus (1 μg/kg over 10 minutes) followed by an infusion (0.3–0.7 μg/kg/h) because of its short half-life (2 hours). It may be useful as intraoperative sedation with peripheral nerve blocks (infusion of 0.7 μg/kg/h equivalent to propofol 35 μg/kg/min), but its hypotensive effect may make it undesirable in conjunction with neuraxial blockade. It has no amnestic effects.

F. **Ketamine** has been used in low doses (20–30 mg intravenously) as a sedative during performance of regional blockade because of its **analgesic properties** in this dose range. Larger doses are associated with hallucinations on emergence. This drug has the advantage of **maintaining cardiovascular stability** and producing less respiratory depression and obtundation of airway reflexes. It is most useful for sedation during spinal anesthesia for fractured hip repair in the elderly, where the analgesia and cardiovascular support are beneficial.

G. **Oxygen.** Although not a sedative drug, oxygen is appropriate as a supplemental drug when most of these sedatives and analgesics are used. Opioids particularly produce respiratory depression, and this is potentiated by the addition of benzodiazepines. Oxygen desaturation is frequent, and nasal prongs or a face mask are useful, especially in the elderly (6).

H. **Other adjuvants**

1. The preoperative visit has been shown to be extremely effective in reducing anxiety in patients.
2. Kind attention to the patient's concern and situation will reduce the need for any of the preceding medications. Small gestures, such as comfortable positioning of the table and the offer of a warm blanket, are greatly appreciated.
3. **Music** also has sedative properties. Selected tapes can be provided through a portable cassette player or a piped-in music system. This will not only distract and pacify most patients, but the headphones will also eliminate many of the anxiety-provoking sounds and conversations of the induction room and the operating room.

I. **General anesthetic agents** are sometimes helpful and occasionally necessary. When **upper abdominal surgery** is being performed under intercostal, paravertebral, spinal, or epidural block, supplemental general anesthesia with an endotracheal tube is advisable to obtund diaphragmatic sensation, protect the airway, and provide controlled ventilation. The presence of a regional block **reduces the minimum alveolar concentration (MAC)** of inhalational anesthesia, and when the endotracheal tube is the most significant stimulus the patient may perceive, a fraction of MAC is usually sufficient (7). As mentioned elsewhere, performance of regional blocks in an unconscious adult may increase the risk of nerve injury.

III. Monitoring

A. Intraoperatively, patients undergoing regional anesthesia require the **same standards of monitoring** as those receiving general anesthesia, including electrocardiogram (ECG), blood pressure device, and a pulse oximeter, as per standard American Society of Anesthesiologists (ASA) guidelines.

B. The patient undergoing regional anesthesia must also be monitored closely for the **expected hemodynamic changes** of blocks, and especially for the signs of potential systemic toxicity.

1. Specific monitoring to detect increasing blood levels of local anesthetic must focus on the patient's **mental status** and therefore requires constant verbal contact. The anesthetist or assistant should engage in conversation with the patient and be alert for the first signs of a change in mental concentration or slurring of speech, especially in the first 20 minutes following injection of a large quantity of local anesthetic.
2. A **pulse oximeter** is the most frequently applied monitor in an induction area. Providing information about heart rate as well as oxygen saturation, it is useful during regional anesthesia, particularly when sedation may produce respiratory depression. It is also an effective pulse counter for monitoring heart rate changes with an epinephrine-containing test-dose solution.
3. **Blood pressure** monitoring is essential following spinal, epidural, or sympathetic blocks. An automatic noninvasive device with a short cycling time is ideal because it leaves the anesthesiologist's hands free to make interventions during the early stages of hypotension. A baseline blood pressure value should be established before performing any blocks that will produce sympathetic blockade.
4. The **block level** should also be monitored, especially when a sympathectomy is produced. Block level and blood pressure should be measured every 3 to 5 minutes for the first 15 minutes following the block to warn of unexpected high levels. Block level should be monitored during the course of epidural or spinal anesthesia, because both of these techniques may demonstrate a change of level over the first hour.
5. **A final note.** All blocks involving significant quantities of local anesthetic must be administered in a location that provides **immediate resuscitation equipment**.

REFERENCES

1 Mulroy MF, Neal JM, Mackey DC, et al. 2-Chloroprocaine and bupivacaine are unreliable indicators of intravascular injection in the premedicated patient. *Reg Anesth Pain Med* 1998;23:9.

2 Bernards CM, Carpenter RL, Rupp SM, et al. Effect of midazolam and diazepam premedication on central nervous system and cardiovascular toxicity of bupivacaine in pigs. *Anesthesiology* 1989;70:318.

3 **Benumof JL. Permanent loss of cervical spinal cord function associated with interscalene block performed under general anesthesia. *Anesthesiology* 2000;93:1541.**

4 **Smith I, Monk TG, White PF, et al. Propofol infusion during regional anesthesia: sedative, amnestic and anxiolytic properties. *Anaesth Analg* 1994;79:313.**

5 **Kamibayashi T, Maze M. Clinical uses of α2-adrenergic agonists. *Anesthesiology* 2000;93:1345–1349.**

6 Smith DC, Crul JF. Oxygen desaturation following sedation for regional analgesia. *Br J Anaesth* 1989;62:206.

7 Hodgson PS, Liu SS. Epidural lidocaine decreases sevoflurane requirement for adequate depth of anesthesia as measured by the Bispectral Index monitor. *Anesthesiology* 2001;94:799–803.

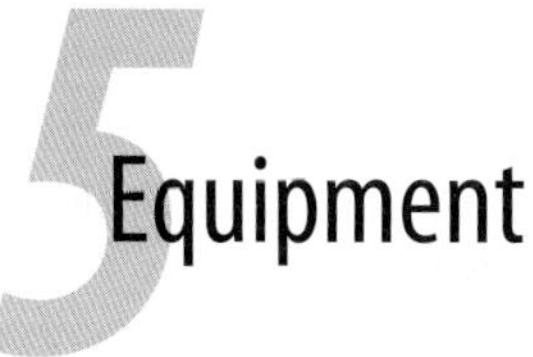

5 Equipment

Michael F. Mulroy

Regional techniques can be performed with almost any syringe and needle. Success depends more on the skill of the operator than on the quality of the instrument. Nevertheless, there are differences in equipment that make some devices more effective than others and, in experienced hands, can optimize the performance of regional techniques.

I. General principles

Equipment for regional blocks is usually stocked in **prepared sterile trays**. These include skin-preparation swabs, drapes, needles, syringes, solution cups, and a sterility indicator. The choice of equipment will be dictated by the specific blocks attempted and by personal preference, but some general comments are warranted.

A. Disposable versus reusable equipment. Reusable block trays allow maximum flexibility in choosing specific needles, syringes, and catheters. They allow for the purchase of products that are manufactured to more exact specifications than those usually found in disposable trays. However, reusable trays represent a significant initial capital investment and require additional technician time to maintain, as well as a perception of a greater risk of transmission of infectious diseases.

Concern about infectious diseases, especially newer ones that are resistant to conventional sterilization techniques, has created a greater reliance on disposable equipment. The quality of disposable trays has improved, and the willingness of the manufacturers to "*customize*" trays to the needs of individual institutions is widespread. They remove the burden of sterilization from the local department or hospital (although not the responsibility of checking for sterility).

B. Sterilization. If presterilized disposable trays are not used, reusable equipment must be both cleaned and sterilized between uses. Detergents are not desirable for cleaning reusable needles and syringes because of the chance of chemical contamination of local anesthetic solutions from residual cleansing agents left on the syringe or needle. Blood and other foreign material must be removed with water only. Significant bacterial or viral contamination is removed by heat sterilization at 121°C or above for 20 minutes (steam under pressure). Appropriate indicators of adequate heat exposure must be placed both in the center of each sterilized packet and on the outside.

Plastic and rubber will not tolerate heat treatment and must be sterilized with **ethylene oxide gas** exposure. A long period of aeration is required to remove residual gas. A different indicator strip is used to document sterility. Disposable trays usually have such an indicator in their central compartment. This indicator must be checked before using the tray.

If **local anesthetic** drugs are added to trays after they are opened, they must be wrapped sterilely and handled in an aseptic manner.

C. Skin preparation (asepsis) requires meticulous attention to reduce the chance of introduction of microorganisms, especially when neuraxial techniques are employed. A consensus panel of the American Society of Regional Anesthesia and Pain Medicine has published a summary of recommendations, outlined here **(1)**.

1. The current recommended solution is **chlorhexidine gluconate,** a potent broad-spectrum germicide, preferably in 80% alcohol. It has immediate germicidal properties that persist for several hours and are not impaired by the presence for organic compounds such as blood. Skin reactions are also less common than with iodine-containing preparations. One major challenge is that standard chlorhexidine is **colorless;** the addition of a pigment may reduce the chance of unintentional confusion with local anesthetic solutions.
2. **Povidone-iodine** is an iodophor preparation with good antimicrobial action against gram-positive and -negative organisms. The activity of this solution is based on the release of free iodine, which is dependent on the water dilution of the solution. Careful adherence to the manufacturer's instructions for dilution and use is important. Activity of these solutions depends on the release of iodine, and therefore requires **several minutes of contact and drying** for effectiveness. Like chlorhexidine, potency is significantly improved by **addition of alcohol**. Unlike previous iodine–alcohol solutions, these preparations are not likely to burn tissues, although excessive quantities in body folds can cause irritation, and should be washed off after completion of the block. Single-use containers are preferable because of the potential of contamination of larger bottles. A few patients are truly **allergic** to topical iodine preparations and require alternative solutions. Although both povidone-iodine and chlorhexidine are approved by the U.S. Food and Drug Administration (FDA) for surgical skin preparation, neither has received official endorsement due to the lack of sufficient studies. Neither has been implicated in neurologic damage, but, again, there are insufficient data to ensure their "safety."
3. **Isopropyl alcohol** (70%) is a third satisfactory alternative as a skin preparation, and does not require scrubbing. Like chlorhexidine, it carries a potential risk of unrecognized contamination of anesthetic solutions if used as a colorless solution. Alcohol alone or in any of these solutions is **flammable,** and increases the potential for operating room fires.
4. Regardless of the agent used, total sterility of the skin is rarely achieved, and careful attention to **aseptic technique** is needed. A wide area should be prepped, and sterile towels or plastic drapes should be placed on the skin to extend the working field.

D. Aseptic technique. In addition to chemical preparation, other steps are necessary to reduce the introduction of pathogens during regional anesthetic techniques.

1. **Hand washing** is essential to reduce transmission of organisms by health care workers, and should be performed before each block, before donning gloves. A traditional soap and water washing is adequate, as well as the use of alcohol-containing skin cleansers.
2. Removal of **jewelry** and watches is controversial, but has been shown to reduce bacterial count after hand washing in health care workers. The role of artificial or long fingernails is unclear.
3. The use of **gloves** is strongly recommended, although the addition of gowns does not appear to add additional safety.
4. The use of **masks** during regional techniques also remains controversial. Data in the surgical literature is ambiguous about the role of masks in

reducing infection, although there are case reports of nosocomial infections that appeared to be transmitted by anesthesiologists not wearing masks.

5. Appropriate **sterile draping** for the injection site is also necessary to reduce contamination. The use of a set of sterile towels is often sufficient for single injection techniques, but a wider continuous drape with a central opening is preferred for insertions of catheters or use of ultrasonographic probes, where contamination of the lengthy catheters is more likely. Clear plastic drapes are ideal to allow visualization of the anatomy or motor response to nerve stimulation.
6. The use of **bacterial filters** appears justified for long-term catheter insertions, but not warranted for short-term use of catheters.

II. Syringes

Although syringes are generally considered only as carrying instruments for the local anesthetics, their features are important.

A. The **resistance between the barrel and the piston is critical** when using the "loss of resistance" technique for identifying the epidural space. Glass syringes have been superior to most plastic material in allowing free movement. New lubrication techniques have produced plastic products with low friction, but generally the disposable products rely on a gasket to provide a seal, which gives firm resistance in the movement of the piston and will obscure changes in resistance to injection as the needle is advanced. **Glass syringes** have the disadvantage that a small amount of powder from sterile gloves can cause the piston to stick in the barrel, but generally these syringes provide better appreciation of resistance.

B. The **size of the syringe** also affects performance.

1. The **smallest syringes** (1 mL) **give the greatest accuracy in measurement,** as is required in adding epinephrine to the anesthetic solution. A small diameter (3–5 mL) syringe gives a better feel of resistance during epidural insertion but is impractical for injection of large volumes.
2. For injection, a 10-mL **syringe is most comfortably held in the hand;** larger syringes are heavy and bulky and usually require two hands for good control. They do not allow the fine control needed for localizing nerves. **Disconnecting and reconnecting** the needle can also be awkward with large syringes if one hand is occupied in fixing the needle in place on the nerve. Larger syringes also add more weight and are more likely to cause an unwanted advancement of the needle. A 10-mL **syringe appears to be a practical compromise**. It is inconvenient to refill frequently, but use of a 10-mL syringe limits the quantity injected at any one time and therefore serves to encourage incremental injection of large volumes of local anesthetic.
3. If a larger syringe (20 or 30 mL) is used, it is desirable to avoid direct connection to the needle by using a short length of **flexible intravenous tubing** as a connector. This allows for finer control of the needle, but may require an assistant to handle aspiration and injection with the syringe.
4. A **three-ring adapter** is useful on the 10-mL syringe (control syringe, Figure 5.1). It allows greater control in injecting solution and also allows the solo operator to refill the syringe with one hand while holding the needle in place in the patient with the other. These adapters are available on plastic as well as glass syringes.

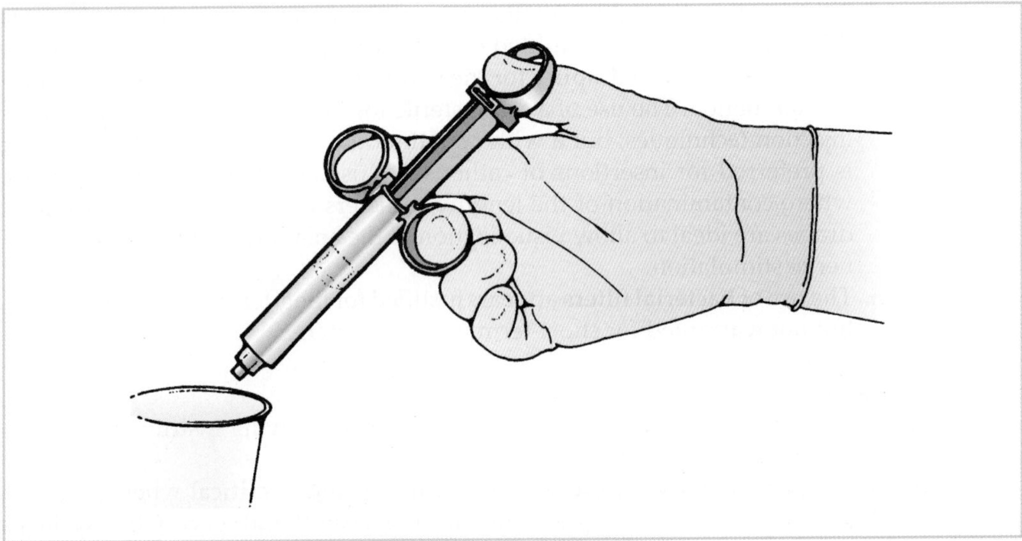

Figure 5.1. The three-ring ("control") syringe. This adaptation to the plunger of a standard 10-mL syringe allows greater control of injection, easier aspiration, and the opportunity to refill the syringe with one hand.

5. The connection to the hub of the needle affects the ease of fixation of the needle. The **Luer-Lok adapter,** which screws tightly onto the matching needle hub, does not require forceful friction to provide a seal and is therefore less likely to cause unwanted movement of the needle when attaching the syringe. This coupling also provides a connection less likely to leak on injection. A tight seal is critical when using resistance to identify the epidural space.
6. Therefore, an **ideal tray** would have Luer-Lok syringes in 1-, 3-, and 10-mL sizes with a three-ring adapter on the latter, plus a glass syringe for epidural localization.

III. Needles

Although local infiltration can be performed with almost any needle, special adaptations can facilitate success with regional techniques.

A. Regional-block needles

1. Peripheral nerve blocks are most commonly performed with special needles adapted for **use with nerve stimulators** (see subsequent text). These needles are usually approximately 22 gauge in size, with a specially adapted Luer-Lok hub or side-arm extension that includes a 20- to 40-cm (8- to 16-in.) wire connection for attachment to the negative lead of the nerve stimulator (Figure 5.2). The needles are also **sheathed** with a nonconducting cover to concentrate the electrical current at the tip, which is most commonly a **short-beveled design**. The incidence of nerve injury is presumed to be less with shorter-bevel needles (16 versus 12 degrees) (Figure 5.2). The short-bevel needle may offer more resistance to advancement. Larger (19 gauge) insulated stimulating needles are also available with curved tips that allow passage of catheters.
2. Regional anesthetics can also be performed with traditional unsheathed needles using the paresthesia technique or localization with other landmarks.

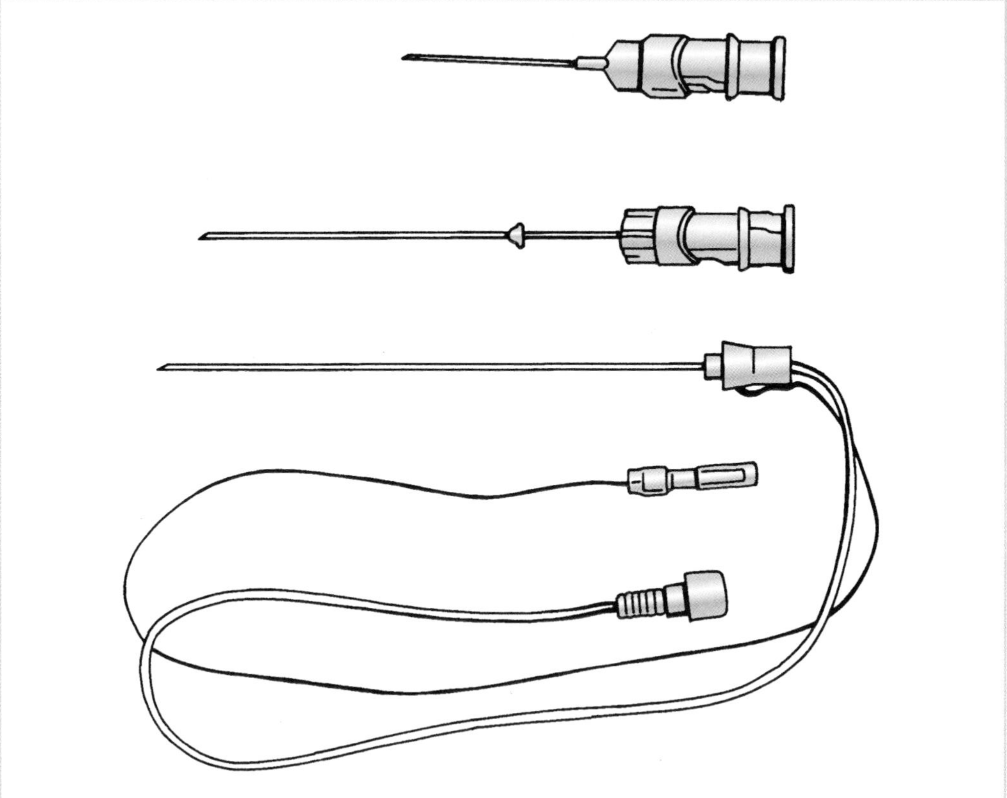

Figure 5.2. Regional anesthesia needles. For superficial blocks, such as the axillary, short 25-gauge needles (*top*) with a shorter-bevel angle (compared to standard Quincke-type needle points) are very effective. For deeper injections, longer needles may be equipped with a "safety bead" on the upper shaft (*middle*) to prevent loss of the needle in the subcutaneous tissue if it separates from the hub. Needles used for peripheral nerve stimulator blocks (*bottom*) include the direct attachment for the nerve stimulator connection and the short tubing for the injection syringe. This tubing serves to remove the weight of the syringe from the needle hub, allowing finer control.

The gauge employed is a **compromise between ease of injection and discomfort caused**. Smaller needles (25 to 32 gauge) are best for skin infiltration because their insertion is less uncomfortable. The 23-gauge size is suitable for **superficial blocks,** such as axillary or intercostals on thin patients. A larger, more rigid shaft is usually required for any deeper needle insertions. The **22-gauge 38 or 50 mm (1.5- or 2-in.) size is needed for most** regional techniques. A 127 or 152 mm (5- or 6-in.) 20-gauge needle is used for **deep blocks,** such as the celiac plexus, where free aspiration is desired.

B. Spinal needles

1. Spinal needles are necessarily **longer** (90–127 mm [3.5–6 in.]) and usually **styletted** to prevent occluding the lumen with a plug of skin or subcutaneous tissue before the dura is punctured. A number of **bevel designs** have been introduced since the original Quincke (sharp bevel) style was first used, and most are designated by the name of their inventor (Figure 5.3). The **rounded** Greene and Whitacre points are designed to be **less traumatic** to the dura itself, apparently splitting or spreading rather than cutting the longitudinal

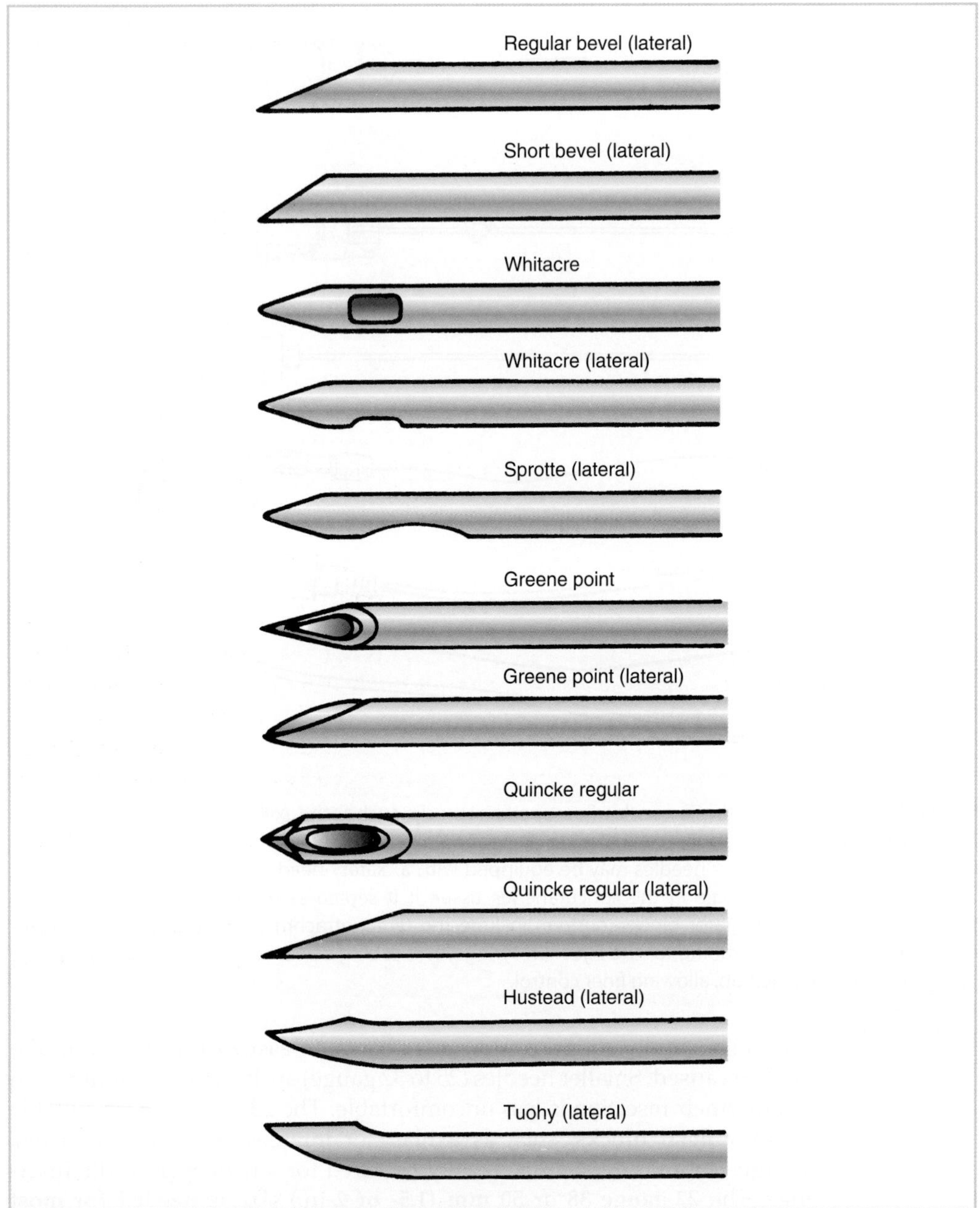

Figure 5.3. Standard regional anesthesia needle bevels.

fibers, thereby promoting more rapid sealing of the dural hole. Experience with the rounded-bevel design (especially the Whitacre and the Sprotte derivation of it) has shown an impressive **reduction in the incidence of postdural puncture headache**.

2. The gauge of spinal needles is also important in terms of the probability of a headache, although it is apparently not as important as the needle type (see Chapter 6). **Smaller needles create smaller holes** and less transdural

leak, but they are more difficult to insert and to aspirate. The **25-gauge rounded-bevel needle is the size most frequently chosen as a reasonable compromise.**

C. **Epidural needles**

1. Epidural needles are of a larger gauge, both to permit better **assessment of loss of resistance** and to **allow the passage of catheters**. An 18-gauge thin-walled needle is the smallest that will pass a 20-gauge catheter, and 16- or 17-gauge needles are commonly used for catheters. A 19-gauge needle is satisfactory for single injections. A 22-gauge needle has been used, but the perception of resistance is more challenging through the narrower opening.
2. A conventional **Quincke-point** needle can be used for a single injection technique, although some practitioners prefer the blunter, short-beveled **Crawford** needle for epidural or caudal insertion. The **Tuohy** needle with a curved point was first introduced to facilitate the passage of catheters. **Hustead** modified this needle to reduce the bevel angle slightly in the hope of reducing the chance of shearing the catheter during passage (Figure 5.3). The angle of both of these bevels may allow better direction of the catheter into the main axis of the epidural canal, but the greater curvature and the offset of the point of the needle from the mid axis of the shaft also make them more likely to **deviate from the intended path** during advancement. The longer bevel also creates the possibility that the tip of the needle may communicate a loss of resistance before the full opening of the bevel is completely through the ligamentum flavum. These needles may need to be advanced another 2 to 3 mm beyond their initial penetration of the ligament before a catheter will pass. Most of these needles are manufactured with 1-cm **markings** along the shaft to allow better appreciation of the needle depth or movement.
3. Tuohy needles have also been manufactured with additional channels and end holes to facilitate simultaneous insertion of spinal needles for **combined spinal–epidural (CSE) anesthesia** (2).
4. The hubs of epidural needles have also been adapted in some cases with "*wings*" to allow better control of the depth of advancement, particularly in the thoracic region (Figure 5.4).

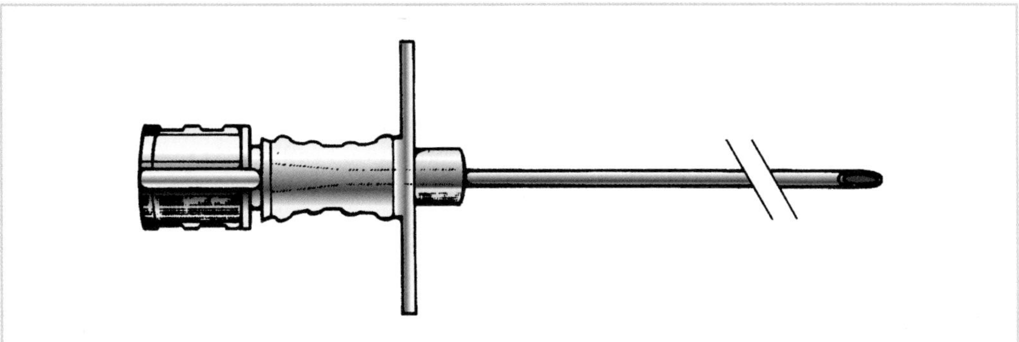

Figure 5.4. Wing adapters on needle hub. The flanges attached to the hub of a standard epidural needle allow greater control of the advancement of the tip when the flanges are grasped between the thumb and forefinger while the other fingers rest on the skin and control the depth of insertion. These flanges come in several modifications.

D. **Introducers** are useful in spinal and epidural anesthesia. These are short, large-bore, sharp-pointed needles. For spinal anesthesia, these can be inserted through the skin and into the interspinous ligament. They create a rigid path to guide the more flexible small-gauge spinal needles. They offer the added advantage of allowing the tip of the spinal needle to **bypass the skin** and therefore avoid contamination with preparatory solution or residual skin bacteria. For epidural use, a skin hole made with these needles reduces the resistance to insertion of the epidural needle and allows more sensitive appreciation of the ligaments themselves.

IV. Catheters

A. A multitude of catheters is available for insertion through epidural or peripheral nerve block needles.

1. For **basic catheters,** the primary difference among them is the construction material, which gives different performance characteristics. Newer catheters of **nylon, polyamide, or polyvinyl** offer **compromises between flexibility (increased risk of kinking) and rigidity (risk of puncturing dura or veins),** and the appropriate balance is a matter of personal choice among the wide selection available.
2. Another feature offered in epidural catheters is the presence of **lateral injection ports** proximal to a closed, soft-tip end. This may reduce the chance of dural puncture, and the presence of multiple holes reduces the chance of occlusion of the catheter by tissue or blood clot blocking a single hole. However, multiple holes may also allow unrecognized dural or venous puncture, because a test dose may not give a reliable response if only one hole is in a vessel or into the dura. Many practitioners prefer a single-port catheter for this reason. On the other hand, aspiration is more likely to be an effective test with multiple-orifice catheters (3).
3. **Marks** at 1- or 5-cm (0.5–2 in.) intervals along the first 20 cm (8 in.) are useful in guiding insertion of the catheter to the correct depth. **Radiopaque markers** on the catheter are useful in documenting position of chronic indwelling catheters or catheters for injection of neurolytic agents. The selection of any or all of these features is again a matter of personal experience and choice.
4. A **spring-wire reinforced flexible** catheter combines the ideal features of easy passage, minimal trauma, and low risk of occlusion or migration. If the catheter is to remain in place for several days for postoperative analgesia, these devices allow adaptation of the catheter to patient movement, and **may reduce the frequency of catheter migration.**
5. The most complex version of the continuous catheter is the addition of a **stimulating wire to the tip** of a catheter for continuous peripheral nerve block. Use of such catheters allows continuous identification of the nerve as the catheter is advanced, and may increase the probability of effective location of the tip after full insertion (4), although at a higher cost.

B. **Adapters** are needed to allow injection from a syringe into a catheter. These are usually of the **Tuohy-Borst type, where screwing one fitting onto another** tightens a rubber sleeve around the catheter and holds it in place. There are **as many connectors available as there are catheters,** and the selection is again a personal choice based on cost, reliability, and ease of use. All connectors should have a **Luer-Lok adapter** for fitting a syringe and a cap to provide sterility of the fitting between injections. All catheters used for repeated injections on surgical wards should be **clearly labeled** as epidural or peripheral nerve catheters, ideally with a colored label, to prevent unintentional injection of intravenous drugs.

C. Epidural catheters can also be inserted into the **subarachnoid space,** although the larger needles used for the standard catheters may increase the risk of headache. At one point, smaller microcatheters (27 gauge or smaller) were employed through smaller needles to reduce this problem. Unfortunately, problems with neurotoxicity (see Chapter 3) led to their withdrawal from the market.

V. Infusion devices

In the last 10 years, anesthesiologists have become more actively involved in the continuation of regional techniques in the postoperative period for pain relief (see Chapter 23). There are several continuous-infusion devices available to assist in the delivery of local anesthetics or local anesthetic–opioid mixtures for postoperative pain relief (5).

A. For **inpatient** use, there are **small electrically driven pumps** that provide, in addition to a continuous infusion, a **patient-controlled option** that allows supplemental doses at times of increased need. These devices are **individually programmable** and demonstrate a high degree of flexibility. They usually contain a **locked chamber** for the infusion itself, because opioids are used commonly in this setting. It is important that such devices have the potential for a continuous infusion, as well as a lockout interval to prevent excessive dosage by the patients. Mechanical **failures with such devices are rare,** and they are highly effective for inpatient postoperative analgesia.

B. The use of continuous catheters for **peripheral nerve blocks** also benefits from the attachment of a continuous-infusion pump. Several modalities are available.

1. The simplest are **elastomeric** bulbs that contain a fixed amount of local anesthetic under a constant pressure, which is then delivered at a fixed rate through a flow valve connected to the catheter. These pumps can provide continuous infusions for 24 to 48 hours for brachial plexus and lower-extremity analgesia. The limitation of the elastomeric pumps is the fixed delivery volume, although newer devices have added a bolus capacity.
2. There are also **spring-loaded mechanical pumps** that are similar to the bulbs in their simplicity. They also rely on a constant tension to deliver the solution, and have been equipped with bolus capability.
3. Alternatively, **small battery-operated, programmable, mechanical pumps** are available, which have the same options as the inpatient infusion devices; that is, they can deliver both continuous infusion and incremental additional boluses on patient demand. Again, mechanical problems with these pumps are rare and they appear to provide a useful option for prolonging postoperative analgesia in both inpatients and outpatients.

VI. Nerve localization

Although many blocks can be performed using simple injection around an easily identified landmark (saphenous nerve at the knee, perivascular axillary block), deeper injections require confirmation of nerve localization. The historical method is to elicit a paresthesia. Recent advances allow easier identification, and may reduce the chance of unintentional nerve injury.

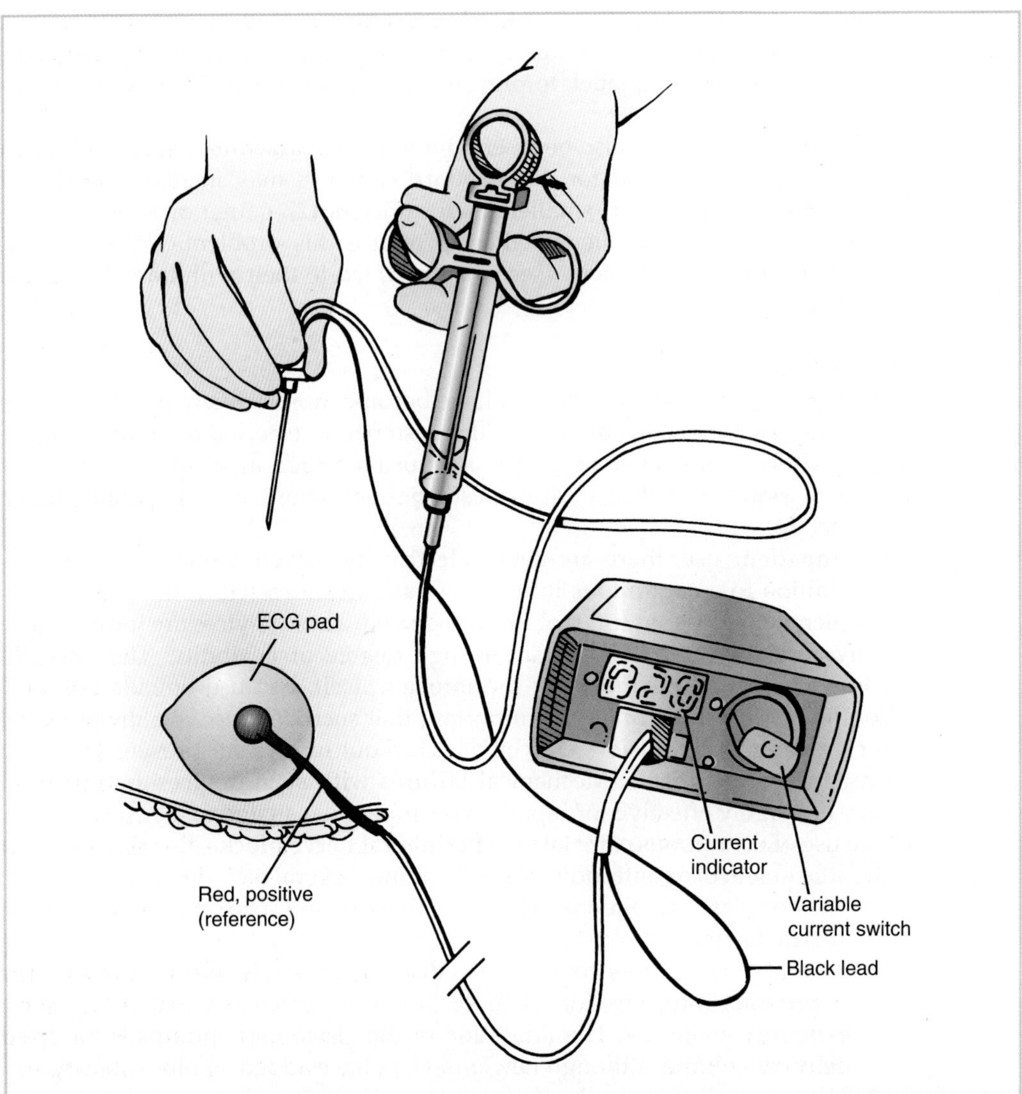

Figure 5.5. Nerve stimulator attached to regional-block needle. The negative (black) lead is attached to the exploring needle, whereas the positive (red) is connected to a reference electrocardiogram (ECG) pad used as a "ground." The stimulator is set to deliver 1 to 2 mA of current to detect the nerve. The current is reduced further as the needle is advanced closer to the nerve. Motor stimulation at a current of 0.5 mA or less suggests that the needle is adjacent to the nerve.

A. **Nerve stimulators.** The peripheral nerve stimulator delivers a **pulsed electric current** to the tip of an **exploring needle** (Figure 5.5). As the needle approaches a nerve, depolarization is produced. Efferent **motor nerves (A-α fibers) are most easily depolarized,** so these devices have the advantage of identifying mixed peripheral nerves by producing a muscle twitch rather than eliciting uncomfortable sensory paresthesias.

1. The degree of stimulation is dependent on the total current (amperage) and (presumably) the distance between the current source and the nerve. This principle led to the development of nerve stimulators with variable

outputs. A **high current (approximately** 1–2 mA) **can be used to identify the approach** to a nerve. A progressively lower current may document increasing proximity of needle to nerve. In practice, 2 mA will produce depolarization of a motor nerve at a distance. As the needle is moved closer to the nerve, a **smaller current** (0.5–0.6 mA) **suggests adequate proximity to the nerve**. Recent reports have questioned the relationship between the current and the distance to the nerve, bringing into question whether any correlation can be assumed. Specifically, needles in direct contact with nerves (based on paresthesias) may require currents from 0.1 to greater than 1 mA to produce a response, so the relevance of the final stimulating current is unclear (6,7). Current practice suggests that a **current of 0.5 mA is ideal,** but adequate anesthesia is produced with greater and lesser current, and there is no evidence of greater risk of nerve injury with lower currents.

2. The **characteristics of the stimulating current** can also be modified to produce a sensory response. The short-**duration** impulse commonly used (0.1 ms) is effective in stimulating motor fibers, but a longer-duration pulse (0.3 ms) will also stimulate sensory fibers, a useful feature if a pure sensory nerve is being sought.
3. The ideal nerve stimulator has a **variable linear output** with a clear display of current delivered. The positive (red, ground) lead of the stimulator is connected to a skin electrode. The negative (black, cathode) lead is attached to the exploring needle. The connection can be made with an "alligator"-type clamp, but commercial sheathed needles with electrical connectors incorporated in their design are more commonly used (Figure 5.6).
4. **Electrically insulated** (sheathed, Teflon-coated) **needles** concentrate more current at the needle tip and will increase the accuracy of nerve localization. The electrical isolation of the needle shaft causes the depolarization to decrease after the needle point passes the nerve, which is not the case with unsheathed needles. Sheathed needles are more expensive, but are the best choice.
5. **Nerve stimulators are not a substitute for knowledge of anatomy and proper initial needle placement.** They will only help document the proximity of the needle to the nerve once it is already near. The stimulator cannot find the nerve for the novice who has not reviewed anatomy. Although it is speculated that their use may reduce the potential for nerve damage, no study has shown an increased safety margin when nerve stimulators are used, and nerve injuries occur despite their use (8). Stimulators are useful for teaching residents in a heavily premedicated patient, and they are particularly useful in pediatric practice, where blocks are usually performed on a sedated or anesthetized patient. Stimulators are useful in the obtunded or uncooperative patient in whom motor stimulation may be a needed substitute for identification of a paresthesia. But the use of a nerve stimulator does not eliminate the risk of nerve injury when blocks are performed on unconscious adults (9).
6. Another challenge is that the use of a stimulator may require **two individuals**—one sterilely gloved for the procedure and the other operating the device, although there are new foot control pedals available that will obviate this obstacle.

B. Ultrasonography. Transcutaneous ultrasonography is the latest addition to nerve localization techniques **(10,11)**. It employs images produced by

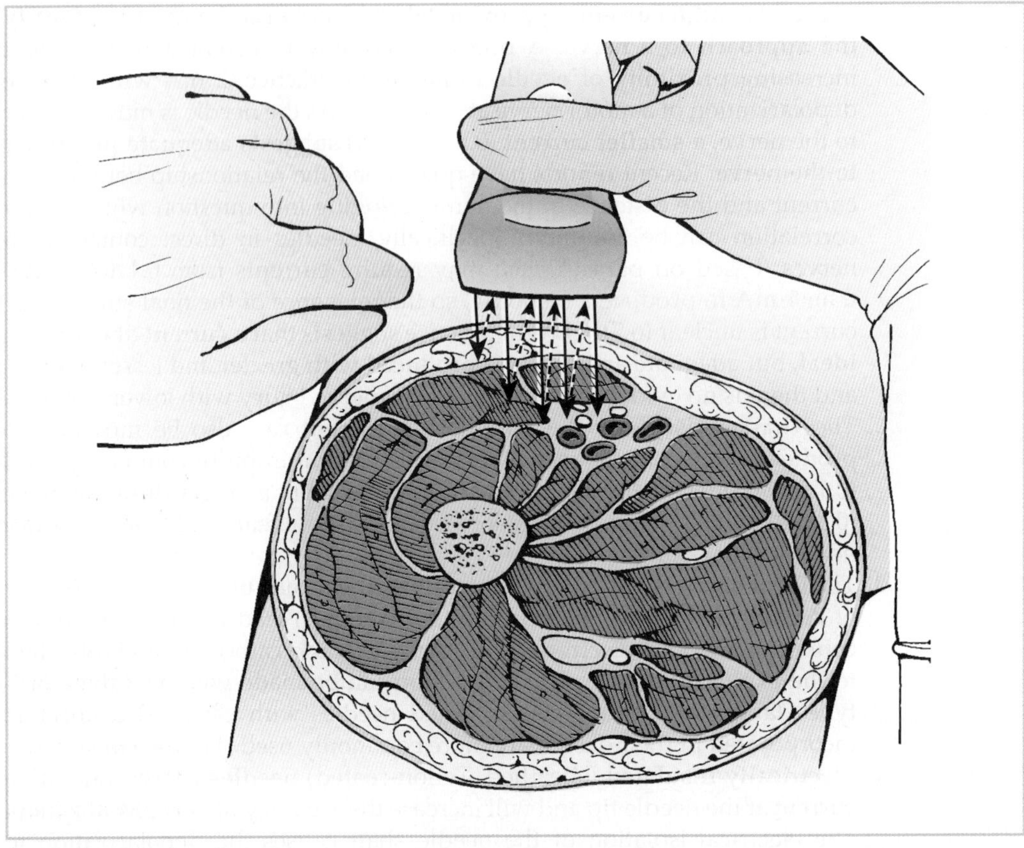

Figure 5.6. Relationship of transducer, waves, and needle for nerve block. Sound waves penetrate tissue are reflected back from tissue interfaces and recorded by the transducer. Metallic needles are easily visualized when in the narrow beam of the transducer.

high-frequency sound waves to provide real-time imaging of peripheral nerves and the surrounding fascial planes and to guide needle insertion and distribution of injected local anesthetics **(12, 13)**.

1. **Ultrasound waves** (greater than 20 MHz frequency) are generated by passing an alternating electrical current across piezoelectric crystals. The waves easily penetrate skin, and propagate away from the transducer. They are **absorbed** by tissues **or reflected** back to the ultrasonographic probe when they strike structures of varying densities. The degree to which ultrasound waves are reflected or absorbed determines the signal intensity on an arbitrary black and white scale. Tissues that allow easy passage of sound waves (water, blood, air) appear as **dark areas ("hypoechoic")**. Tissues that strongly reflect the waves (such as bone, tendons, and nerves) generate large signal intensities and appear **white, or "hyperechoic**." The returned waves are captured by the transducer head, and amplified by software to calculate the **depth** of the echo and compensate for the loss of signal energy with distance ("attenuation"). Therefore, sharper images of nerves and vessels are available, even at depth. Careful placement of the probe, with the appropriate angulation and frequency, can give excellent visualization of nerve and vascular structures (Figure 5.6). Metal needle

shafts, especially if scored, are also easily identified when they lie directly in the reflective plane of the ultrasonographic probe.

2. The **quality** of images relates to the **frequency of the sound wave,** with the **higher frequencies (**10–15 MHz**) giving the best resolution,** but at the price of a **limited depth of penetration** (a maximum of 3–4 cm). Nevertheless, the choice of the appropriate frequency, focus, and angulation of the ultrasonographic probe can be arranged to provide visualization of even the deepest peripheral nerves, such as the sciatic and the infraclavicular brachial plexus. Manufacturers of ultrasonic devices have recently focused their attention on improving the identification of peripheral nerves by improved hardware and software resolution of the images, including probes that sample with multiple frequencies and several waves, to allow "compound" derivation of the images. These innovations produce increasingly high quality visualization of nerves.
3. Several probes types are available.
   a. **Linear array** probes of 4 cm (1.6 in.) width give best visualization of shallow nerves and are ideally suited for following the path of an "in-plane" needle advancement.
   b. **Narrower flat probes** (1.5 cm [0.7 in.]) can fit more easily in **constricted spaces,** such as the supraclavicular fossa, and avoid the loss of signal from discontinuous contact between the probe and the skin.
   c. **Curved array probes** usually generate **lower frequencies,** and are best suited for wide views of **deeper structures,** such as the sciatic nerve in the subgluteal area. For all the probes, the use of the gel both inside and outside of protective sterile plastic sheaths is also important.
4. In practical terms, nerves can be visualized either in a **transverse section (short axis)** when the transducer is placed perpendicular to the path of the nerve, or in **longitudinal view (long axis)** when the transducer is parallel to the path of the nerve (Figure 5.7). Generally, depending on the angle of the transducer, the short axis view gives the appearance of a tubular structure with a dark (hypoechoic) center, or a series of such tubular structures within a peripheral nerve, compared to a long axis view which is often a brighter, hyperechoic picture of the nerve. With either approach, an injecting needle can be introduced **perpendicular to the plane of the transducer ("out of plane")** or **parallel to the beam of the transducer itself ("in-plane"),** so that the length of the needle and its exact depth can be easily visualized. Out-of-plane injections require more adjustments of the transducer angle or small test injections of local anesthetic to help identify the tip of the needle. In-plane injections are slightly more difficult because of the constant attention necessary to maintain the shaft of the needle in the narrow beam of the transducer, but they allow for visualization of the spread of the local anesthetic around the nerves when they are used in conjunction with the transverse (short axis) approach to the nerves. Both techniques are useful and have been employed successfully. Both have also been used for the positioning of the needle and the subsequent insertion of continuous catheters.
5. Another useful feature of ultrasonography is the ability to **identify flow,** usually represented by "color-flow" Doppler images of blood in a vessel or heart chamber. This feature is useful for confirming blood vessels. It can also be used to confirm flow of anesthetic from a catheter or needle tip.

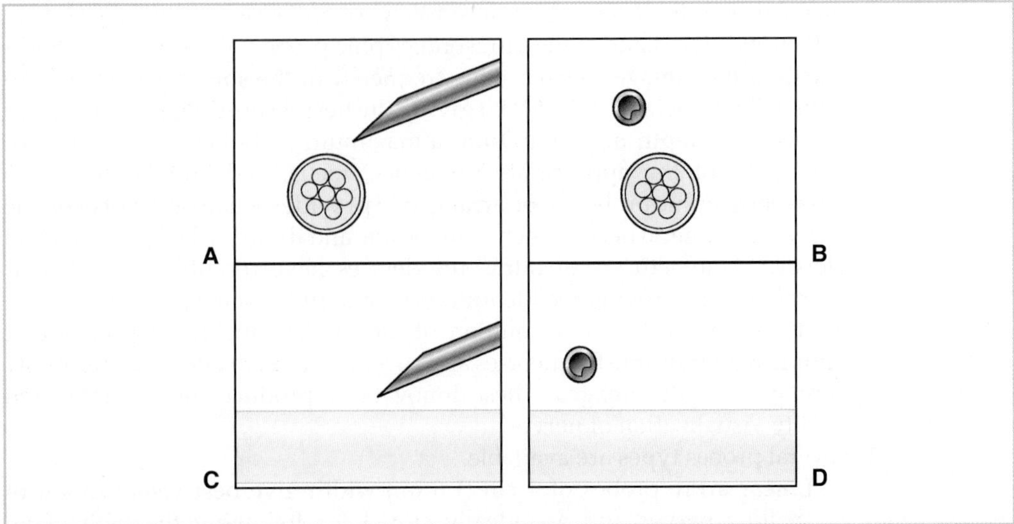

Figure 5.7. Various angles of visualization of nerve and needle. **A:** Nerve in cross-section (short axis) and needle out of plane. **B:** Nerve in short axis, needle "in plane." **C:** Nerve in longitudinal (long axis) view, needle out of plane. **D:** Nerve in long axis, needle in plane.

6. Comparative studies show that in experienced hands ultrasonographic localization can be **faster and more reliable** than other techniques, even with novices (14–16). Time to identification of the nerve is reduced, required volume of local anesthetic appears to be reduced, and onset time is faster. Overall reliability is also higher in some series. The question of whether nerve injury is reduced is not yet resolved.
7. Still, there is an undeniable "*learning curve*" associated with this new technology, as well as considerable expense for current machines. The equipment is bulky (compared to a nerve stimulator) and requires adjustment of ambient light for maximum efficiency. The increasing use of ultrasonography for central line placement and surgical lesion localization may, however, make the machines more available in many settings. The advantages of this technique and the continuing improvements in quality and affordability of equipment may help overcome these obstacles.
8. Despite the enthusiasm of many advocates, ultrasonographic guidance, like nerve stimulation, still requires a **basic knowledge of anatomy** and a presumed location of the nerves by the operator. The ultrasonograph operator must learn to use the more easily discernable hyperechoic (bone, clavicle, transverse process) and hypoechoic (veins and arteries) landmarks that will help guide him/her to the location of the nerves themselves. Because the nerves can often appear similar to tendons in their ultrasonographic image, knowledge of anatomy and relative positioning of the structures is still essential. With appropriate adjustments, ultrasonographic guidance can provide rapid and reliable identification of nerve structures. It is particularly useful in identifying patterns of variable anatomic distribution. Because of the hyperechoic nature of the bones surrounding the central neuraxis, ultrasonographic techniques are less helpful for neuraxial blockade (17). Its future in the specialty is still unclear, but the early experience

suggests a positive role for peripheral nerve blockade and for peripheral catheter insertion (18). This technique is particularly useful in the pediatric patient where heavy sedation or general anesthesia is often used to facilitate neural blockade, and the direct visualization of local anesthetic injection facilitates the process.

Each of the chapters of this manual describes the appropriate approach and images obtained with ultrasonography for peripheral nerve blockade.

REFERENCES

1 **Hebl JR. The importance and implications of aseptic techniques during regional anesthesia. *Reg Anesth Pain Med* 2006;31:311–323.**

2 Birnbach DJ, Stein DJ, Murray O, et al. Povidone iodine and skin disinfection before initiation of epidural anesthesia. *Anesthesiology* 1998;88:668.

3 Norris MC, Fogel ST, Dalman H, et al. Labor epidural analgesia without an intravascular "test dose." *Anesthesiology* 1998;88:1495–1501.

4 Salinas FV, Neal JM, Sueda LA, et al. Prospective comparison of continuous femoral nerve block with nonstimulating catheter placement versus stimulating catheter-guided perineural placement in volunteers. *Reg Anesth Pain Med* 2004;29:212–220.

5 Ilfeld BM, Morey TE, Enneking FK. Portable infusion pumps used for continuous regional analgesia: delivery rate accuracy and consistency. *Reg Anesth Pain Med* 2003;28:424–432.

6 Choyce A, Chan VW, Middleton WJ, et al. What is the relationship between paresthesia and nerve stimulation for axillary brachial plexus block? *Reg Anesth Pain Med* 2001;26:100.

7 Urmey WF, Stanton J. Inability to consistently elicit a motor response following sensory paresthesia during interscalene block administration. *Anesthesiology* 2002;96:552–554.

8 Borgeat A, Ekatodramis G, Kalberer F, et al. Acute and nonacute complications associated with interscalene block and shoulder surgery: a prospective study. *Anesthesiology* 2001;95:875.

9 Benumof JL. Permanent loss of cervical spinal cord function associated with interscalene block performed under general anesthesia. *Anesthesiology* 2000;93:1541.

10 **Gray AT. Ultrasound-guided regional anesthesia: current state of the art. *Anesthesiology* 2006;104(2): 368–373.**

11 **Marhofer P, Chan VW. Ultrasound-guided regional anesthesia: current concepts and future trends. *Anesth Analg* 2007;104:1265–1269.**

12 **Sites BD, Brull R, Chan VW, et al. Artifacts and pitfall errors associated with ultrasound-guided regional anesthesia. Part I: understanding the basic principles of ultrasound physics and machine operations. *Reg Anesth Pain Med.* 2007;32:412–418.**

13 **Sites BD, Brull R, Chan VW, et al. Artifacts and pitfall errors associated with ultrasound-guided regional anesthesia. Part II: a pictorial approach to understanding and avoidance. *Reg Anesth Pain Med.* 2007;32:419–433.**

14 Williams SR, Chouinard P, Arcand G, et al. Ultrasound guidance speeds execution and improves the quality of supraclavicular block. *Anesth Analg* 2003;97:1518–1523.

15 Sites BD, Gallagher JD, Cravero J, et al. The learning curve associated with a simulated ultrasound-guided interventional task by inexperienced anesthesia residents. *Reg Anesth Pain Med* 2004;29:544–548.

16 Chan VW, Perlas A, McCartney CJ, et al. Ultrasound guidance improves success rate of axillary brachial plexus block. *Can J Anaesth* 2007;54:176–182.

17 Arzola C, Davies S, Rofaeel A, et al. Ultrasound using the transverse approach to the lumbar spine provides reliable landmarks for labor epidurals. *Anesth Analg* 2007;104:1188–1192.

18 Horlocker TT, Wedel DJ. Ultrasound-guided regional anesthesia: in search of the holy grail. *Anesth Analg* 2007;104:1009–1011.

6 Spinal Anesthesia

Francis V. Salinas

I. Introduction

Spinal anesthesia remains one of the **simplest and most effective** regional anesthesia techniques available to the anesthesiologist. Administration of the appropriate choice and dose of local anesthetic into the intrathecal (or subarachnoid) space results in **rapid onset** of **dense surgical anesthesia** with a **high degree of success**. Despite the relative simplicity of the technique, a thorough knowledge of the functional anatomy of the central neuraxis, the factors that determine local anesthetic distribution within the intrathecal space (which ultimately determines the spread or extent of surgical anesthesia), as well as the factors that determine duration of anesthesia are critical to optimizing the success of spinal anesthesia in the inpatient and outpatient setting. Lastly, an understanding of the physiological effects and potential complications of spinal anesthesia are key elements to ensure patient satisfaction and safety.

II. Anatomy

An understanding of the functional anatomy of spinal anesthesia not only provides a basis for successful technique, but also provides the basis for understanding the clinical evaluation of intrathecal local anesthetic distribution. Therefore, the anesthesiologist must be familiar with the **surface anatomy** of the spinal column and then develop a mental picture of the underlying three-dimensional topography of the **vertebral column** and supporting ligaments that surround the spinal canal containing the **spinal cord and nerves**, with their associated **meninges** and **cerebrospinal fluid (CSF)**.

A. Vertebral column. The vertebral column is composed of the 33 bony vertebra and 5 ligaments that provide the supporting and protective conduit for the spinal cord and spinal nerves.

1. There are **7 cervical, 12 thoracic, 5 lumbar, 5 sacral, and 4 coccygeal** vertebral segments (Figure 6.1). Spinal anesthesia is typically performed in **the lower lumbar region.** The typical lumbar vertebra is composed of the anterior vertebral body and posterior bony elements (two pedicles project posteriorly from the vertebral body and two flattened lamina that connect the pedicles to form the vertebral arch) that together form the **vertebral foramen** (Figure 6.2). The vertebral foramina of the adjoining vertebrae combine to form the longitudinal spinal canal that contains the spinal cord. The adjoining paired pedicles of each vertebra are characterized by superior and inferior notches, which form the **intervertebral foramina**, through which the paired segmental spinal nerves exit the spinal canal (Figure 6.2). Paired **transverse processes** project posterolaterally from the junctions of the pedicles and lamina. A single **spinous process** projects posteriorly (and typically slightly inferiorly, thereby overlapping the vertebra below) from the posterior aspect of the vertebral arch at the midline junction of the paired lamina. The bony elements provide sites for muscle and ligamentous attachments.
2. The vertebral column is held together and stabilized by **five ligaments** (Figure 6.3). The **supraspinous ligament** connects the apices (tips) of the

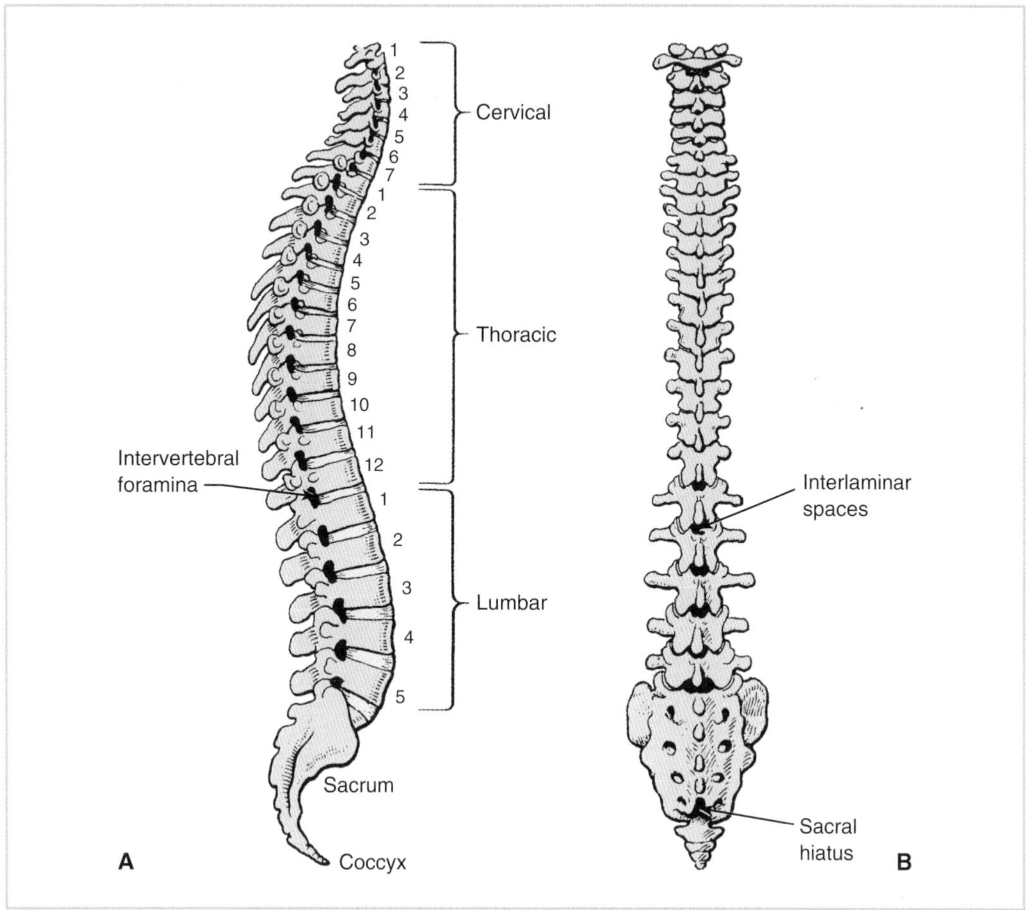

Figure 6.1. Vertebral column, lateral **(A)** and posterior **(B)** views, illustrating the cervical, thoracic, lumbar, sacral, and coccygeal segments. Note the curvatures, intervertebral foramina, and interlaminar spaces. (Adapted from Cousins MJ, Bridenbaugh LD, eds. *Neural blockade in clinical anesthesia and management of pain*, 3rd ed. Philadelphia: Lippincott Williams & Wilkins, 1998:205.)

spinous processes from the seventh cervical vertebra to the sacrum. The **interspinous ligament** connects adjoining spinous processes, attaching from the root to the apex of each spinous process, thereby blending anteriorly with the ligamentum flavum and posteriorly with the supraspinous ligament. The laminas of adjacent vertebral arches are connected by the **tough, wedge-shaped ligamentum flavum**, which is composed primarily of elastin. The ligamentum flavum binds the paired vertebral lamina of adjoining vertebra together, thereby forming the **posterior wall of the vertebral spinal canal**. It is through this posterior ligamentous "opening" (the interlaminar space) in the spinal canal that the subarachnoid space is reached with a spinal needle. Entry into the spinal canal is protected by the dense ligamentum flavum and by the spinous process of the cephalad lumbar vertebra at each level, which angles inferiorly to protect the space below.

3. The vertebral column has **characteristic curves in the lumbar and thoracic regions** that (Figure 6.4), in conjunction with patient position and baricity

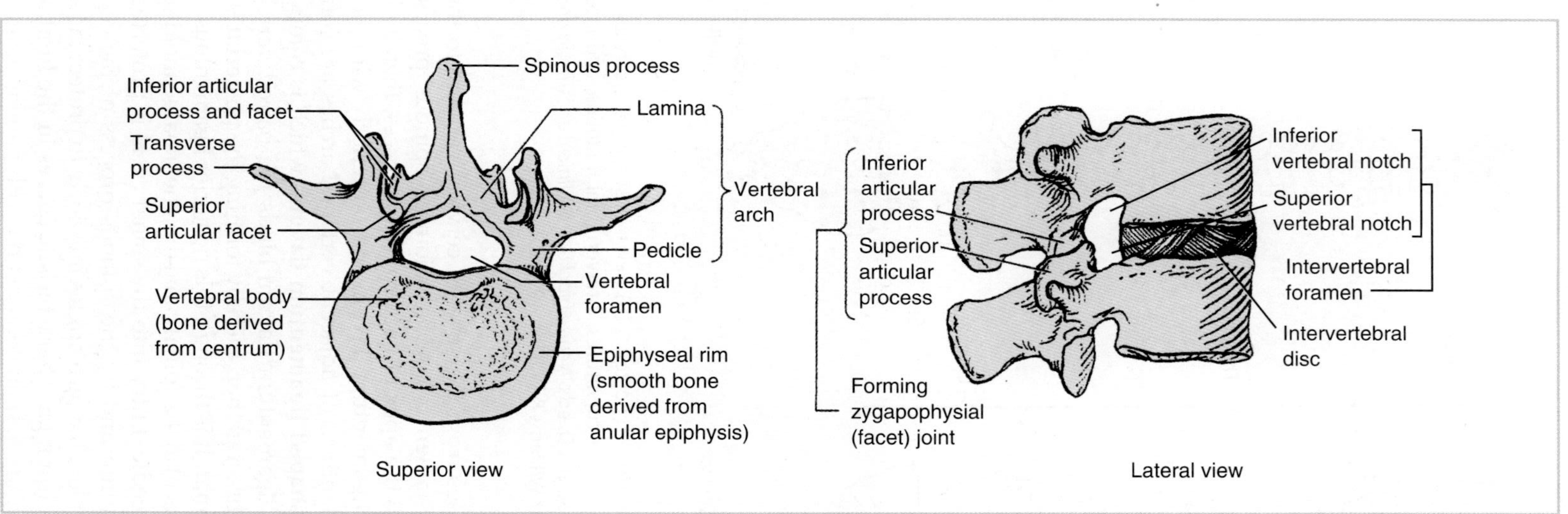

Figure 6.2. Typical lumbar vertebra illustrating superior and lateral views of the anterior vertebral body, the elements that form the vertebral arch (the paired pedicles and paired lumina), and single midline spinous process. Note the superior and inferior vertebral notches of the adjoining pedicles, which form the intervertebral foramen. (Adapted from Moore KL, Dalley AF. *Clinically oriented anatomy*, 5th ed. Philadelphia: Lippincott Williams & Wilkins, 2006:480.)

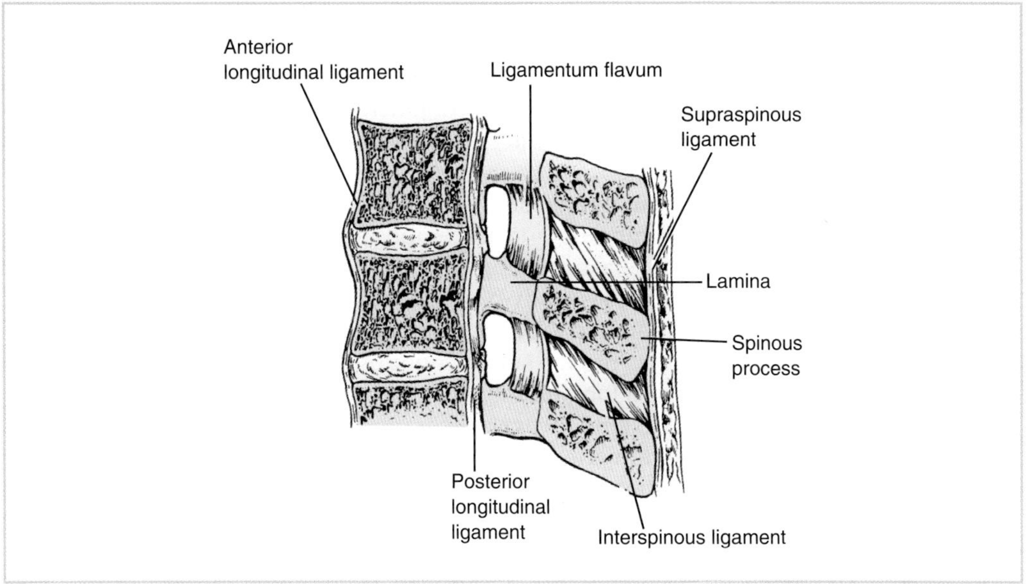

Figure 6.3. Sagittal section of vertebral column illustrating the supporting ligaments and their bony attachments. The interspinous ligaments connect adjacent spinous processes, and the ligamentum flavum connects adjacent lamina. (Adapted from Cousins MJ, Bridenbaugh LD, eds. *Neural blockade in clinical anesthesia and management of pain*, 3rd ed. Philadelphia: Lippincott Williams & Wilkins, 1998:205.)

of local anesthetics, influence the distribution of local anesthetics within the subarachnoid space in patients placed in the supine horizontal position. Local anesthetic solution injected at the peak height of the lumbar anterior convexity (lumbar lordosis) will distribute both caudad and cephalad to varying degrees depending on the baricity of the local anesthetic. The cephalad spread of hyperbaric local anesthetic solutions is limited to

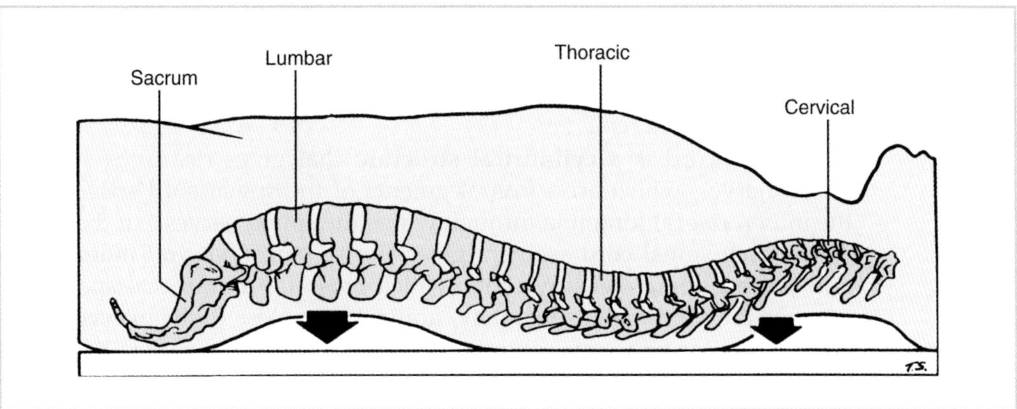

Figure 6.4. Normal curvature of the spinal column in the supine horizontal position. Hyperbaric solutions injected at the peak of lumbar lordosis will distribute (through gravity) to the lower sacral and thoracic concavities. (Adapted from Raj PP. *Handbook of regional anesthesia*. New York: Churchill Livingstone, 1985:225.)

the mid-to-upper thoracic dermatomes by encouraging pooling within the thoracic concavity (thoracic kyphosis).

B. **Meninges.** The spinal meninges consist of **three membranes (the** *dura mater, arachnoid mater*, **and** *pia mater***)** that in conjunction with the CSF in the intrathecal space envelop, support, and protect the spinal cord and nerve roots (Figure 6.5).
   1. The spinal **dura mater** ("tough mother") is the outermost and thickest meningeal membrane and is composed primarily of collagen fibrils, interspersed with elastic fibers and ground substance in an anatomic arrangement that allows ready passage of drugs (1). Therefore, the dura has been incorrectly assumed to be the primary barrier to diffusion of epidurally administered drugs into the subarachnoid space. The dura mater forms the **dural sac**, which is a long tubular sheath contained within the surrounding spinal canal that extends from the foramen magnum to the lower border of the second sacral vertebra, where it fuses with the filum terminale. The dura extends laterally along the spinal nerve roots, becoming continuous with connective tissue of the epineurium of the spinal nerve at the level of the intervertebral foramina.
   2. The **arachnoid mater** is closely applied to the inner surface of the dura mater, and is composed of overlapping layers of flattened epithelial-like cells that are connected by frequent tight junctions and occluding junctions (2). Although much thinner than the dura, it is the anatomic arrangement of the arachnoid that accounts for the vast majority of the resistance to drug diffusion through the spinal meninges.
   3. The **pia mater** closely invests the surface of the spinal cord and nerve roots and is composed of three to six layers of cells. There is underlying subpial tissue composed primarily of collagen that separates the pial cellular layer from the neural tissues. Scanning electron photomicrograph examination demonstrates fenestrations on the pial surface of the spinal cord and nerve roots that allow direct contact with the subarachnoid space (3). The **intrathecal (or subarachnoid) space, which lies between the arachnoid mater and the pia mater**, is the target compartment for spinal anesthesia. Additionally, the spinal nerve roots and rootlets traverse the intrathecal space, allowing for local anesthetic uptake. The pia mater extends to the tip of the spinal cord where it becomes the filum terminale, which anchors the spinal cord to the sacrum (Figure 6.5).

C. **Spinal cord**
   1. The spinal cord is a **cylindrical structure** that gives rise to 31 pairs of spinal nerves, which arise from segments of the spinal cord specified by the intervertebral foramina through which the spinal nerves exit the spinal canal. Each spinal cord segment gives rise to paired **ventral motor roots and paired dorsal sensory roots**, which cross the intrathecal space and traverse the dura mater separately, uniting in or close to the intervertebral foramina to form the corresponding paired mixed spinal nerves. Although consistently larger than the corresponding ventral nerve roots, anatomic studies have demonstrated that dorsal nerve roots commonly divide into two to three separate bundles upon exiting the spinal cord, whereas most ventral nerve roots exit as a single bundle (4). Additionally, as the dorsal nerve root bundles course further laterally, they further subdivide into as many as one to ten fascicles before the dorsal root becomes the dorsal

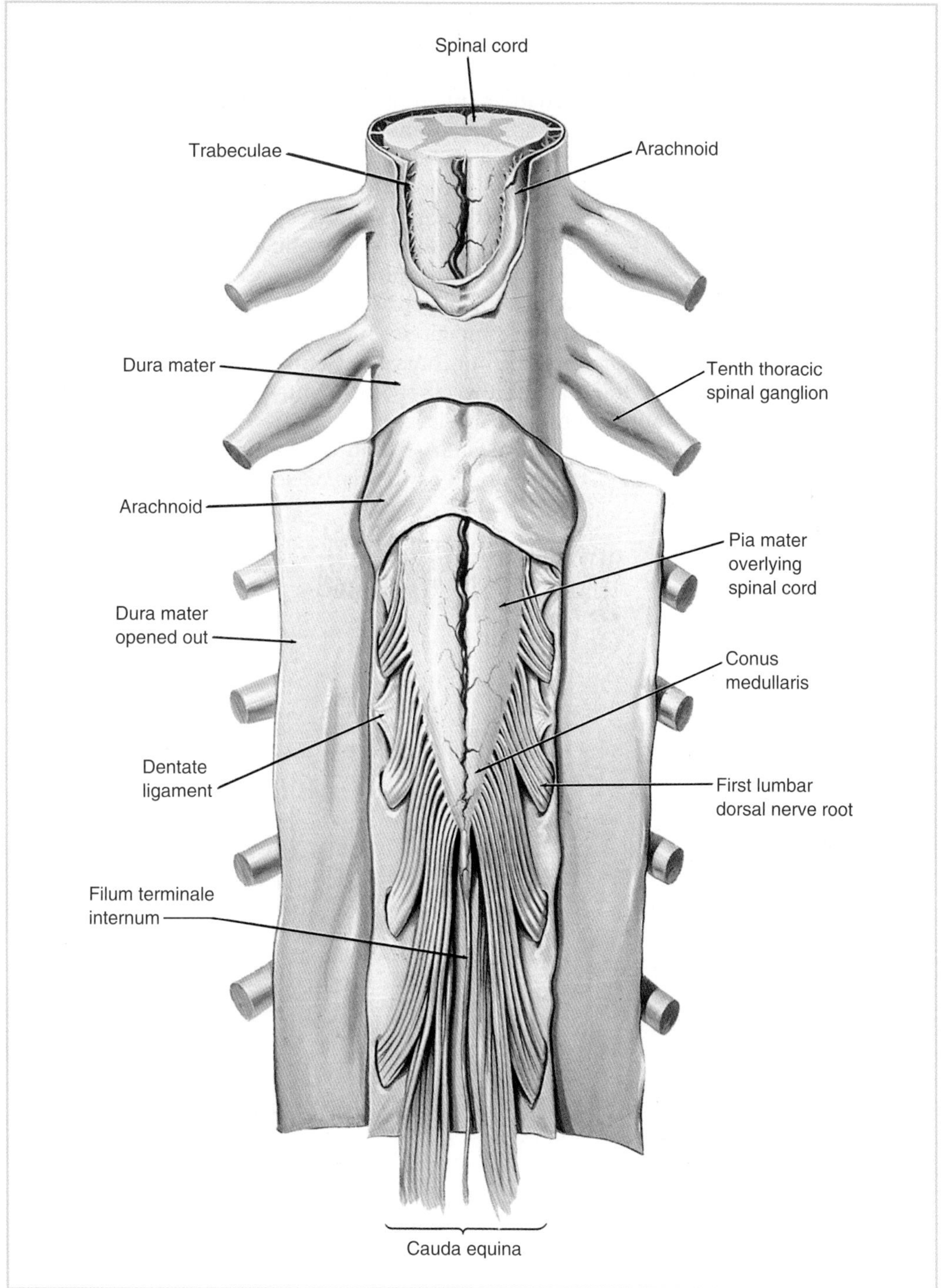

Figure 6.5. Lumbosacral spinal cord and the spinal meninges (dura, arachnoid, and pia). Note also the terminal portion of the spinal cord (conus medullaris) and the nerve roots of the lower lumbar and sacral spinal cord segments, giving rise to the cauda equina. (Adapted from Cousins MJ, Bridenbaugh LD, eds. *Neural blockade in clinical anesthesia and management of pain*, 3rd ed. Philadelphia: Lippincott Williams & Wilkins, 1998:209.)

root ganglion (5). Therefore, the larger, but typically multistranded dorsal nerve roots offer a substantially larger surface area for local anesthetic uptake compared to the smaller, single ventral nerve roots. This anatomic arrangement may partially explain the relatively faster onset and ease of obtaining sensory blockade versus motor blockade.

2. The portion of the spinal cord that gives rise to paired nerve roots and spinal nerves is called a *spinal cord segment*. The skin area supplied by a given spinal nerve and its corresponding cord segment is called a *dermatome* (Figure 6.6). Because measuring local anesthetic concentration within the subarachnoid space is impractical, and dermatomes can be considered the sensory projections of the spinal cord segments, qualitative assessment of the loss of afferent sensory functions (such as temperature, pinprick, and touch) provides an indirect, but clinically useful estimate of local anesthetic distribution within the intrathecal space, and more importantly, an estimate of the extent of surgical anesthesia.
3. In adults, the **spinal cord is shorter than the vertebral column** and typically, the caudal extent (known as the *conus medullaris* [Figure 6.5]) most

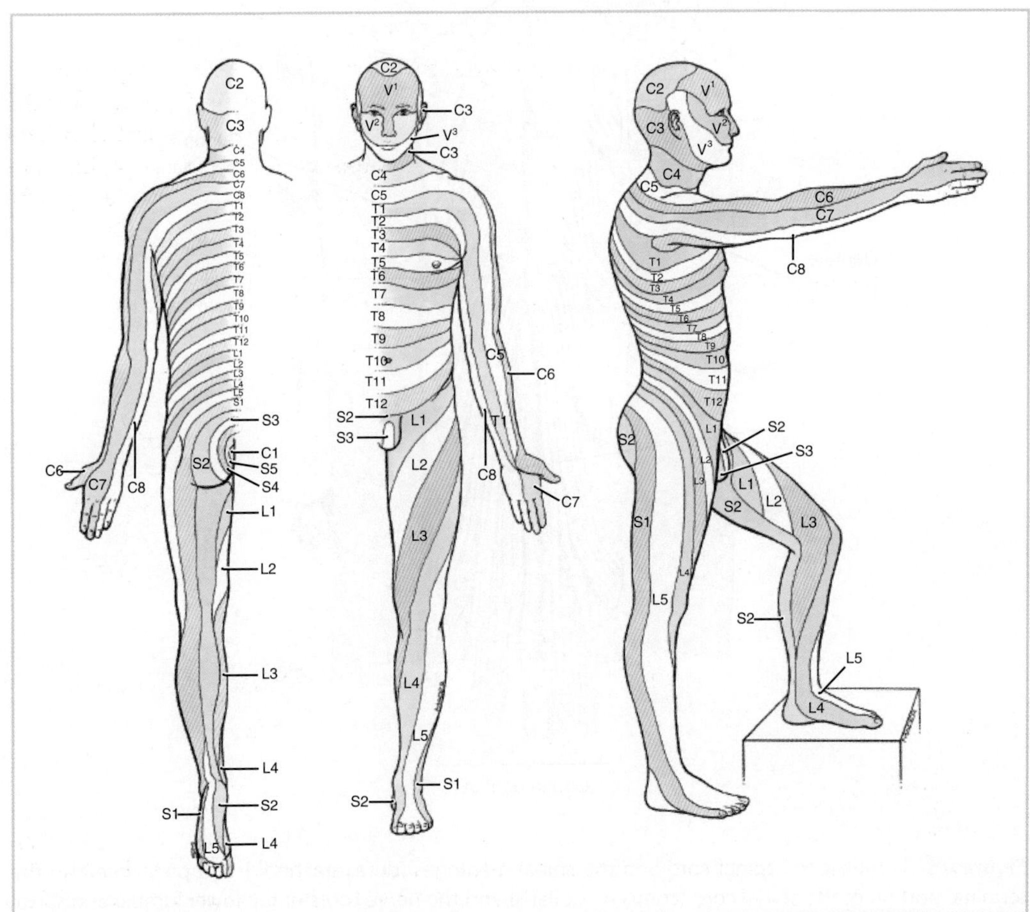

Figure 6.6. Sensory dermatomes. (Adapted from Agur AMR, Lee MJ, eds. *Grant's atlas of anatomy*, 10th ed. Philadelphia: Lippincott Williams & Wilkins, 1999:296.)

commonly extends to the **lower third of the first lumbar vertebral body**, but may be as low as the upper third of the third lumbar vertebral body (6). Therefore, attempting spinal anesthesia at or above the L2-3 intervertebral space (IVS) may potentially increase the risk of mechanical trauma (with the spinal needle) to the spinal cord in a small number of patients.

4. Because the spinal cord is shorter than the vertebral column, there is **progressive obliquity of the lower thoracic, lumbar, and sacral spinal nerve roots**, which makes them travel increasingly longer distances within the subarachnoid space (from their spinal cord segments of origin) to the intervertebral foramina through which they exit as the corresponding spinal nerve. The collection of spinal nerve roots within the intrathecal space caudal to the conus medullaris is collectively termed the *cauda equina* due to it resemblance to a horse's tail (Figure 6.5). The enlargement of the intrathecal space containing the cauda equina is termed the *lumbar cistern*. It is within the lumbar cistern where local anesthetics are initially injected for spinal anesthesia.

D. **Surface anatomy**

1. When preparing for spinal anesthesia, it is critical to accurately identify surface landmarks on the patient. Identification of the lumbar vertebral (or more correctly, **intervertebral space level**) **level is the initial step** during the performance of spinal anesthesia. The desired level is determined by inspection and palpation of surface landmarks. A **line connecting the iliac crests (the intercristal or Tuffier's line) most commonly intersects the vertebral column at the L4-5 IVS** (Figure 6.7) (6). There is substantial patient variability and the intercristal line may intersect with vertebral column as cephalad as the L3-4 IVS and as caudad as the L5-S1 IVS **(Figure 6.8)**.

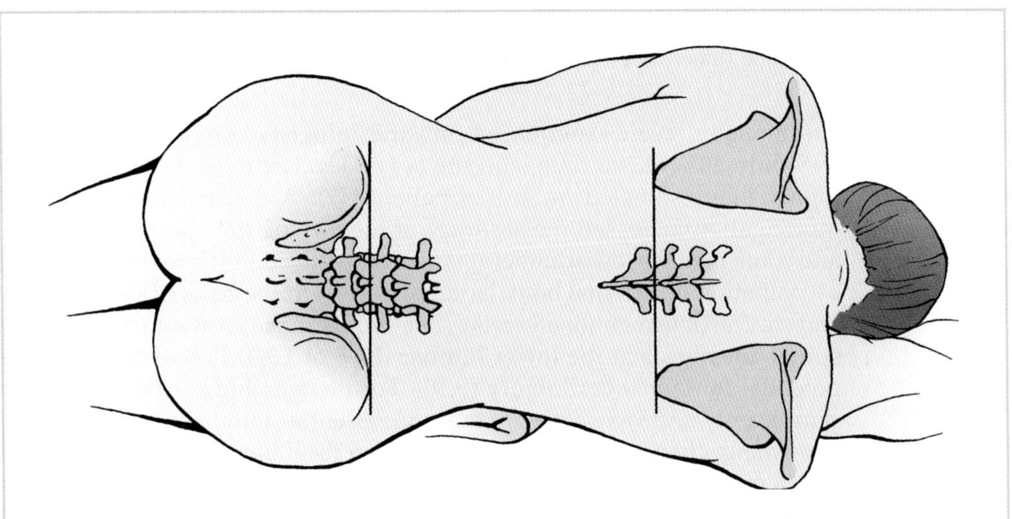

Figure 6.7. Patient position for spinal or epidural blockade. The patient's knees are drawn up toward the chest and the head flexed downward to provide the maximum anterior flexion of the vertebral column. The pillow should be placed under the head but not under the shoulders to avoid rotation of the spine. The hips and shoulders should be perpendicular to the surface of the bed, resisting the usual inclination of the patient to roll the superior shoulder forward. A line drawn between the posterior iliac crests usually crosses the spinal column at the L4-5 interspace or L4 spinous process. Similarly, for thoracic epidural injection, a line between the inferior tips of the scapulae crosses the T9 spinous process.

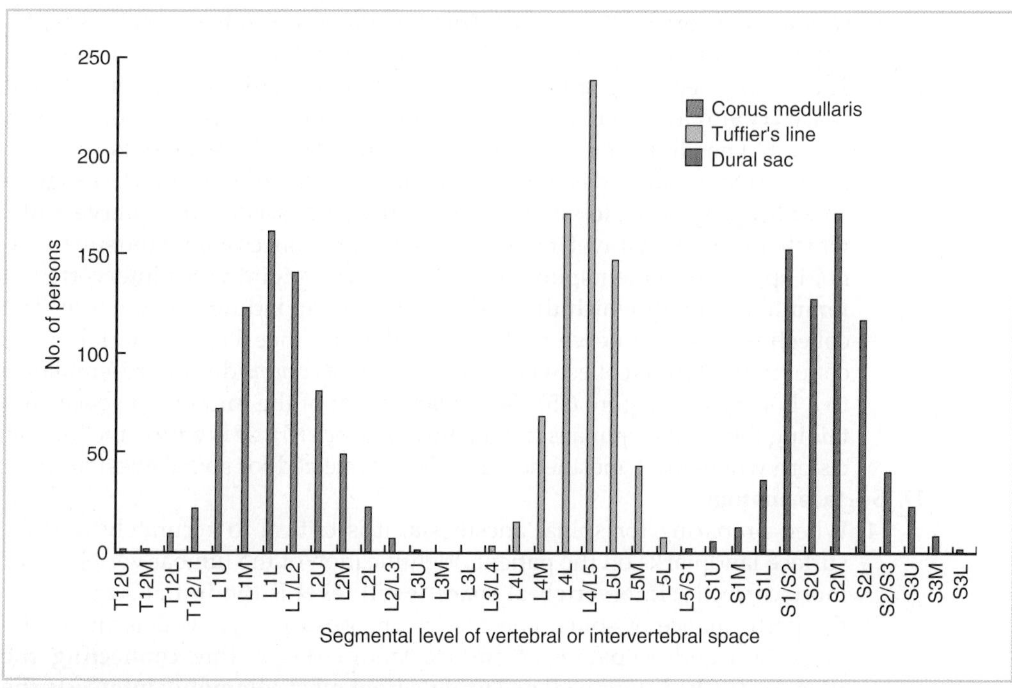

Figure 6.8. Distribution of the vertebral level in segments at which the conus medullaris, the intercristal (Tuffier's) line, and the dural sac cross. The segmental levels where the spinal cord ends, Tuffier's line crosses, and the dural sac ends follow a normal distribution. Each vertebra was divided into four segmental thirds of the vertebral body—upper (U), middle (M), and lower (L)—and the intervertebral space (IVS). The most caudal distribution of the conus should not cross with the most cephalad level of the actual intercristal line in this patient population. (Adapted from Kim JT, Bahk J, Hung JH. Influence of age and sex on the position of the conus medullaris and Tuffier's line in adults. *Anesthesiology* 2003;99:1359–1363.)

Additionally, **even experienced anesthesiologists correctly identify the IVS only 30% of the time**, and the actual level of the IVS was one space higher than estimated in 50% of patients **(7)**. A recent ultrasonographic investigation increased the accuracy of identifying the correct IVS to 70% and confirmed the low accuracy (30%) of correctly identifying the correct IVS by palpation of external bony landmarks (8). On the basis of the anatomic and clinical data mentioned earlier, one should make an **attempt to perform spinal anesthesia at the lower lumbar (L4-5 or L3-4) IVS** to minimize the potential for spinal cord injury (9,10). Fortunately, lumbar flexion (which significantly improves access to the intervertebral–interlaminar space) does not usually change the position of the intercristal line, and even in cases in which change occurs (with full flexion), the intercristal line does not move beyond the next level (11).

III. Indications and Contraindications

A. Local anesthetics injected into the intrathecal space generally produce sensory afferent blockade and varying degrees of efferent motor block cephalad and caudad to the site of intrathecal injection. The **cephalad extent of spinal anesthesia is dependent on the baricity of the local anesthetic solution** relative to patient position at the time of intrathecal injection and patient position during the

Table 6.1 Classification of afferent and efferent nerve fibers

Fiber class	Axon diameter (μm)	Myelin	Conduction velocity (m/s)	Innervation	Function
Aα	12–20	+++	75–120	Afferent from muscle spindle propioceptors Efferents to skeletal muscle	Motor and reflex activity
Aβ	5–12	+++	30–75	Afferent from cutaneous mechanoreceptors	Touch and pressure
Aγ	3–6	++	12–35	Efferent to muscle spindles	Muscle tone
Aδ	1–5	++	5–30	Afferent pain and temperature nociceptors	"Fast" pain, touch, and temperature
B	<3	+	3–15	Preganglionic sympathetic efferents	Autonomic function
C	0.2–1.5	–	0.5–2.0	Afferent pain and temperature	"Slow" pain, temperature

surgical procedure. There is a gradually decreasing concentration of local anesthetic within the CSF as a function of distance from the initial site of intrathecal injection, which causes a gradient of afferent and efferent conduction block due to the differential sensitivities of spinal nerve fibers based on their axon diameter and conduction velocity **(Table 6.1). Preganglionic efferent fibers are the most sensitive to local anesthetic** conduction block and therefore may be anesthetized **two to six dermatome segments higher than afferent sensory block** (most typically assessed as loss of pinprick sensation), which in turn extends **two to three dermatomes higher than efferent motor block** (12). A more clinically relevant assessment is the extent of surgical anesthesia, both in terms of the sensory extent (local anesthetic distribution within the CSF) and the density (local anesthetic concentration within the CSF). A clinically useful assessment of the dermatomal level of surgical anesthesia is the use of transcutaneous electrical stimulation (TES). Tolerance to TES (of pain or discomfort) of 10-mA, 50-Hz continuous square wave (easily produced with most peripheral nerve stimulators) for 5 seconds has been shown to be a **reliable predictor of tolerance to surgical stimulation** (13).

B. Knowledge of the correlation between surface anatomy and dermatomal projections of the spinal cord segments is essential to assess whether the extent (or peak block height) of sensory block is adequate for the planned surgical procedure, as well as assessment of regression of sensory block to plan discharge from the recovery room. For example, the **fourth thoracic dermatome corresponds to the nipples**, the **sixth** thoracic dermatome to the **xyphoid process**, the **tenth** thoracic dermatome to the **umbilicus**, and the perineum to the second through fourth sacral dermatome (**Table 6.2 and Figure 6.6**). It is also essential to know that the internal organs are innervated differently and anesthesia of an overlying cutaneous region does not necessarily confer surgical anesthesia to an underlying visceral organ (**Table 6.3**).

1. For example, a low level of spinal anesthesia (S4-L1) is useful for perianal or **perineal surgery**.

Table 6.2 Surface anatomy and dermatome levels

Surface anatomy	Sensory dermatome
Perineum	S2-S4
Lateral foot	S1
Knee and distal thigh	L3-L4
Inguinal ligament	T12
Umbilicus	T10
Tip of xyphoid process	T6
Nipple	T4
Inner aspect of forearm	T1-T2
Thumb and index finger	C6-C7
Shoulder and clavicle	C5-C4

2. Although **foot-ankle** (S1-L5) and **knee** surgery (L3-4) occur at the lumbosacral dermatomes, the use of thigh tourniquet (and tolerance to tourniquet pain) will often require a peak sensory block height to T10-T8 (14).
3. A peak block height of T10 is ideal for transurethral **prostatectomy** or **hysteroscopy** procedures because it provides excellent surgical anesthesia while preserving sensation in the abdomen and dome of the bladder, allowing earlier warnings signs and the diagnosis of **extravasation** of fluid into the abdominal cavity.
4. Higher peak sensory levels of spinal anesthesia (T6-T4) are required for **lower abdominal surgery** such as inguinal herniorrhaphy, appendectomy, abdominal hysterectomy, or cesarean delivery. In such procedures, however, patients may perceive an unpleasant discomfort associated with traction on the peritoneum or abdominal viscera. In this case, higher levels of spinal anesthesia are required (although usually impractical) and judicious use of supplemental intravenous sedation and analgesia are indicated.
5. Higher levels of spinal anesthesia (T1) have been advocated for **upper abdominal procedures** (such as open cholecystectomy, bowel resection, and exploratory laparotomy. This level of spinal anesthesia provides the surgeon with a contracted bowel because of the complete sympathetic efferent block. However, this level of spinal anesthesia is associated with changes in both **cardiovascular and pulmonary function**. The complete efferent sympathetic efferent block will decrease resting arterial vascular tone (afterload), significantly decrease venomotor tone (preload) resulting in variable degrees of hypotension, which may be exacerbated in the patient who is hypovolemic. Additionally, this level of sympathetic efferent blockade may result in severe bradycardia (due to blockade of the cardiac accelerator fibers at T1-4). This may exacerbate any vagally mediated reflex decrease in heart rate secondary to peritoneal traction. Although high levels of spinal anesthesia do not have clinically significant effects on pulmonary function in patients without respiratory disease, motor blockade of the diaphragm and abdominal muscles does result in clinically relevant decreases in peak

Table 6.3 Common surgical procedures appropriate for spinal anesthesia and recommended peak sensory block height

Surgical procedure	Recommended minimum peak block height
Perirectal and perineal	
Incision and drainage of rectal abscess	S4-L1
Hemorrhoidectomy	
Transvaginal slings	
Lower extremity surgery with tourniquet use	
Knee replacement	T10-T8
Knee arthroscopy	
Below-knee amputation	
TURP	
Cystoscopy and hysteroscopy	T10
Vaginal delivery	
Total hip replacement	
Femoral–popliteal bypass	
Varicose vein stripping	
Lower abdominal	
Hysterectomy (low transverse incision)	T4
Cesarean delivery	
Inguinal herniorrhaphy	
Appendectomy	
Upper abdominal[a]	
Open cholecystectomy	T1
Abdominal exploration	

TURP, transurethral resection of the prostrate.
[a]Requires concomitant general anesthesia.

expiratory flow rate and peak expiratory pressure. Therefore, high levels of spinal anesthesia are not appropriate for patients who are dependent on abdominal muscles to maintain adequate ventilation.

C. There are **absolute and relative contraindications** to spinal anesthesia. Absolute contraindications include **patient refusal, infection at proposed site of skin puncture and injection, severe untreated hypovolemia,** intrinsic or iatrogenic (systemic anticoagulation and platelet inhibitors) **defects in hemostasis**, and **increased intracranial pressure** (as this may potentially increase the risk of uncal herniation when intracranial pressure is decreased as CSF is lost through the needle). Performance of spinal anesthesia in patients with **preexisting neurologic deficits** such as radiculopathies or peripheral neuropathies (**15**, 16), demyelinating diseases such as multiple sclerosis (17) is **controversial**. Although no clinical study has demonstrated that spinal anesthesia worsens preexisting neurologic disease, the vast majority of anesthesiologists would consider it a significant contraindication. **Aortic stenosis**, once considered an absolute contraindication to spinal anesthesia, does not necessarily preclude a carefully conducted spinal anesthetic (18). Despite conflicting results in the literature, except in the most extraordinary circumstances (where the benefits of regional anesthesia outweigh the potential risk of central neuraxial infection);

spinal anesthesia should not be performed in patients with untreated systemic infection. In contrast, available data suggest that patients with evidence of **systemic infection** may safely undergo spinal anesthesia, provided appropriate antibiotic therapy is initiated before dural puncture and the patient has demonstrated response to therapy, such as decrease in fever and decrease in granulocystosis **(19)**.

IV. **Determinants of local anesthetic distribution and duration of action**

A. The **physiochemical properties** and **clinical pharmacology** of local anesthetics and analgesic adjuvants (to local anesthetics) are addressed in more detail in Chapters 1 and 2. This section will discuss the determinants of local anesthetic distribution within the subarachnoid space as well as duration of action. Application of spinal anesthesia into daily clinical practice requires a block of sufficiently rapid onset to facilitate the timely start of surgery and more importantly a block of adequate duration for the planned (type and anatomic) surgical procedure, as well predictable (and prompt when needed) return of neurologic function to facilitate a timely discharge from either the recovery room or to home. Conversely, a spinal anesthetic with an unnecessary cephalad spread may increase the risk for cardiovascular complications of hypotension and bradycardia. A basic definition of a few terms is essential for understanding the determinants of the clinical efficacy of spinal anesthesia. *Distribution* of local anesthetics within the intrathecal space determines the spatial extent of sensory, motor, and sympathetic block. *Uptake* of local anesthetics into the neuronal tissues determines which neuronal functions **(Table 6.1)** are affected during spinal anesthesia. Uptake into neuronal tissues is a function of CSF concentration relative to the neuronal and perineuronal tissue concentration, which is largely determined by distribution, as the CSF concentration of local anesthetic will progressively decrease from the area of initial highest concentration (injection site) as a function of distance. *Elimination* of local anesthetics from the intrathecal space determines duration of action.

B. **Determinants of intrathecal local anesthetic distribution.**Many factors have been proposed to influence the distribution of local anesthetic solutions with the intrathecal space (20, **21**). After injection, the local anesthetic will initially spread simply by **bulk flow** created by displacement of CSF. Subsequently, the most important factor in determining intrathecal local anesthetic distribution is the **baricity** of the local anesthetic solution relative to the influence of gravity (patient position). Other clinically relevant factors include **total dose** given, the IVS chosen for injection, and several patient characteristics.

1. **Baricity.** Baricity is defined as the ratio of the density of the local anesthetic solution relative to the density of the patient CSF at 37°C. Local anesthetic solutions that have the same density as CSF are termed *isobaric*. Local anesthetic solutions that have a greater density than CSF are classified as *hyperbaric*, whereas solutions that have a lower density than CSF are classified as *hypobaric*. Hyperbaric solutions will distribute (sink) to the most dependent areas of the intrathecal space, whereas hypobaric solutions will distribute toward (rise upward) the nondependent areas of the intrathecal space. The effects of gravity are determined by the choice of patient position (supine, prone, lateral, and sitting), and in the supine position, by the curvatures of the spinal column. The mean density of CSF varies significantly among specific patient population subgroups (**Table 6.4**). Because

Table 6.4 Density and baricity of cerebrospinal fluid (CSF) in different patient subgroups and commonly used local anesthetics

	Mean (SD) density at 37°C	Range within 3 SD of the mean
Patient population		
Men	1.00064 (0.00012)	1.00028–1.00100
Older women	1.00070 (0.00018)	1.00016–1.00124
Younger women	1.00049 (0.00004)	1.00037–1.00061
Pregnant/postpartum	1.00030 (0.00004)	1.00018–1.00042
Hyperbaric solutions[a]		
Lidocaine 5% in dextrose 7.5%	1.02650	1.01300–1.0142
Tetracaine 0.5% in dextrose 5%	1.0136 (0.0002)	1.01300–1.0142
Bupivacaine 0.5 to 0.75% in dextrose 8.25%	1.02426 (0.00163)	1.01935–1.029131
Chloroprocaine 3%	1.00257 (0.00003)	1.00248–1.00266
Hypobaric solutions[b]		
Lidocaine 0.5% in water	0.99850	Hypobaric
Bupivacaine 0.35% in water	0.99730	Hypobaric
Tetracaine 0.2% in water	0.99250	Hypobaric
Bupivacaine 0.5%	0.99944 (0.00012)	0.99908–0.99980
Isobaric solutions (plain)		
Lidocaine 2%[c]	1.00004 (0.0006)	0.99986–1.00022
Tetracaine 0.5%[d]	1.0000 (0.0004)	0.99880–1.00120

SD, standard deviation.
[a]Local anesthetic solutions with a baricity of >1.0015 can be expected to predictably behave in a hyperbaric manner.
[b]Local anesthetic solutions with a baricity of <0.9990 can be expected to predictably behave in a hypobaric manner.
[c]May act in an isobaric or hypobaric manner depending on patient population.
[d]Tetracaine 1% diluted 1:1 with 0.9% saline.

of the wide variability in CSF density, hyperbaric and hypobaric solutions must have densities three standard deviations above or below a patient population mean CSF density, respectively to predictably behave in a hyperbaric or hypobaric manner. Therefore, based on patient variability and the known density of local anesthetic solutions, commonly used local anesthetics (specifically, plain bupivacaine 0.5% and plain lidocaine 2.0%) classified as "isobaric" may in fact behave in a hypobaric manner depending on patient position. **Table 6.4** lists the density range and classification of commonly used local anesthetics.

a. **Hyperbaric spinal anesthesia.** Hyperbaric solutions are commonly prepared by mixing the local anesthetic solutions with **dextrose**. When the patient is placed in the supine horizontal position after injection of a hyperbaric solution (in the lumbar region), the curvatures of the spinal column will influence the subsequent distribution within the intrathecal space. Hyperbaric solutions will tend to distribute by force of gravity toward the **lowest points of the thoracic (T6-7) and sacral (S2) curvatures** (Figure 6.4) (22). Therefore, pooling of hyperbaric local anesthetic solutions within the thoracic kyphosis has been postulated to explain the clinical observation that they tend to produce spinal anesthesia with an average peak sensory block height in the midthoracic region. Individual anatomic variations in the lowest point of the thoracic kyphosis, the maximum angle of decline of the lumbar spinal canal, and the maximum

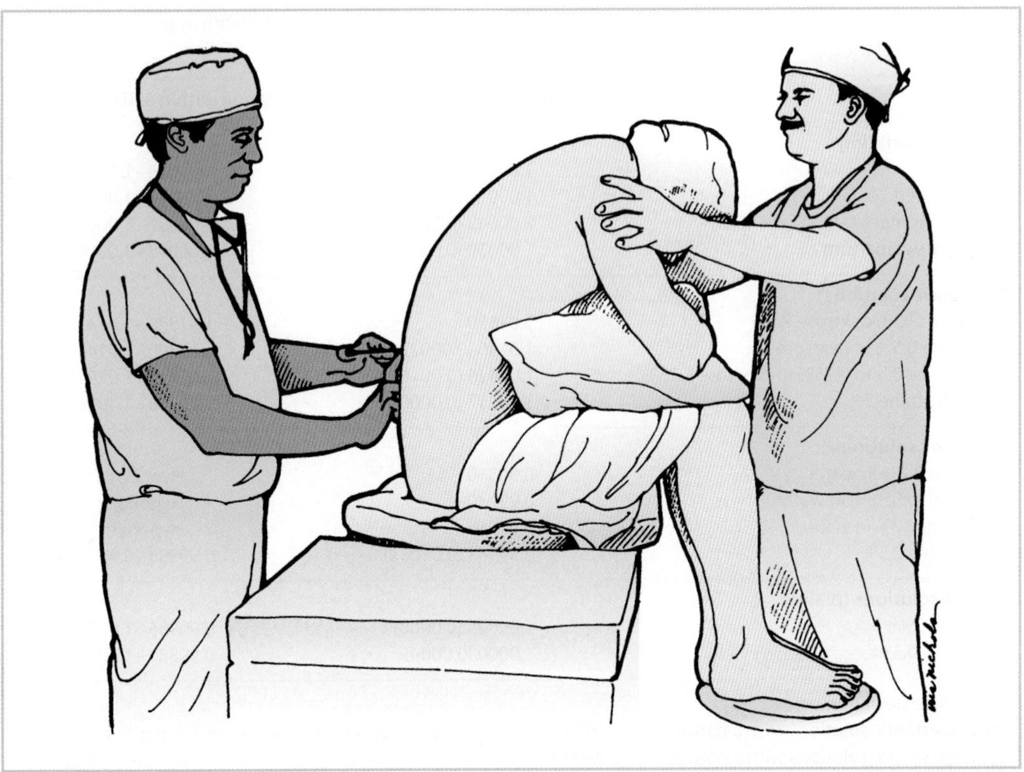

Figure 6.9. Sitting position for spinal anesthesia. The patient's legs are allowed to hang over the edge of the bed, and the feet are supported on a stool to encourage flexion of the lower spine. The shoulders are hunched forward and the patient is encouraged to grasp firmly onto a pillow held over the abdomen. If sedation is given, an assistant should maintain the position and monitor the vital signs. This position is optimal for identifying the midline in obese patients or those with unusual spinal anatomy.

angle of incline of the upper thoracic spinal canal, may also contribute to the variability in peak sensory block height of hyperbaric solutions (23).

(1) Injection of hyperbaric local anesthetic solutions with the patient in the sitting position (for 5–10 minutes) has been advocated as a means to restrict distribution to the lumbosacral dermatomes, producing a *"saddle block"* **(Figure 6.9)**. However, this practice is based on the misconception that hyperbaric solutions will then behave in an "isobaric manner" as they become diluted sufficiently in the CSF and are no longer influenced by gravity once the patient is placed in the supine (or supine lithotomy) position. Clinical studies, however, have demonstrated that a hyperbaric spinal anesthetic block initially restricted to the lumbosacral dermatomes will eventually distribute to the peak thoracic sensory block height equivalent to that which would have been obtained had the patient been immediately placed in the horizontal supine position (24).

(2) Similar to the concept of obtaining a saddle block (by restricting the distribution of hyperbaric local anesthetic solution based on gravity), injection of hyperbaric solutions with a patient in the lateral position (with the operative side dependent) and maintaining the operative side in the dependent position for 10 to 15 minutes has also been advocated as a means to achieve "unilateral spinal anesthesia". One of the proposed advantages of unilateral spinal anesthesia is that limiting the sympathetic blockade to one side may decrease the incidence of hypotension (25). The major disadvantage of unilateral spinal anesthesia is that it requires at least 15 minutes in the lateral position after injection to predictably obtain a unilateral blockade.

b. **Hypobaric spinal anesthesia.** Hypobaric local anesthetic solutions are typically prepared by diluting commercially available plain local anesthetic solutions with **sterile distilled water**. For example, lidocaine 2% diluted with sterile water to lidocaine 0.5% (26) or bupivacaine 0.5% diluted with sterile water to 0.35% (27) will reliably result in "clinically hypobaric" spinal anesthesia. Although less commonly used, hypobaric spinal anesthesia is ideally suited for perineal and perirectal surgical procedures performed with the patient in the prone jackknife position (**Figure 6.10**). The advantages of this technique are twofold.

   (1) First, the local anesthetic is injected with the patient in the operative position, thereby minimizing the need to change patient position.

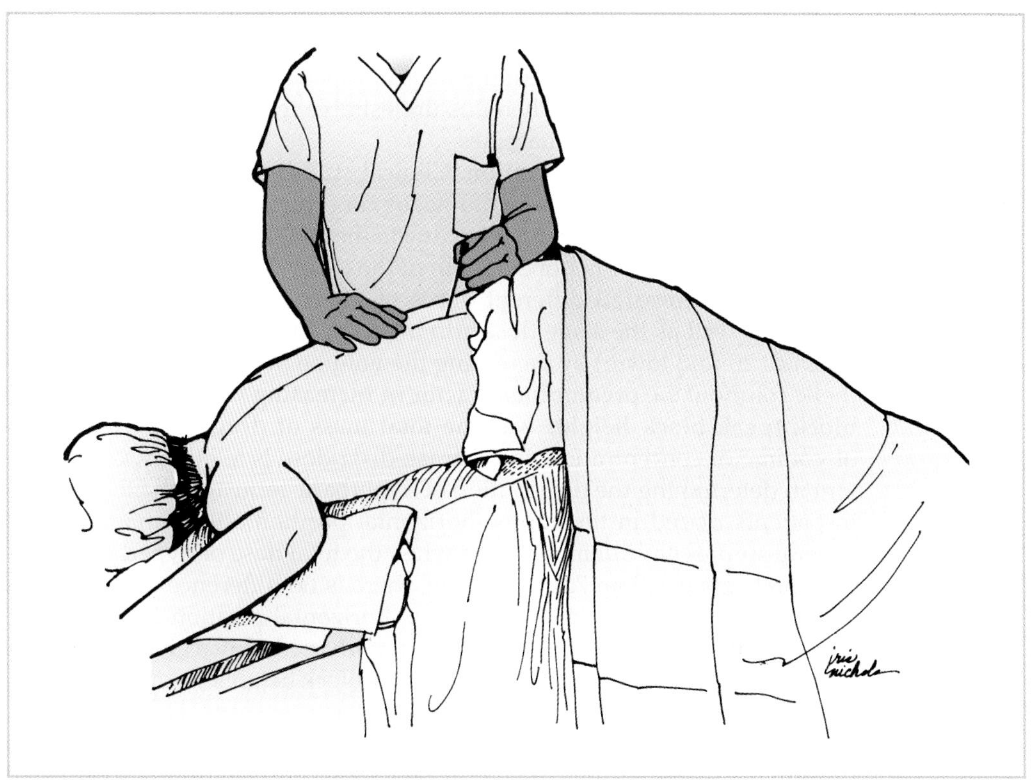

Figure 6.10. Jackknife position. Hypobaric spinal anesthesia can be administered with the patient positioned on a flexed operating table, such as for rectal procedures. The flexion point of the table should be directly under the hip joint, and the use of a pillow under the hips will help accentuate the flexion needed to identify the lumbar spinous processes. Aspiration of the spinal needle is often necessary to confirm dural puncture, because the lower cerebrospinal fluid (CSF) pressure in this position will not necessarily generate a spontaneous flow of fluid.

(2) Second, the local anesthetic distribution will be restricted to lumbosacral dermatomes as long as the patient is maintained in the operative position.

Care must be taken when recovering the patient who still has a functional block, as placing the patient in the head-up position during the recovery period may cause the block to rise to the thoracic dermatomes (26). Hypobaric spinal anesthesia may also provide significant advantages for major hip surgery performed in the lateral position (with operative side uppermost). Compared with isobaric bupivacaine spinal anesthesia, hypobaric bupivacaine spinal anesthesia demonstrated a significantly **delayed onset of sensory regression on the operative side** and more importantly, time needed until need for analgesia after surgery (27).

c. **Isobaric spinal anesthesia.** An isobaric local anesthetic solution is most easily prepared by mixing equal volumes of **tetracaine** 1% solution with either CSF or sterile saline. As stated before, plain bupivacaine 0.5%, commonly referred to as *isobaric*, is clearly a hypobaric mixture (Table 6.3). Therefore, depending on the patient position at the time of injection and during surgery, this solution will behave "unpredictably" if one expects it to behave in an isobaric manner. The major advantage of truly isobaric solutions is that **patient position during and after injection should have no effect on intrathecal distribution.** Isobaric solutions tend not to distribute far from the site of initial injection and are particularly useful when it is undesirable to obtain sensory block in the higher thoracic dermatomes.

2. **Dose, volume, and concentration.** Clinical studies attempting to separate the individual effects of dose, volume, or concentration on local anesthetic distribution are difficult to interpret due to the fact that manipulating one of these factors affects either one or both of the other factors. In two well-done studies that compared different doses of plain local anesthetic solutions (28,29), as well as the same dose administered in lower concentrations (as much as 20-fold lower) by increasing the volume of the injected local anesthetic solution, the **predominant factor in increasing the extent of sensory block (peak block height) was the total mass of drug** given, regardless of volume or concentration. In contrast, drug dose is relatively less important in determining the distribution of hyperbaric local anesthetic solutions in patients placed in the supine horizontal position after initial injection. Several studies have demonstrated when the total dose of hyperbaric bupivacaine is greater than 7.5 to 10.0 mg; there is no difference in peak block height in patients placed in the supine horizontal position (30, **31**). Conversely, in a dose–response study of hyperbaric bupivacaine 0.75%, 3.75 mg, 7.5 mg, and 11.25 mg, the peak sensory block heights obtained were T9, T7, and T4 **(32)**.

3. **IVS injection site.** The location of the lumbar IVS injection site has been proposed to have a clinically significant effect on peak sensory cephalad distribution of plain local anesthetic solution. Conflicting studies can be explained by the use of plain bupivacaine 0.5% in these studies. In one study, the mean peak block height was decreased from T6 to T10 when plain bupivacaine 0.5% was injected initially at L3-4, followed by a repeat injection in the same patients at the L4-5 IVS (33). In this study, plain bupivacaine 0.5% solutions were injected at ambient room temperature with

the patient in the lateral position and then immediately placed in the supine horizontal position. In a conflicting study (34), when plain bupivacaine 0.5% solutions adjusted to 37°C are injected into patients in the sitting position and maintained in the sitting position for 2 minutes before placing them supine, there was no difference in peak sensory block height when injections at the L2-3 versus L3-4 IVSs were compared. These seemingly conflicting data can be explained as follows. First, plain bupivacaine 0.5% is clearly hypobaric and not isobaric as these previous studies assumed. Second, there were differences in the baricity of the plain bupivacaine solutions, as the density of local anesthetic solutions is inversely proportional to temperature. Third, there were differences in patient position during initial injection. Therefore, it appears that when hypobaric solutions are injected with the patient in the sitting position, the effect of the IVS is outweighed by the effect of gravity (as the hypobaric solutions will float cephalad within the intrathecal space) relative to local anesthetic baricity.

4. **Needle aperture direction.** The use of a pencil point needle (such as a Whitacre or Sprotte, see Chapter 5) results in **directional flow out of the needle aperture,** diverting the direction of local anesthetic direction from the longitudinal aspect of the needle (35). In a study of plain lidocaine 2%, patients were randomly assigned to local anesthetic injection (in lateral position) with the needle aperture either oriented in a cephalad direction or a caudad direction (36). The group with the local anesthetic injection directed in the cephalad direction had a mean higher peak sensory block height (T3 versus T7), as well as a shorter duration of lumbar (L1-5) sensory anesthesia (149 versus 178 minutes), and shorter time to spontaneous urination and discharge. Therefore, it appears that with plain-isobaric solutions, needle aperture direction does influence local anesthetic distribution. Additionally, by presumably providing sacral sparing in this study, there was a faster return of sacral autonomic function, thereby, facilitating a more timely discharge.
5. **Patient factors.** Although there is significant variation in the extent of local anesthetic distribution among patients using a standard technique, spinal anesthesia is **very reproducible in the individual patient** (37). However, individual patient factors such as **age, height, body mass index, and gender have little if any clinically relevant significance in accurately predicting local anesthetic distribution differences from patient to patient.**

C. **Determinants of duration of action of spinal anesthesia.** Clinically, spinal anesthetic blockade **recedes in a cephalad to caudad manner from peak block height to the sacral dermatomes.** Depending on the criteria chosen in any given study, duration of action can be defined as time to onset of **two-dermatome regression** from peak sensory block height, or as **time to complete regression** to sacral dermatomes. More clinically relevant, the **duration of surgical anesthesia** is dependent on the interaction of the spatial extent of the block, time-course regression, and anatomic location of the surgical procedure. Additionally, time course to complete regression of sensory and motor block are important considerations for ambulatory spinal anesthesia. Resolution of blockade after spinal anesthesia occurs when the neural tissue concentration of local anesthetic falls below the minimum blocking concentration for given neural function. Elimination **does not involve metabolism** of local anesthetics with the intrathecal space, but occurs completely through vascular absorption within both the intrathecal and epidural space. Therefore, the **duration of spinal anesthesia is primarily determined by the physiochemical properties** of the specific local anesthetic agents that determines it availability for vascular absorption, the total mass of local anesthetic administered, and the degree of vascular absorption.

1. **Local anesthetic choice.** One of the primary determinants of duration of action is the choice of local anesthetics. The physiochemical properties of lipid solubility and to a lesser extent, protein binding largely influences the time course of vascular absorption **(see Table 1.1 in Chapter 1)**.
   a. **Procaine** is the **shortest acting** local anesthetic for spinal anesthesia. Its short duration of action can be largely attributed to its very low lipid solubility and protein binding, relative to the longer-acting agents.
   b. **2-Chloroprocaine** is also a **short-acting** local anesthetic agent that has been shown in volunteer and clinical studies to have a comparable anesthetic profile to equivalent doses of lidocaine, with the notable exceptions of lack of transient neurologic symptoms (TNS) and a 20% faster time to complete recovery of sensorimotor function (14,38).
   c. **Lidocaine** is considered a **short-to-intermediate duration** local anesthetic agent, and has historically been the most extensively used local anesthetic for spinal anesthesia. Plain lidocaine of dose 50 mg will produce a peak block of T6 with onset of 2-dermatome regression of 50 to 60 minutes, 100 minutes of lumbar anesthesia, and complete regression in 120 to 140 minutes. The use of lidocaine has fallen dramatically due to concerns regarding **TNS** (see discussion on complications). Depending on the type of surgery, the incidence of TNS ranges from 15% to 33%.
   d. **Mepivacaine** is also a **short-to-intermediate duration** local anesthetic agent and provides a similar anesthetic profile compared to equivalent doses of lidocaine, with a lower incidence of TNS (3%–6%) compared to lidocaine.
   e. **Bupivacaine** is the prototypical and most widely used l**ong-acting aminoamide local anesthetic** agent. The extent and duration are **dose related** (32). Within a clinically relevant dose range of 3.75 to 11.25 mg of hyperbaric bupivacaine 0.75%, it appears that for every additional milligram, there is an increase in the average duration of surgical anesthesia by 10 minutes and an increase until complete recovery of 21 minutes. There is, however, a **wide degree of variability**, largely due to its high degree of lipid solubility. Lower doses (5–7.5 mg) have been used for ambulatory anesthesia as an alternative to lidocaine, but are hampered by a higher degree of block failure and wide interpatient variability in complete resolution.
   f. **Ropivacaine and levobupivacaine** are **long-acting** aminoamides developed as alternatives to bupivacaine as "less cardiotoxic" alternatives for epidural and peripheral regional anesthesia. Levobupivacine is less cardiotoxic by virtue of its formulation as the pure L-stereoisomer of bupivacaine, but is no longer commercially available in the United States. Ropivacaine is less cardiotoxic due to combination of its formulation as a pure L-stereoisomer and chemical structure (lower lipid solubility) conferring a lower potency. Because cardiotoxicity is not a clinically relevant concern when using bupivacaine for spinal anesthesia (given the doses used for spinal anesthesia and the doses required to

produce significant cardiotoxicity), neither local anesthetic has gained widespread use.

g. **Tetracaine** is the prototypical **long-acting aminoester** local anesthetic agent. Its increased lipid solubility (compared to bupivacaine) confers greater potency and the dose can be decreased by 20% to 30% for equivalent blockade.

h. Although local anesthetic agents may be classified as short, intermediate, and long-acting, it is evident from Table 6.5 that there is wide interpatient variability. In a study (39) comparing 12 volunteers who underwent spinal anesthesia on three separate occasions with three different hyperbaric local anesthetic agents (lidocaine 100 mg, bupivacaine 15 mg, and tetracaine 15 mg) in random order and in double-blind manner, the average time until complete sensory resolution was not only different between the three agents, but was also highly variable within each local anesthetic agent group: lidocaine (234 minutes, range 137–360 minutes), bupivacaine (438 minutes, range 180–570 minutes), and tetracaine (546 minutes, range 120–720 minutes).

2. **Local anesthetic dose.** For any given local anesthetic agent, **increasing the dose increases the duration** of action. See Table 6.5 for details.
3. **Block distribution.** For a given dose of local anesthetic, spinal blockade with a **higher peak sensory block will completely regress faster** compared to a lower peak cephalad distribution (40). The most likely pharmacokinetic explanation for this phenomenon is based on the wider distribution within

Table 6.5 Doses and duration of commonly used local anesthetic solutions for spinal anesthesia

Local anesthetic solution	Dose (mg)	Mean peak block	Onset of two dermatome regression (min) (SD)	Time to regression to L1-L2 (min) (SD)	Complete regression (min) (SD)
Hyperbaric chloroprocaine	40	T7	45 (20)	64 (10)	14 (140)
Plain lidocaine	50	T6	56 (5)	104 (5)	130 (18)
Hyperbaric lidocaine	50	T4	50 (16)	104 (5)	130 (18)
Plain mepivacaine	60	T4	95 (21)	150 (32)	210 (18)
	80	T4	100 (20)	160 (20)	225 (23)
Plain bupivacaine	10	T7	33 (16)	127 (41)	178 (20)
Hyperbaric bupivacaine	8	T5	59 (13)	135 (51)	198 (33)
	12	T5	65 (32)	123 (44)	164 (30)
	15	T10[a]	159 (49)	253 (64)	>360
	15	T4	110 (30)	216 (46)	360

SD, standard deviation.

[a]Hyperbaric bupivacaine with 15 mg with two patient groups (supine position with peak block of T4 compared with 30-degree head elevation position with peak block restricted to T10). Note the significant difference in onset of two-dermatome regression, duration of lumbar anesthesia, and complete regression with the same dose of hyperbaric bupivacaine but with different initial peak blocks.

(Kooger-Infante NE, Van Gessel E, Forster A, et al. Extent of hyperbaric spinal anesthesia influences duration of block. *Anesthesiology* 2000;92:1319–1323.)

the CSF with a higher peak sensory block height. The wider CSF distribution presumably results in a lower local anesthetic CSF concentration throughout the intrathecal space, as well as a larger surface area leading to more rapid vascular absorption (41). Consequently, it requires less time for the local anesthetic concentration within the neural tissue to fall below the minimum blocking concentration. As noted earlier, the use of hypobaric spinal anesthesia for unilateral hip surgery performed with operative side uppermost not only prolongs the duration of anesthesia on the operative side (as compared to the dependent nonoperative side), but also prolongs the duration of postoperative analgesia (28).

4. **Anesthetic adjuncts.** The two most commonly used class of anesthetic adjuncts added to local anesthetic solutions to prolong (as well as intensify the depth of block) of spinal anesthesia are α-adrenergic agonists and opioids.
   a. **α-Adrenergic agonists.** The primary mechanism by which intrathecal administration of **epinephrine** prolongs the duration of action is believed to be due to α-adrenergic–mediated **vasoconstriction**, thereby leading to decreased vascular absorption thus allowing for increased neural tissue uptake of local anesthetics. Clinically, the effectiveness of intrathecal epinephrine is dependent on the local anesthetic agent to which it is added. Although epinephrine 0.2 mg does not prolong the duration of thoracic anesthesia when added to lidocaine, it clearly prolongs the duration of lumbosacral anesthesia by 25% to 30%, which would be clinically relevant for lower extremity and perineal surgery (42). Similarly, epinephrine 0.2 mg added to plain bupivacaine 15 mg did not prolong thoracic anesthesia, but increased the duration of lumbar anesthesia by 20% (43). In contrast, epinephrine 0.2 to 0.3 mg significantly prolongs the duration of tetracaine spinal anesthesia by 30% to 50% at all dermatomal levels, with slightly greater effect in the lumbosacral dermatomes (44,45). Despite its usefulness in reliably prolonging the duration of spinal anesthesia, epinephrine **significantly prolongs the return of sacral autonomic function (the ability to spontaneously void)** and increases the risk of urinary retention (and possibly bladder overdistention) (46). Therefore, the use of epinephrine is not recommended for outpatient spinal anesthesia.
   b. **Opioids.** Opioids interact **synergistically** when combined with local anesthetic solutions by blocking noxious afferent stimuli at a different site of action than local anesthetics. Specifically, opioids interact with and bind to opioid receptors located within the gray matter of the substanstia gelatinosa in the dorsal horn of the spinal cord. Spinally mediated analgesia is mediated by several mechanisms: (i) increased K^+ conductance, which hyperpolarizes ascending postsynaptic second-order projecting neurons, (ii) release of spinal adenosine, and (iii) inhibition of the release of excitatory neurotransmitters including glutamate and substance P from primary afferent neurons (47,48).
      (1) Fentanyl is by far the most commonly used intrathecal opioid. The lipophilic profile of fentanyl allows it to have a **rapid onset** of action (5–10 minutes) and an **intermediate duration** of action (60–120 minutes), which makes it a suitable agent as an analgesic adjunct to local anesthetic solutions to augment the efficacy of spinal

anesthesia. Clinical studies have demonstrated that 20 to 25 μg of fentanyl added to lidocaine (49) or bupivacaine (50) for spinal anesthesia prolongs the duration of anesthesia without prolonging the time to complete recovery of sensorimotor function and bladder function.

(2) **Morphine** is the most commonly used hydrophilic opioid. Its physiochemical characteristics results in a **slow onset of action** (30–60 minutes), but also a **prolonged duration** of action, which makes it well suited for extended postoperative analgesia. Doses of preservative-free morphine in the range of 100 to 200 μg provide extended spinally mediated analgesia (up to 24 hours) for a variety of common lower abdominal and lower extremity procedures such as cesarean delivery, abdominal hysterectomy, radical prostatectomy, and total hip arthroplasty **(51)**. At these lower doses, the risk of respiratory depression is very unlikely. In contrast, the minimum effective analgesic dose required after total knee arthroplasty is typically 300 to 500 μg (52,53). At these doses, the occurrence of **side effects such as nausea, vomiting, urinary retention, and pruritus** increase significantly compared to lower doses (53,54). The risk of respiratory depression with intrathecal morphine is dose related, with a few instances of clinically significant respiratory depression with doses in the 300 to 500 μg range (54,55).

V. Technique

The successful technique of spinal anesthesia begins with proper preparation well before insertion of the spinal needle. Because the induction of spinal anesthesia results in numerous physiological changes as well the occurrence of rare, but potentially serious complication, immediate detection, and corrective action must be taken to minimize significant morbidity and even mortality. The location where spinal anesthesia is induced must be equipped with an **oxygen** source, a means to administer positive pressure ventilation, airway management equipment, as well as immediate access to **emergency drugs for resuscitation** and intubation. Patient preparation includes proper **monitoring**, including continuous monitoring of heart rate and oxygen saturation and intermittent noninvasive blood pressure monitoring. Finally, intravenous sedation may be administered to facilitate patient cooperation to a degree that the patient is comfortable but cooperative and communicative.

A. Patient position. Proper patient positioning is critical to making spinal anesthesia efficient and successful. The choice of which position to perform spinal anesthesia is influenced by a combination of the preference of the anesthesiologist, patient characteristics (obesity, hemodynamic status, and the presence of painful conditions such as hip fracture), and the baricity of local anesthetic solution in conjunction with the site and position of surgery. The three positions in which spinal anesthesia may be performed are lateral decubitis, sitting, and prone jackknife.

1. **Lateral decubitus position (Figure 6.7).** The lateral decubitis position is especially useful for **lower extremity surgery**, depending on the baricity of the local anesthetics solution. The use of hyperbaric solutions with the operative side dependent allows initial preferential distribution to the surgical site depending on the duration of time spent in the lateral position

after intrathecal injection. Hypobaric solutions are ideally suited for hip surgery performed in the lateral position as the position is then maintained for the duration of the surgical procedure. Ideally, the patient's back is positioned parallel to the edge of the operating table (or hospital gurney) to allow the anesthesiologist easy access to the lower back. The hips and knees are flexed so as to draw the patient's knees toward the abdomen and lower chest. The neck may also be flexed forward. The hips and shoulders should be aligned so that they are perpendicular to the edge of the bed, thereby preventing the spine from rotating. The head and lower legs may need to be supported with pillows or blankets, especially if the patient's hips are broad. It is often very helpful to have a trained assistant help attain and maintain this ideal position. The patient should be encouraged to actively curve the lower back toward the anesthesiologist. All of these maneuvers will contribute to widening the lumbar intervertebral and interlaminar spaces.

2. **Sitting position (Figure 6.9)**. Many anesthesiologists prefer the sitting position as this **facilitates identification of the midline**, especially in obese patients. The patient should be seated with the legs hanging off the operating table and the feet supported by a footrest to facilitate forward flexion at the hips and maintain position stability. A pillow placed on the patient's thighs will also help encourage the patient to maintain forward flexion of the lumbar spine. Once again, an assistant can prove invaluable to encourage and help the patient maintain this position. Depending on the surgical site, the patient may need to be positioned supine immediately after intrathecal injection. If the patient is left in this position for several minutes after intrathecal injection of a hyperbaric local anesthetic solution, **preferential lumbosacral anesthesia** is produced, creating a classically referred to *saddle block*. Careful attention must be paid to the patient's blood pressure if left in the sitting position for any length of time after intrathecal injection, as this will only enhance the degree of expected venous pooling in the lower extremities (and significant decreases in venous return) due to the sympathetic effects of the spinal anesthetic.
3. **Prone jackknife position (Figure 6.10)**. For surgical procedures that require the patient to be in the prone jackknife position (such as **rectal or perineal procedures)** the efficient induction of spinal anesthesia may be accomplished by injection of a **hypobaric** local anesthetic solution with the patient already placed in this position. The patient is positioned prone on the operating table with the hips placed directly over the break in the operating table to facilitate flexion at the hips **(Figure 6.10)**. Additionally, a pillow placed under the lower abdomen helps flexion of the lumbar spine.

B. **Anatomic approach to the subarachnoid space.** Spinal anesthesia should be performed in the mid-to-lower lumbar IVSs, ideally at L4-5 IVS or L3-4 IVS. Spinal anesthesia attempted at or above the L1-2 IVS should be avoided to minimize the risk of needle trauma to the conus medullaris, as it may be located as low as the upper part of the L3 vertebral body in a small percentage of patients (Figure 6.8). After the patient is positioned and the desired IVS is located, there are two key steps to minimize the risk of infection: First, the anesthesiologist should clean his or her hands by either careful hand washing or preferably, with an alcohol-based hand rub. Next, wide and uniform application of skin disinfectant with either povidone-iodine (PI) solution or chlorhexidine-alcohol solution to the skin around the intended puncture site should be performed and then allowed to dry. All antiseptic solutions are neurotoxic, and care must be taken to prevent contamination of spinal needles or local anesthetic solutions with the disinfectant.

1. **Midline approach.** After the appropriate monitors and supplemental oxygen are applied, intravenous sedation is titrated to patient comfort, the appropriate patient position is obtained, the IVS space is chosen and marked, and sterile preparation and draping are completed, the technique of subarachnoid puncture is begun. In the midline approach, the spinal needle **insertion is located in between the adjacent spinous processes (Figures 6.3 and 6.11)**.
   a. After the patient is warned, a 25- to 27-gauge needle is used to slowly and gently raise a **skin wheal** of local anesthetic over the intended spinal needle insertion site. Next, a 22- to 25-gauge needle is then inserted and advanced with a 10 to 15 degree of cephalad angulation (while injecting local anesthetic) through the subcutaneous tissue, supraspinous ligament, and then, the interspinous ligament (**Figure 6.11**).
   b. After local anesthetic infiltration, the patient position is rechecked, as the patient may pull away if there is discomfort associated with the initial local anesthetic infiltration and reduce the flexion of the lower back.

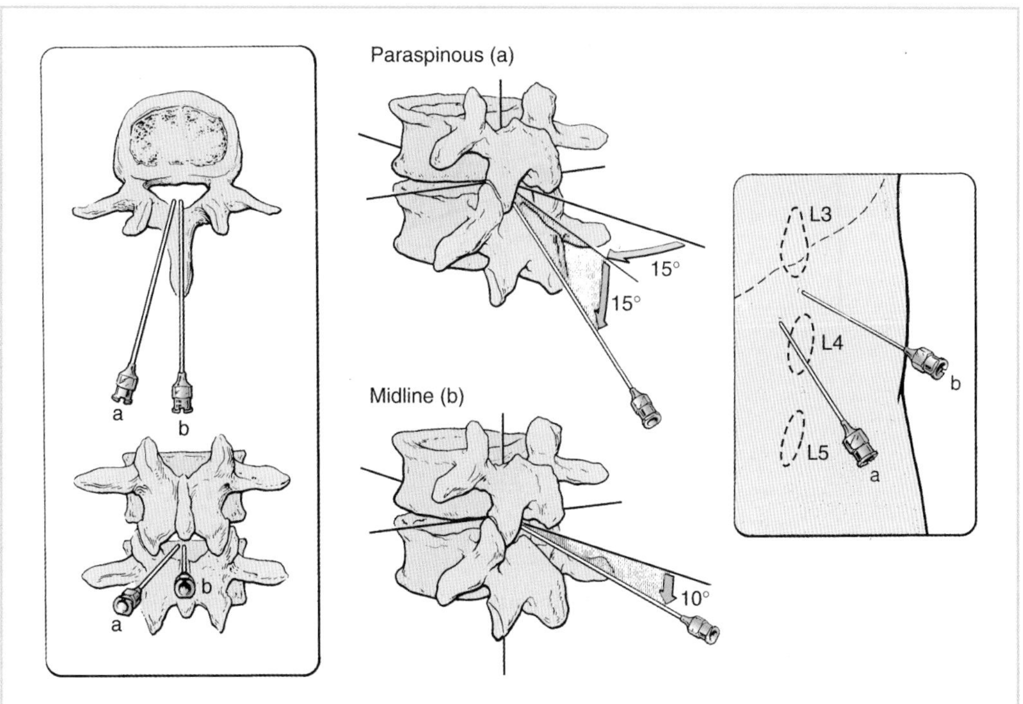

Figure 6.11. The needle insertion point and angulation of needle advancement are illustrated for paraspinous (*a*) and midline (*b*) approaches. (Adapted from Cousins MJ, Bridenbaugh LD, eds. *Neural blockade in clinical anesthesia and management of pain*, 3rd ed. Philadelphia: Lippincott Williams & Wilkins, 1998:231.)

c. The needle used for local anesthetic infiltration may also serve to **verify the midline approach** in between the interspinous space. If bone is encountered with the needle used for local anesthetic infiltration, the appropriate maneuvers can be taken (see subsequent text) to relocate the needle in the proper orientation for a midline approach. Care should be taken not to insert the local anesthetic infiltration needle too deeply in thin patients, as the needle tip may penetrate the dura-arachnoid membrane, leaving a dural puncture with a cutting needle, and potentially increasing the risk of a postdural puncture headache (PDPH).

d. Next, the **introducer needle** is inserted at the site of skin infiltration with a **slight cephalad angulation** through the skin, subcutaneous tissue, supraspinous ligament, and should then be seated in the interspinous ligament **(Figures 6.11 and 6.12)**. In the lumbar region, the spinous

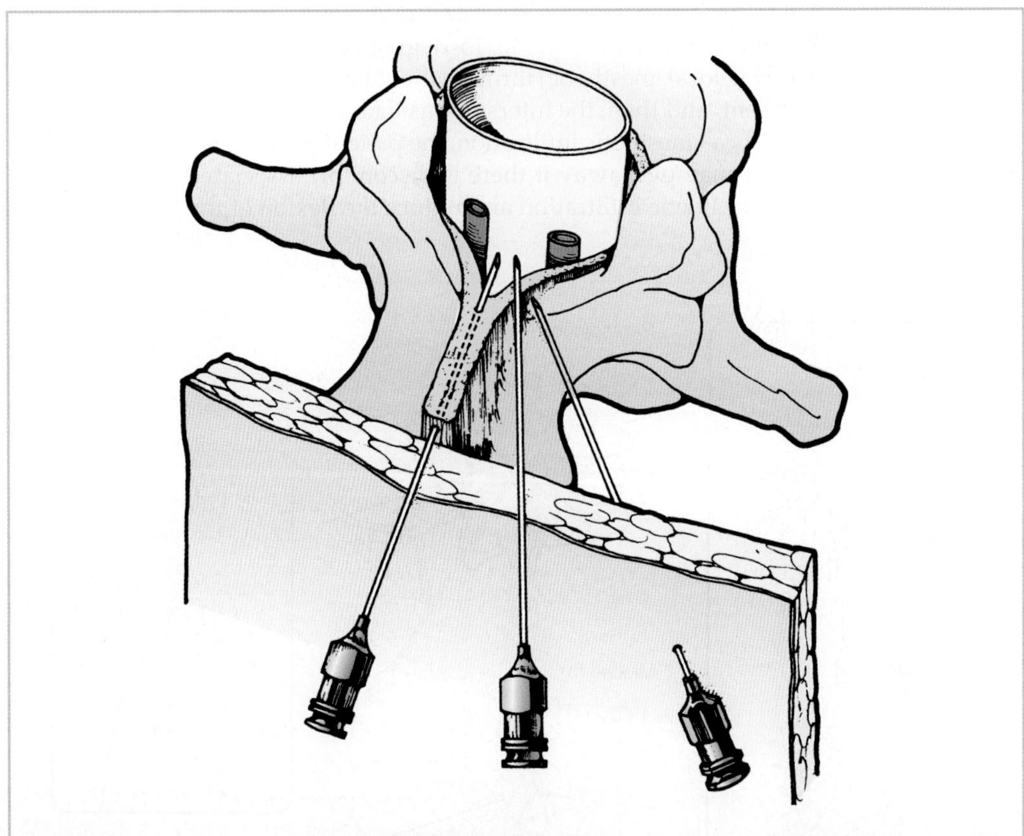

Figure 6.12. Spinal needle insertion, lateral and paramedian approach. In the classic midline approach, the needle traverses the entire interspinous ligament in a slight cephalad direction and exits through the triangular ligamentum flavum into the epidural space before puncturing the dura. In elderly patients with calcified interspinous ligaments, the entry point can be moved one fingerbreadth lateral to the ligament, still passing in the midline of the interspace, but approaching the ligamentum flavum from a slightly oblique angle. A third alternative is to enter the skin much further laterally and inferior to the interspace (a fingerbreadth opposite the inferior spinous process) and pass the needle directly perpendicular onto the lamina, and then "walk" superior and medially until the ligament is contacted. All three of these approaches are suitable for spinal or epidural blockade.

process angulates slightly caudad at the tips and the interlaminar space is slightly cephalad to the interspinous space. The use of an introducer is required when using smaller-gauge (typically 24- to 25-guage) spinal needles to reduce the deflection of the spinal needle tip away from the midline (56). Additionally, an introducer needle **reduces contamination** of the spinal needle with disinfectant solution, epidermis, and skin bacteria. If properly positioned, the introducer will be firmly seated in the interspinous ligament. If the introducer deviates when released, then it is likely that it is not in the midline interspinous space. In this case the introducer needle should be repositioned.

e. Once the introducer needle is correctly positioned, it should be stabilized by grasping the hub between thumb and index finger of the nondominant hand. Additional stability can be provided by placing the back of the grasping hand against the patient's back. The hub of the **24- to 25-gauge pencil point spinal needle** is grasped with thumb and index finger of the dominant hand and inserted through the introducer following the cephalad angulation but otherwise midline approach to the interlaminar space **(Figure 6.13)**.

f. If the needle is on the correct course, two changes in resistance to advancement will be perceived. The firm **ligamentum flavum** will be encountered, followed by the **dura-arachnoid membrane** interface. After

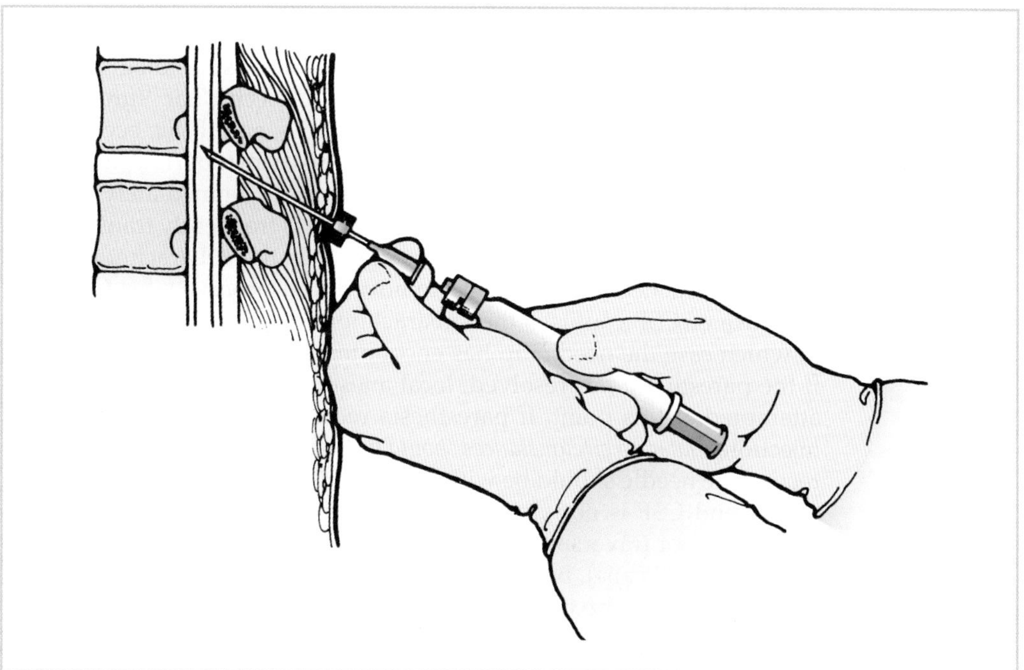

Figure 6.13. Spinal needle and introducer. The spinal needle is inserted through a larger-gauge introducer. The use of the introducer avoids the problem of contamination of the tip of the spinal needle with prep solution, epidermis, or skin bacteria, and allows a rigid channel for the smaller-gauge needles frequently used to reduce the incidence of headaches. Whenever the syringe is attached or removed from the needle hub, the opposite hand rests firmly against the back and grasps the hub firmly, preventing unintentional advancement or withdrawal.

this second change in resistance (often perceived as a loss of resistance or "pop"), needle advancement should stop as this usually indicates that the needle tip is now in the subarachnoid space. After the pop is felt, the nondominant hand releases the introducer needle and grasps the hub of the spinal needle to stabilize its position in the subarachnoid space. The stylet of the spinal needle is withdrawn with the dominant hand to allow for **flow of CSF**. If free flow of CSF does not occur, the hub of the spinal needle is rotated 90 degrees, in the event that a small flap of dura or arachnoid is obstructing the orifice. The stylet may also be reinserted to clear any obstruction. There is sometimes a "false pop" as the needle tip enters the epidural space and further advancement through the dura-arachnoid membranes is required. If no fluid is obtained, the stylet is replaced and the needle is gently advanced slightly further until another "pop" is appreciated and then the stylet is removed. The preceding steps are repeated until CSF is identified when the stylet is removed.

g. Occasionally, the subarachnoid space is completely traversed by the spinal needle without being appreciated by the anesthesiologist and the needle tip "pops" out through the anterior dura-arachnoid membrane to enter the anterior epidural space. When the needle is advanced further, the posterior surface of the vertebral body is encountered. In this case the stylet is removed and the needle withdrawn incrementally in 3 mm steps, with rotation of the hub 90 degrees at each increment until CSF is identified in the spinal needle hub.

h. Before initiating the procedure, the anesthesiologist should warn the patient of the possibility of a **paresthesia**. The anesthesiologist should explain to the patient that he or she may feel an "electric" or "funny bone" sensation in their buttocks or lower extremities, and if this occurs, they should communicate this immediately. If the patient reports a paresthesia at any time, the needle advancement is stopped immediately and the needle position immobilized. The paresthesia is frequently transient and mild and simply serves as an indication that the subarachnoid space has been reached. The stylet is removed and observed for CSF. The presence of CSF confirms the subarachnoid position of the needle tip, in which case the needle tip has encountered part of the cauda equina. If the paresthesia has resolved, local anesthetic injection may be safely attempted at this point. If paresthesia recurs with either aspiration or injection, *under no circumstances should an injection be made*! If paresthesia recurs, the needle should be withdrawn and repositioned. If paresthesia occurs and CSF is not visible, then it likely results from contact with the nerve root traversing the epidural space, indicating that the needle is in the spinal canal, but has deviated away from midline. In this case, the needle should be withdrawn and redirected to the side opposite the paresthesia.

i. Once free flow of CSF is obtained, the syringe containing the local anesthetic solution is attached to the hub of the spinal needle. During injection, the hub is fixed in position with the nondominant hand by placing the back of the hand firmly against the patient's back and then grasping the hub with thumb and index finger (Figure 6.13). **Gentle aspiration of 0.1 to 0.2 mL of CSF** confirms subarachnoid position before injection. The **local anesthetic solution is injected slowly (0.5 mL/s).**

Some anesthesiologists repeat aspiration midway through the injection or at the end of injection to confirm that the needle tip remained in the subarachnoid space during the entire injection process. Whether this process improves the success rate of spinal anesthesia is unknown. Once the injection is complete, the spinal needle and introducer are removed together as a unit.

j. If bone is encountered, a mental note of the depth is made and the spinal needle (hub) is partially withdrawn and repositioned in a slightly more cephalad direction and advanced. If bone is encountered again, the depth is compared to the first encounter **(Figure 6.14)**. If bone **contact is deeper** than previously encountered, the needle is most likely advancing along the superior crest of the spinous process below the IVS and it should be angled more cephalad and advanced further. **If bony contact is shallower** than previously encountered, it is most likely that inferior surface of the spinous process above the IVS and less cephalad angulation is indicated before advancing further. If bony contact is repeatedly encountered at the **same depth,** it is most likely the lamina, indicating that the needle is not in the true midline. The direction of the

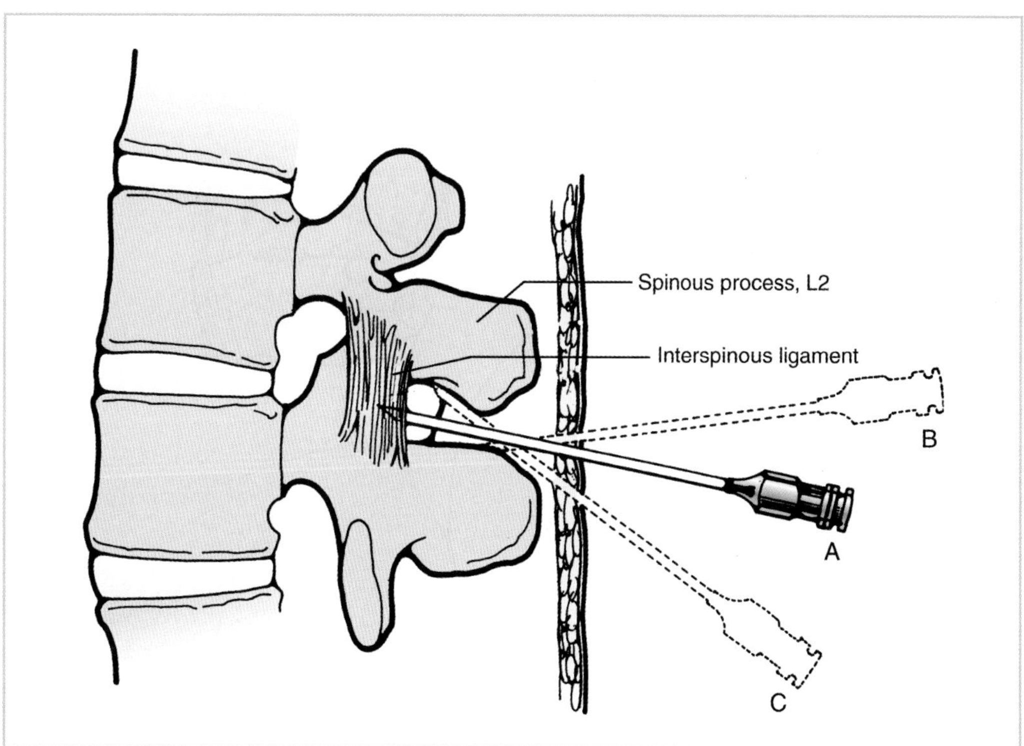

Figure 6.14. Spinal needle insertion, lateral view. For the classic midline approach, the needle is introduced in the middle of the interspace and advanced with a slight cephalad angulation. If correctly angled (*A*), it will enter the interspinous ligament, ligamentum flavum, and epidural space. If bone is contacted, it may be the inferior spinous process (*B*), and cephalad redirection will identify the correct path. If angling cephalad causes contact with bone again at a shallower depth (*C*), it is probably the superior spinous process. If bone is encountered at the same depth after several attempts at redirection (not shown), the needle is most likely on the lamina lateral to the interspace, and the position of the true midline should be reassessed.

needle (and introducer) is reevaluated to ensure that they are midline and perpendicular to the long axis of the spinal column. Occasionally, the patient may be able to communicate which side the needle tip has deviated from the midline. In this case, the needle is withdrawn and advanced in the opposite direction. Regardless of whether the patient can communicate which side he or she feels the needle is on, a logical and systematic approach will result in the minimum number of readjustments. The most frequent misdirection occurs when the patient rolls slightly forward away from the anesthesiologist during attempts to flex the spine. In this case, although the needle may be advanced parallel to the floor, it will not be perpendicular to the spinal column leading the needle tip to deviate away from the midline. In general, the needle direction will need to be oriented slightly toward the floor to compensate for this rotation of the spine (Figure 6.15).

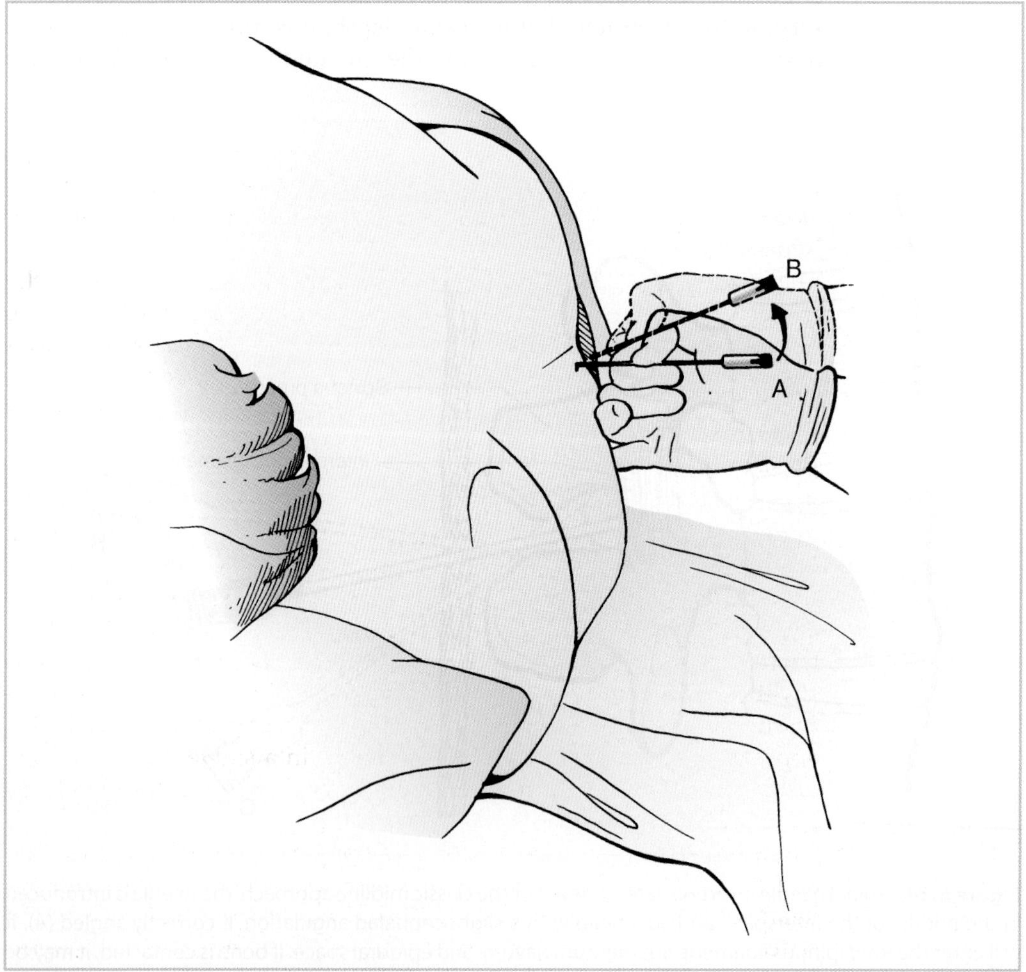

Figure 6.15. Patient position lateral view. Most patients will rotate their body anteriorly in an attempt to flex their back, and the initial spinal (or epidural needle) orientation (*A*) will therefore need to be redirected slightly downward towards the plane of the floor (*B*) to be truly perpendicular to the midline of the patient.

k. The technique for the midline approach is similar for when patients are either in the **sitting** or **prone jackknife** position. When the subarachnoid space is encountered with the prone jackknife position, CSF flow may not be apparent due to the relatively lower CSF pressure in this position. To augment the CSF pressure, the operating table position can be adjusted to raise the head temporarily

2. **Paramedian.** The classic midline approach is adequate for most patients, and has the advantage of being simple to learn. However, if the patient has a heavily calcified interspinous ligament (elderly patients) or has difficulty flexing the spine to increase (patients with hip fractures or the prone jackknife position) the interspinous space, the ligament or spinous processes can be bypassed with the paramedian approach. The paramedian approach may be performed **just slightly lateral from the midline or further away from the midline**.
   a. In the paramedian-lateral approach, the initial spinal introducer insertion site is simply **one to one-half fingerbreadths from the midline** while staying in the **same IVS**. The needle is introduced with a slight medial angle as well as the usual cephalad angulation **(Figures 6.11 and 6.12)**. The anesthesiologist must develop a **three-dimensional image** of the tissues as he or she advances the needle so that the tip ends up in the midline interlaminar space as it reaches the depth of the dura-arachnoid. From here, the advancement and injection process proceeds as before as before but, the supraspinous and interspinous ligaments have been bypassed.
   b. The **paramedian-lateral oblique approach** also starts lateral to the midline, but from a **level opposite the spinous process below the interspace (Figure 6.11 and 6.12)**. From here, the needle is advanced almost 45 degrees to the midline and 45 degrees cephalad to enter the subarachnoid space in the midline. The oblique approach also provides a better angle for catheter insertion as the exit angle at the skin is less likely to lead to kinking of the catheter.
   c. A variation of the paramedian approach involves advancing the needle in two separate steps. First, from the lateral insertion point, the needle is advanced in the parasagittal plane parallel to the midline until the ipsilateral lamina of the vertebra is encountered. Next the spinal needle tip is incrementally "marched cephalad" over the cephalad edge of the lamina into ligamentum flavum. From here, the needle is advanced slightly further until one appreciates the "pop" through the dura-arachnoid membrane as the needle enters the subarachnoid space. This approach allows for moving the needle tip in a single plane at a time rather than the three-dimensional single step approach for the classic paramedian approaches.
   d. Occasionally, the anesthesiologist may angle the needle too medially and the tip of the needle encounters or even traverses the interspinous ligament and crossing the midline to end up in the contralateral epidural space. In this case the spinal needle should be withdrawn and angled less medially. The needle tip may also encounter the root of the spinous process, at which point, the needle will not advance further. In this case, the needle is simply withdrawn and the needle is angled less medially and then advanced.

3. **Lumbosacral (Taylor) approach.** In an occasional patient, none of the approaches previously described allows entry to the spinal canal because of calcification or fusion of the IVS or extensive scarring. In such case, the lumbosacral (L5-S1) vertebral foramen may still be passable, because it is the **largest of the interlaminar openings** to the spinal canal. The lateral oblique approach to the L5-S1 IVS is referred to as the *Taylor approach* in recognition of the urologist who popularized this technique.
   a. This approach can be utilized with the patients **lateral, prone, or sitting**.
   b. The **posterior–superior iliac spine (PSIS)** is identified and a skin mark is made **1 cm medial and 1 cm caudad to the PSIS**. The midline L5-S1 IVS is also identified and marked. A longer spinal needle (120–125 mm) is usually required because the oblique angle creates a greater distance to reach the subarachnoid space.
   c. After the appropriate local anesthetic infiltration the introducer is inserted and directed approximately 45 degrees cephalad and 45 degrees medially, visualizing and aiming for the midline L5-S1 IVS **(Figure 6.16)**.
   d. The changes in resistance as the needle traverse the ligamentum flavum and the dura-arachnoid membrane is the same as for the midline approach.

C. **Patient management after intrathecal injection.** After successful intrathecal injection, and when required, the patient is positioned appropriately for the

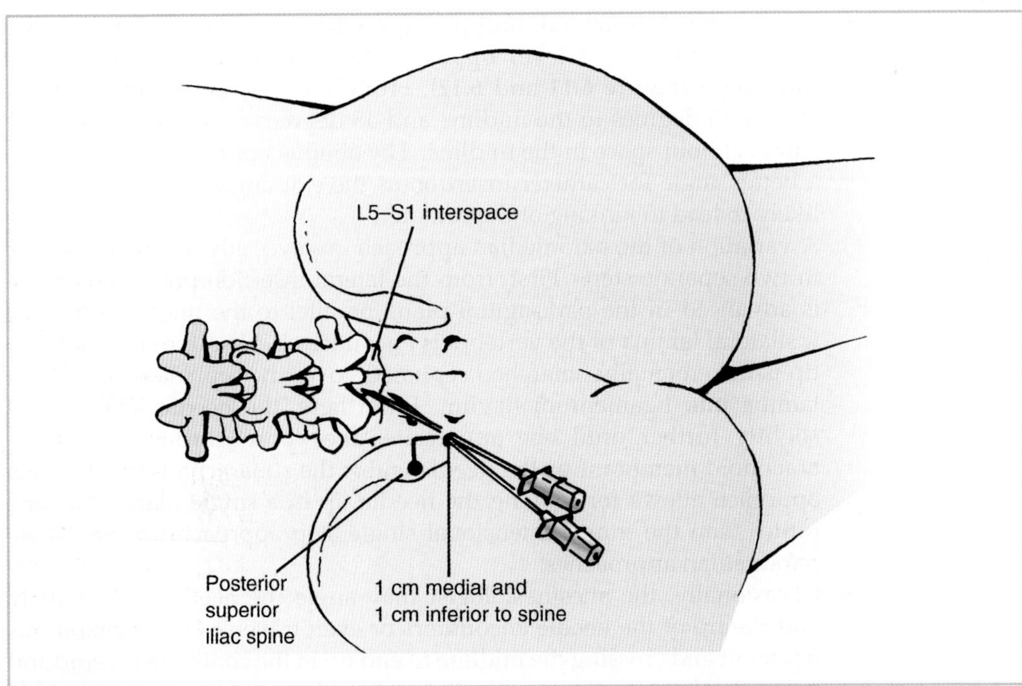

Figure 6.16. Taylor approach for spinal anesthesia. The needle is introduced 1 cm medial to and 1 cm inferior to the posterior–superior iliac spine and advanced at an angle 45 degrees to the midline and 45 degrees cephalad. On contacting the lamina, the needle is then walked upward and medially to enter the L5-S1 interspace.

planned surgical procedure. When positioning the patient, care must be taken to **avoid pressure on peripheral nerves or bony prominences**, as the patient will no longer be able to warn of uncomfortable pressure points. When a hypobaric local anesthetic technique is utilized for the prone jackknife or lateral position (for hip surgery), the patient simply remains in the same position. If a hyperbaric or isobaric local anesthetic technique is used for a supine or supine lithotomy position, the patient is positioned accordingly.

1. The **heart rate and blood pressure are checked** as soon as possible after intrathecal injection as the sympathetic fibers are anesthetized earliest, and venous pooling in the lower extremities begins immediately. The loss of venous return can produce a decrease in blood pressure and heart rate, particularly in elderly or volume-depleted patients. The **peak sensory block height may continue to gradually increase even 30 to 60 minutes** after initial injection resulting in blockade of the upper thoracic sympathetic efferent fibers, often manifest as profound **bradycardia** as the loss of venous return and blockade of the cardiac accelerator fibers (at T1-4) combine to reduce the heart rate. Therefore, frequent readings of blood pressure and continuous heart rate monitoring are mandatory during the conduct of spinal anesthesia.
2. The level of **temperature sensation is tested** with an alcohol swab approximately 2 to 3 minutes after injection, as afferent temperature sensation is anesthetized as rapidly as afferent pain sensation. This early assessment will confirm the presence of spinal anesthesia and provide an estimate of the ultimate peak sensory block height. If temperature sensation is difficult to assess, a **pinch or pinprick may be employed** to assess sensory block distribution.
3. Depending on the cephalad extent of the surgical procedure (when employing a hyperbaric technique), the level of sensory block may be adjusted by utilizing the Trendelenburg (to increase the peak sensory height) or reverse Trendelenburg (to limit the peak sensory height) position. If the lumbar IVS level of injection is caudad to the peak of the lumbar lordosis, the Trendelenburg maneuver may not be adequate to facilitate a cephalad spread of hyperbaric local anesthetic, as a larger percentage of the local anesthetic solution may preferentially pool in the sacral kyphosis. Because hip flexion can flatten the normal degree of lumbar lordosis, this should limit the degree of pooling of local anesthetic in the sacral kyphosis. Therefore, if a lower than expected level peak sensory block height is obtained after injection of a hyperbaric local anesthetic solution, combining hip flexion with Trendelenburg position has been shown to effectively increase the peak sensory height of spinal anesthesia compared to Trendelenburg position alone (57). The early use of reverse Trendelenburg position may limit the cephalad spread of solutions, but will not provide regression of a hyperbaric solution once it has already spread to higher thoracic segments. In this situation, use of this maneuver may aggravate the hypotension associated with high blockade.
4. Intraoperatively, **supplemental oxygen** is recommended, especially for older patients or those with high blocks or deeper levels of sedation. **End-tidal carbon dioxide monitoring** to constantly assess the rate of spontaneous ventilation may be performed either by a face mask or nasal cannula. Although patients may not feel pain at the surgical site, they may still be

uncomfortable (in nonanesthetized areas of their body) or apprehensive. Supplemental intravenous **opioids, benzodiazepines, or hypnotics** may be titrated to patient comfort. A warming blanket is indicated for longer procedures as cutaneous vasodilatation aggravates the heat loss associated with cold operating rooms. Comforting reassurance from an attentive, caring, and empathetic anesthesiologist can also facilitate more favorable intraoperative experience by the patient.

5. Postoperatively, the patient should continue to be monitored until the spinal anesthetic recedes. Sympathetic efferent block may reliably be expected to have dissipated when all sensory and motor function has returned, including return of proprioception in the great toe. In contrast, **postural control functional balance required to stand and ambulate unassisted may be impaired for as long as 90 to 120 minutes after recovery of gross motor function** (58). Therefore, ambulation without assistance should be a major factor in determining home readiness after outpatient spinal anesthesia. **Bed rest** for 24 hours has been traditionally recommended after spinal anesthesia to prevent PDPH. There is no evidence to support this recommendation, although it will delay the appearance of symptoms. **Heavy lifting and straining** are best avoided, spinal anesthesia is quite compatible with outpatient surgery and early ambulation (provided functional balance has returned).

VI. **Continuous spinal anesthesia**

A. Insertion of a catheter into the subarachnoid space increases the **flexibility** and **usefulness** of spinal anesthesia by allowing continuous or repeated local anesthetic administration to extend the distribution or duration of anesthetic blockade. The technique is similar to continuous epidural anesthesia, except that a needle than can accommodate a catheter is advanced until CSF is obtained; then the catheter is passed through the lumen. There are currently no spinal microcatheters marketed in the United States that have been specifically approved by the U.S. Food and Drug Administration (FDA). Most commonly, 18-gauge epidural needles and 20-gauge epidural catheters are used. Unfortunately, needles and catheters of this size may increase the risk of PDPH, especially in younger patients and parturients (59). This technique is well suited for elderly patients, who have a lower risk of PDPH. Because of the increased risk of PDPH, smaller needle/catheter combinations had been developed with spinal catheters in the range from 24- to 32-gauge. The FDA has subsequently advised against using catheters smaller than 24 gauge, as they are associated with an increased risk of sacral pooling of larger doses of local anesthetics that is thought to be the mechanism for cauda equina syndrome (CES) (60).

B. After subarachnoid placement of the needle and confirming the presence of CSF, the **catheter is threaded 2 to 3 cm** into the subarachnoid space with the needle bevel facing cephalad or caudad to facilitate catheter advancement beyond the needle tip.

C. The same local anesthetic agents are used as for a single-injection technique. **Extreme care should be taken to avoid injecting excessive doses** of local anesthetic as this increases the possibility of **sacral pooling**, which potentially increases the risk of CES. There are several guidelines for local anesthetic administration for continuous spinal anesthesia.

1. Use the **lowest effective anesthetic concentration**. The use of more dilute solutions is also desired for convenience of more accurate administration.
2. Administer a **test dose and assess the extent of sensory block. Sufficient time must be allowed for onset of anesthesia** before additional injections are administered. After appropriate intervals (45–90 minutes) depending on local anesthetic agent used, supplemental local anesthetic can be administered, starting with **half of the original dose**. This is usually administered at a time equal to two-thirds the expected duration of the orginal dose. Place a limit on the total amount of local anesthetic to be administered.
3. Because the catheter and connector "dead space" account for a large volume relative to the volume of anesthetic administered, the **catheter should be flushed with previously aspirated CSF after each injection**.
4. The continuous technique represents a **theoretic risk of infection**, because a foreign body is introduced into the subarachnoid space. Although this has not proved to be the case, the drug and flush syringes can be arranged on a three-way stopcock to enhance the preservation of sterility.
5. If **sacral misdistribution** of local anesthetic is suspected, use maneuvers to increase the intrathecal distribution of local anesthetic (place the patient in Trendelenburg position, with or without hip flexion).

VII. Complications

Spinal anesthesia is associated with potential complications and these should be considered when deciding the risk-to-benefit ratio for a specific patient and surgical procedure. Awareness of these potential complications, prevention with the appropriate technique, vigilance with early recognition and prompt treatment are foundations for the safe conduct of spinal anesthesia.

A. **Cardiovascular.** Hypotension, bradycardia, and cardiovascular collapse are all potential side effects and complications associated with spinal anesthesia.

1. **Hypotension** is the **most frequent** side effect of spinal anesthesia and is a direct result of venous pooling and arteriolar dilation secondary to sympathetic efferent blockade (61). The frequency of hypotension is dependent on the criteria used to define hypotension and occurs in 16% to 33% of patients. In contrast, if a decrease in mean arterial pressure of 30% within 10 minutes of induction of spinal anesthesia is defined as hypotension, then the frequency decreases to 8.2%. Furthermore, **clinically relevant hypotension** is that which requires treatment (with fluids and vasoactive agents) and is estimated to occur in **5% to 6% of patients** (62). Risk factors for developing hypotension include (62, **63**): peak sensory block height above T5, urgency of surgery, chronic alcohol consumption, age older than 40, baseline systolic blood pressure less than 120 mm Hg, chronic hypertension, combined spinal-general anesthesia, and intrathecal injection at or above the L2-3 IVS **(Table 6.6)**. The severity of decreases in blood pressure is loosely correlated with the extent of sympathetic blockade, as well as intravascular volume of the patient. Maximum decreases in blood pressure typically occur within 20 to 30 minutes, but may occur as late as 45 to 60 minutes after the induction of spinal anesthesia (64).
   a. The decrease in blood pressure may be prevented by **prophylactic volume infusion**, but this is dependent on the timing of the volume infusion. Administration of prophylactic volume loading (20 mL/kg) of lactated

Table 6.6 Spinal anesthesia–associated risk factors and odds ratios for hypotension and bradycardia

Risk factors	Odds ratio
Hypotension	
Peak sensory block height greater than T5	3.8
Chronic alcohol consumption	3.1
Urgency of surgery	2.9
Age older than 40 yr	2.5
Baseline systolic blood pressure <120 mm Hg	2.4
Chronic hypertension	2.2
Combined spinal-general anesthesia	1.9
Intrathecal injection at or above the L2-3 IVS	1.8
Bradycardia	
Baseline heart rate less than 60 bpm	4.9–16.2
ASA physical status 1 (vs. 2 or 3)	3.5
Prolonged PR interval	3.2
β-Adrenergic blockade use	2.9
Peak block height above T5	1.7
Age younger than 37 yr	1.4
Male gender	1.4
Case duration	2.0

IVS, intervertebral space; bpm, beats per minute; ASA, American Society of Anesthesiologists.

Ringers at the time of induction of spinal anesthesia has been shown to be significantly more effective in decreasing the frequency of clinically relevant hypotension compared to the same volume infusion administered 20 minutes before the induction of spinal anesthesia (65). Although fluid loading is the treatment of choice to treat spinal anesthesia–induced hypotension, this approach must be used with caution in those patients with left ventricular dysfunction. A large intravenous load of crystalloid may precipitate pulmonary venous congestion in the susceptible patient when the associated sympathectomy of the spinal anesthetic resolves. In this situation, lower volumes of fluid resuscitation in conjunction with a continuous vasopressor infusion may be more desirable to treat the hemodynamic effects.

b. If the decrease in blood pressure is abrupt, a **vasopressor** is appropriate to support the blood pressure temporarily until additional fluid replacement can be provided.

(1) Ephedrine in 5- to 10-mg increments administered intravenously is the drug of choice because it produces not only vasoconstriction but also increased cardiac output. The duration of action of ephedrine is typically 5 to 10 minutes, and an intramuscular administration of 25 mg may be needed if longer support is indicated. Alternatively, 25 to 30 mg of ephedrine in 1,000 mL of lactated Ringers may also be effective if longer support of hypotension is indicated.

(2) Phenylephrine in 50 to 100 μg intravenously is a reasonable second choice, especially if tachycardia is present, but this drug will primarily result in systemic vasoconstriction with a minimal increase (or decrease) in cardiac output.

c. **Elevation** of the legs will help reverse the undesirable pooling, but lowering of the head (Trendelenburg position), especially during hyperbaric spinal anesthesia, may cause the sensory block to rise to undesirable higher levels. **Flexion of the operating table** is an ideal compromise as the feet can be elevated, thereby increasing venous return while decreasing the further cephalad spread of the sympathetic block. A rapidly rising block occasionally prompts the inexperienced anesthesiologist to place the patient in reverse Trendelenburg position (head up, feet down) to stop the cephalad spread of anesthesia. This may lead to further venous pooling in the lower extremities, potentially leading to marked decreases in blood pressure.

2. **Bradycardia.** Although a decrease in venous return and systemic vascular resistance are the primary mechanisms for decreases in cardiac output and blood pressure, decreases in heart rate also contribute to the hemodynamic effects. As the level of sympathetic block reaches the upper thoracic levels, the **cardiac accelerator fibers are blocked**, resulting in marked degrees of vagal tone. The frequency of moderate bradycardia (defined as heart rate between 40–50 beats per minute [bpm]) is approximately 10% and the frequency of severe bradycardia (defined as heart rate less than 40 bpm) is approximately 1% (66). The risk factors for bradycardia include peak sensory block height above T5, decreasing age, American Society of Anesthesiologists (ASA) physical status 1, baseline heart rate less than 60 bpm, prolonged PR interval, therapy with β-adrenergic blockers, case duration, and male gender **(Table 6.6)**. Severe bradycardia associated with spinal anesthesia may lead to sudden onset of asystole and cardiovascular collapse (see subsequent text). However, prompt treatment with intravenous atropine 0.5 to 1.0 mg and ephedrine 5 to 10 mg (especially when accompanied by hypotension) may abort this downward spiral.

3. **Cardiovascular collapse** associated with spinal anesthesia is not an infrequent event and is often **preceded by bradycardia and hypotension**. As hypotension and bradycardia are not uncommon, adequate volume resuscitation during the induction of spinal anesthesia, continued vigilance with prompt replacement of surgical fluid losses, and pharmacologic treatment of hypotension and bradycardia are essential elements in preventing this potentially catastrophic complication **(67)**. Additionally, **excessive sedation may mask inadequate ventilation**, leading to hypoxia and/or hypercarbia, which potentially exacerbate the effects of hypotension and bradycardia. Therefore, treatment of spinal anesthesia–induced hypotension and bradycardia **must be prompt and aggressive** (see preceding text). If initial treatment steps are ineffective, aggressive stepwise escalation of therapy with **atropine (0.5–1.0 mg), ephedrine (25–30 mg), and the early use of epinephrine (0.2–0.3 mg) are indicated**. In the event of cardiovascular collapse, **external cardiac compression** and the use of epinephrine are critical for maintaining the necessary coronary perfusion pressure gradient. In response to recent animal data and concurrent with the most recent ACLS guidelines, epinephrine 1 mg intravenously every 3 to 5 minutes, or vasopressin 40 mg intravenously as a single dose are recommended, along with treating exacerbating factors such as hypoxia, acidosis, and hypovolemia (68).

B. **Total spinal.** *Total spinal anesthesia* is the term used to describe a spinal anesthetic sensory **block that rises above the cervical region**. This level of blockade is usually unintentional, resulting from unanticipated patient movement, inappropriate positioning, or inappropriate doses of local anesthetic. Total spinal anesthesia manifests as rapidly **ascending motor-sensory block, bradycardia, hypotension, and dyspnea** with difficulty swallowing and phonating. **Respiratory arrest and loss of consciousness may soon follow**. Phrenic nerve blockade, cerebral hypoperfusion leading to ischemia of the brainstem respiratory centers, and direct brainstem depression may all contribute to respiratory arrest. Fortunately, when local anesthetic has spread this far cephalad, the total amount (and therefore CSF concentration) is low and motor paralysis is limited and the **duration is short. Prompt recognition and therapy are essential** to prevent cardiac arrest and hypoxic brain injury. Management of total spinal anesthesia is supportive and consists of basic resuscitation (airway, breathing, circulation), with low threshold for endotracheal intubation and ventilation, along with fluids and vasoactive agents to support blood pressure and cardiac output. The patient will usually lose consciousness, and verbal reassurance that he or she will recover is appropriate. An amnestic agent may be desirable during the period of ventilatory support. Morbidity or mortality should not occur if ventilation and perfusion are maintained until the block resolves. Prevention is ideal and attention to total dose of intrathecal local anesthetic and patient position after induction are recommended. Additionally, induction of spinal anesthesia after failed epidural block may be a significant risk factor for a high or total spinal anesthetic (69).

C. **Subdural anesthesia.** The subdural space is essentially the **potential space between the inner surface of the dura and the arachnoid membrane**. It is usually traversed without notice during the process of entering the subarachnoid space. On rare occasions, local anesthetic is injected through either a needle or catheter tip while in this potential space and the resulting local anesthetic distribution is spread widely throughout this space. If the dose injected is intended as an intrathecal injection (relatively small dose), the resulting distribution of local anesthetic results in **widespread but minimal and patchy anesthesia** of sensory and motor nerves and may explain many cases of "failed spinal anesthesia." If the injected dose was intended for epidural anesthesia, the wider distribution of local anesthetic within the subdural compartment results in an unexpected spread of sensory and motor block and may result in symptoms resembling a total spinal anesthetic. The estimated incidence of subdural anesthesia is 1 in 2,000 attempted epidural blocks. If the result is simply a failed spinal anesthetic, a repeat injection may be attempted but with the concern of possibly causing a high spinal as the effects of the spinal block may combine with the subdural block.

D. **Central neuraxial (spinal or epidural hematoma).** Epidural or spinal hematoma is an **extremely rare but potentially catastrophic** complication of attempted spinal (or epidural) anesthesia. Although the bony elements of the spinal canal serve to protect the spinal cord from trauma, entrapment of a space-occupying lesion such as an expanding hematoma within the spinal canal may lead to direct spinal cord compression and ischemic damage. Although spinal-epidural hematomas can occur spontaneously in normal patients, the risk may be increased in **patients with altered hemostasis**. Spinal-epidural hematoma can potentially be precipitated by inserting a needle (or catheter) into the epidural venous plexus in patients in the absence of altered hemostasis (70), but the risk is increased in those patients who are being treated with drugs that affect either primary (antiplatelet agents) or secondary (systemic anticoagulants) hemostasis. Although the exact incidence of hematomas associated with spinal-epidural anesthesia is unknown, it has been estimated to be less than 1 in 150,000 epidural and less than 1 in 220,000 spinal anesthetics respectively **(71)**. The most recent report of the second American Society of Regional Anesthesia (ASRA) consensus conference on neuraxial anesthesia and anticoagulation evaluated the evidence and provides recommendations on the risks associated with use of various medications, as well as tests and outcomes **(71)**. The need for prompt diagnosis and surgical intervention in the event of a spinal-epidural hematoma was demonstrated in the most recent review of ASA closed claims database, which noted that spinal cord injuries were the leading cause of claims in the 1990s, with hematomas accounting for nearly half of spinal cord injuries. More importantly, the presence of postoperative numbness or weakness was typically attributed to local anesthetic effect, which led to delays in the diagnosis. A hematoma should be suspected when a spinal anesthetic (sensory/motor impairment) is unusually long in duration. Other possible signs and symptoms include new onset and progression of back pain and bowel or bladder dysfunction. Prompt imaging and neurosurgical consultation are required as neurologic outcome is poor if more than 6 to 8 hours are allowed to elapse between onset of paralysis and surgical decompression (72).

E. **Infectious complications.** Bacterial infection after spinal anesthesia may present as a localized skin infection, a **spinal-epidural abscess, or meningitis**. The most common source of infection is believed to be the patient's (or anesthesiologist's) normal skin flora. A spinal-epidural abscess will most commonly present as back pain that may be tender on palpation, accompanied by radicular pain, sensory/motor deficits, and fever. The **diagnosis of an abscess is best performed with a magnetic resonance imaging (MRI) of the vertebral canal** and surrounding structures. Therapeutic options include **intravenous antibiotics and surgical drainage/decompression** of the infected area. Signs and symptoms of bacterial meningitis include headache, nausea/vomiting, photophobia, neck stiffness, and fever. The diagnosis is confirmed by CSF examination and culture. Fortunately, prompt treatment with antibiotics usually results in full recovery. In contrast, chemical (or aseptic) meningitis presents in similar manner and is often attributed to inflammation secondary to skin preparation disinfectants contaminating the CSF.

F. **Nerve injury** secondary to spinal anesthesia can be due to either drug toxicity (from the local anesthetic agent or additives) or from direct needle trauma.

   1. **Drug toxicity.** Although laboratory studies confirm that **all local anesthetics are potentially neurotoxic**, clinical experience and a long history of safety suggests that local anesthetic–induced nerve **injury is rare. CES** has been associated with the use of spinal microcatheters and sacral pooling of extremely large and toxic doses of local anesthetics within the lumbar cistern (60). **Transient neurological symptoms (TNS)** is a syndrome that presents with low back pain that radiates to the buttocks and lower extremities after the uneventful resolution of a spinal anesthetic. The symptoms typically present the following day and may last for up to a week **(73)**. Risk factors include outpatient surgery, surgical

positioning that potentially causes stretching of the lumbosacral roots (such as lithotomy or knee arthroscopy), and obesity. However, the predominant risk factor for TNS is the **use of lidocaine** for spinal anesthesia, and although all local anesthetics have been associated with TNS, the incidence (16%–33%) is highest with lidocaine. Although there is **no evidence of permanent neurologic injury**, the symptoms may be severe enough to impair functional activities of daily living and sleeping (74). Treatment is supportive and primarily consists of anti-inflammatory agents and opioids.

2. **Direct needle trauma** may cause nerve damage to a nerve root or the spinal cord and is **usually associated with severe paresthesia in the dermatomal projection** of the spinal nerve root or spinal cord segment. Intraneural injection heralded by severe paresthesia has been implicated as a contributing factor in nerve injury (9,10). Should a paresthesia present with needle advancement, aspiration, or injection, the local anesthetic should not be injected and the needle repositioned until the paresthesia completely resolves.

G. **Hearing loss** has been increasingly described after spinal anesthesia and audiometrically documented hearing loss has been demonstrated (75). The frequency of occurrence has been reported to be between 0.4% and 0.5%, but most cases are not clinically noticeable and the **duration is typically less than 1 week**. The postulated mechanism involves postdural puncture **loss of CSF**, with the resulting decrease in CSF pressure transmitted to the perilymph within the cochlea leading to disruption of hair cell function and hearing deficits. Consistent with this mechanism is the observation that the use of larger gauge spinal needles led to a significantly higher frequency of postspinal hearing deficits. Additionally, improvements in CSF pressure through either epidural blood patch or positional changes in patients with severe PDPH and associated hearing loss provides additional evidence of the mechanism of hearing loss after spinal anesthesia (76).

H. **Nausea** is a common complication associated with spinal anesthesia. The most common etiologies are hypotension and the use of **intrathecal opioids** in the local anesthetic solution. **Hypotension** is believed to cause nausea due to hypoxemia or hypoperfusion of the chemoreceptor trigger zone (CTZ) in the medulla **(77)**. Consequently supplemental oxygen and treatment of hypotension have been shown to effectively treat perioperative nausea. Additionally, spinal anesthesia also leads to a **sympathetic-vagal imbalance** and the unopposed vagal tone results in gastrointestinal hyperactivity and the efficacy of **vagolytic agents (atropine)** to relieve nausea during spinal anesthesia supports this mechanism. The use of intrathecal opioids has been shown to prolong the duration of spinal anesthesia and provide spinally mediated analgesia. Postoperative nausea is a common side effect, but may be effectively treated with dexmethasone and droperidol, while 5-HT antagonists and opioid antagonists have proved to be much less effective.

I. **PDPH (78)**. PDPH is a **relatively common complication** of spinal anesthesia. The reported incidence of PDPH, with current use of smaller 25- to 26-guage pencil point needles, is approximately 0.4% to 1.0%. The incidence increases significantly with the use of larger cutting needles (17- to 18-gauge, such as those intended for epidural anesthesia) and has been reported to be as high as 75%.

1. The postulated mechanisms for PDPH are that the **loss of CSF leads to decreases in CSF pressure**. The decrease in CSF pressure leads to diminished buoyant support allowing the brain to sag (especially in the upright position), resulting in traction and pressure on pain-sensitive intracranial structures (meninges, cranial nerves, bridging veins, and venous sinuses). The decreased CSF pressure is also believed to result in reflex cerebral vasodilatation to compensate for the increased intracranial volume loss, resulting in a vascular-type headache.
2. PDPH typically **presents within 12 to 48 hours** and rarely more than 5 days of dural puncture. The cardinal feature of PDPH is its positional nature, with symptoms worsening in the upright position and improving with recumbency. PDPH is bilateral, with a predominantly frontal–occipital distribution, typically described as "dull, aching, throbbing, or pressure" in nature, and may be mild to severe. Associated symptoms can include nausea and vomiting, photophobia, with onset of cranial nerve involvement (diplopia and hearing loss) indicating a severe case of PDPH. The frequency of occurrence is **higher in younger patients**. Females have slightly higher risk than males, and parturients appear to be at highest risk, although the increased risk in parturients appears to be related to the increased risk of accidental dural puncture with larger bore cutting needles. Although most headaches following dural puncture (intentional or accidental) are a PDPH, a thorough history and physical is essential to rule out benign etiologies (such as nonspecific headache and pneumocephalus) and serious etiologies (meningitis, subdural hematoma, subarachnoid hemorrhage, and headaches associated with preeclampsia/eclampsia).
3. Treatment of PDPH is **based primarily on severity of symptoms and social conditions** of the patient. For example, a mild to moderate headache in the hospitalized patient requires less urgent treatment than the same headache in a postpartum patient anxious to care for her new baby. Prevention is the least expensive form of therapy and the use of smaller-gauge pencil point needles is associated with an acceptably low incidence of PDPH. Alternatively, if an outpatient lives a sufficient distance from the hospital or ambulatory surgical center, then returning for an epidural blood patch (EBP) would be a major inconvenience. Supportive treatment with **oral analgesics** (anti-inflammatory agents, acetaminophen, and opioids) only provides temporary relief and is often ineffective for severe headaches. **Cerebral vasoconstrictors (caffeine and sumatriptan)** may provide temporary relief but do not target the etiology of the symptoms caused by the low CSF due to continue CSF leak. An EBP (see Chapter 7) remains the current gold standard of therapy as it targets the etiology (persistent CSF leak) and postulated mechanism (low CSF pressure) of PDPH. The **efficacy of a single EBP is 70% to 98%, but may require a second EBP, especially in the event of an accidental dural puncture with larger-gauge epidural needles** (79). The mechanisms by which an EBP relieves the symptoms of PDPH are believed to be due to a combination of the mass effect of the injected blood in the epidural space and the translocation of CSF to the intracranial compartment, as well as the formation of a clot over the dural tear that prevents further loss of CSF. Following a successful EBP, maintenance of the recumbent position for 1 to 2 hours may result in a more complete resolution of symptoms. Avoidance of lifting, straining, and air

travel are commonly recommended for 24 to 48 hours to minimize the risk of disruption of the clot.

REFERENCES

1 Fink BR, Walker S. Orientation of fibers in the human dorsal lumbar dura mater in relation to lumbar puncture. *Anesth Analg* 1989;69:768–772.

2 Vandenabeele F, Creemers J, Lambrichts I. Ultrastructure of the human spinal and dura mater. *J Anat* 1996;189:417–430.

3 Reina MA, De Leon Casasola O, Villanueva MC, et al. Ultrastructural findings in human spinal pia mater in relation to subarachnoid anesthesia. *Anaesth Analg* 2004;98:1479–1485.

4 Hogan Q. Size of human lower thoracic and lumbosacral nerve roots. *Anesthesiology* 1996;85:37–42.

5 Hogan Q, Toth J. Anatomy of the soft tissues of the spinal canal. *Reg Anesth Pain Med* 1999;24:303–310.

6 Kim JT, Bahk JH, Sung J. Influence of age and sex on the position of the conus medullaris and Tuffier's line in adults. *Anesthesiology* 2003;99:1359–1363.

7 Broadbent CR, Maxwell WB, Ferrie R, et al. Ability of anaesthetists to identify a marked lumbar interspace. *Anaesthesia* 2000;55:1122–1126.

8 Furness G, Reilly MP, Kuchi S. An evaluation of ultrasound imaging for identification of lumbar intervertebral level. *Anaesthesia* 2002;57:277–280.

9 Reynolds F. Damage to the conus medullaris following spinal anaesthesia. *Anaesthesia* 2001;56:238–247.

10 Hamandi K, Mottershead J, Lewis T, et al. Irreversible damage to the spinal cord following spinal anesthesia. *Neurology* 2002;59:624–626.

11 Kim JT, Jung CW, Lee JR, et al. Influence of lumbar flexion on the position of the intercristal line. *Reg Anesth Pain Med* 2003;28:509–511.

12 Rocco AG, Raymond SA, Murray E, et al. Differential spread of blockade of touch, cold, and pinprick during spinal anesthesia. *Anesth Analg* 1985;64:917–923.

13 Sakura S, Sakaguchi Y, Shinzawa M, et al. The assessment of dermatomal level of surgical anesthesia after spinal tetracaine. *Anesth Analg* 2000;90:1406–1410.

14 Kouri ME, Kopacz DJ. Spinal 2-chloroprocaine: a comparison with lidocaine in volunteers. *Anesth Analg* 2004;98:75–80.

15 JR, Horlocker TT, Schroeder DR. Neuraxial anesthesia and analgesia in patients with preexisting central nervous system disorders. *Anesth Analg* 2006;103:223–228.

16 Hebl JR, Kopp SL, Schroeder DR, et al. Neurological complications after neuraxial anesthesia or analgesia in patients with preexisting peripheral sensorimotor neuropathy or diabetic polyneuropathy. *Anesth Analg* 2006;103:1294–1299.

17 as A, Chan VW. Neuraxial anesthesia and multiple sclerosis. *Can J Anaesth* 2005;52:454–458.

18 McDonald SB. Is neuraxial blockade contraindicated in patients with aortic stenosis? *Reg Anesth Pain Med* 2004;29:496–502.

19 Wedel DJ, Horlocker TT. Regional anesthesia in the febrile or infected patient. *Reg Anesth Pain Med* 2006;31:324–333.

20 Green NM. Distribution of local anesthetics within the subarachnoid space. *Anesth Analg* 1985;64:715–730.

21 Hocking G, Wildsmith JAW. Intrathecal drug spread. *Br J Anaesth* 2004;93:568–578.

22 Hirabayshi Y, Shimizu R, Saitoh K, et al. Anatomical configuration of the spinal column in the supine position. I. A study using magnetic resonance imaging. *Br J Anaesth* 1995;75:3–5.

23 Hirabayshi Y, Shimizu R, Fukuda H, et al. Anatomical configuration of the spinal column in the supine position. II. Comparison of pregnant and non-pregnant women. *Br J Anaesth* 1995;75:6–8.

24 Veering BT, Immink-Speet TT, Burm AG, et al. Spinal anaesthesia with 0.5% hyperbaric bupivacaine in elderly patients: effects of duration of spent in the sitting position. *Br J Anaesth* 2001;77:738–742.

25 Casati A, Fanelli G, Aldegheri G, et al. Frequency of hypotension during conventional or asymmetric hyperbaric spinal block. *Reg Anesth Pain Med* 1999;24:214–219.

26 Bodily MN, Carpenter RL, Owens BD. Lidocaine 0.5% spinal anesthesia: a hypobaric solution for short-stay perirectal procedures. *Can J Anaesth* 1992;39:770–773.

27 Faust A, Fournier R, Van Gessel E, et al. Isobaric versus hypobaric spinal bupivacaine for total hip arthroplasty in the lateral position. *Anesth Analg* 2003;97:589–594.

28 Sheskey MC, Rocco Ag, Bizzarri-Scgmid M, et al. A dose-response study of bupivacaine for spinal anesthesia. *Anesth Analg* 1983;62:931–935.

29 Van Zundert AA, Grouls RJ, Korsten HH, et al. Spinal anesthesia. Volume or concentration: what matters? *Reg Anesth* 1996;21:112.

30 Brown DT, Wildsmith JAW, Covino BG, et al. Effect of baricity on spinal anesthesia with amethocaine. *Br J Anaesth* 1980;52:589–596.

31 Wildsmith JAW, McClure J, Brown DT, et al. Effects of posture on spread of isobaric and hyperbaric amethocaine. *Br J Anaesth* 1981;53:273–278.

32 Liu SS, Ware PD, Allen HW, et al. Dose-response characteristics of spinal bupivacaine in volunteers. Clinical implications for ambulatory anesthesia. *Anesthesiology* 1996;85:729–736.

33 Touminen M, Pitkanen M, Taivainen T, et al. Predictors of spread of repeated spinal anesthesia with bupivacaine. *Br J Anaesth* 1992;68:136–138.

34 Olson KH, Nielsen TH, Kristofferson E, et al. Spinal anesthesia with plain bupivacaine 0.5% administered at spinal interspace L2/L3 or L4/L5. *Br J Anaesth* 1990;64:170–172.

35 Serpell MG, Gray WM. Flow dynamics through spinal needles. *Anaesthesia* 1997;52:229–236.

36 Urmey WF, Stanton J, Bassin P, et al. The direction of the Whitacre needle aperture affects the extent and duration of isobaric spinal anesthesia. *Anesth Analg* 1997;84:337–341.

37 Taivainen T, Touminen M, Kuulasmaa KA, et al. A prospective study on reproducibility of the spread of spinal anesthesia using plain bupivacaine 0.5%. *Reg Anesth* 1990;15:12–14.

38 Casati A, Fanelli G, Danelli G, et al. Spinal anesthesia with lidocaine or preservative-free 2-chloroprocaine for outpatient knee arthroscopy: a prospective, randomized, double-blind comparison. *Anesth Analg* 2007;104:959–964.

39 Frey K, Holman S, Mikat-Stevens M, et al. The recovery profile of hyperbaric spinal anesthesia with lidocaine, bupivacaine, and tetracaine. *Reg Anesth Pain Med* 1998;23:159–163.

40 Kooger-Infante NE, Van Gessel E, Forster A, et al. Extent of hyperbaric spinal anesthesia influences duration of block. *Anesthesiology* 2000;92:1319–1323.

41 Burm AG, Van Kleef JW, Gladines MP, et al. Plasma concentrations of lidocaine and bupivacaine after subarachnoid administration. *Anesthesiology* 1983;59:191–195.

42 Chiu AA, Liu SS, Carpenter RL, et al. The effects of epinephrine on lidocaine spinal anesthesia: a cross-over study. *Anesth Analg* 1995;80:735–739.

43 Racle JP, Benkhadra A, Poy JY, et al. Prolongation of isobaric spinal anesthesia with epinephrine and clonidine for hip surgery in the elderly. *Anesth Analg* 1987;66:442–446.

44 Armstrong IR, Littlewood DG, Chambers WA. Spinal anesthesia with tetracaine-effect of added vasoconstrictors. *Anesth Analg* 1983;62:793–795.

45 Concepcion M, Maddi R, Francis D, et al. Vasoconstrictors in spinal anesthesia with tetracaine-comparison of phenylephrine and epinephrine. *Anesth Analg* 1984;63:134–138.

46 Moore JM, Liu SS, Pollock JE, et al. The effect on epinephrine on small-dose hyperbaric bupivacaine spinal anesthesia: clinical implications for ambulatory surgery. *Anesth Analg* 1998;86:973–977.

47 Chiari A, Eisenach JC. Spinal anesthesia: mechanisms, agents, methods, and safety. *Reg Anesth Pain Med* 1998;23:357–362.

48 Hamber EA, Viscomi CM. Intrathecal lipophilic opioids as adjuncts to surgical spinal anesthesia. *Reg Anesth Pain Med* 1999;24:255–263.

49 Liu SS, Chiu AA, Carpenter RL, et al. Fentanyl prolongs lidocaine spinal anesthesia without prolonging recovery. *Anesth Analg* 1995;80:730–734.

50 Singh H, Yang J, Thornton K, et al. Intrathecal fentanyl prolongs sensory bupivacaine spinal block. *Can J Anaesth* 1995;42:987–991.

51 Rathmell JP, Lair TR, Nauman B. The role of intrathecal drugs in the treatment of acute pain. *Anesth Analg* 2005;101:S30–S43.

52 Rathmell JP, Pino CA, Taylor R, et al. Intrathecal morphine for postoperative analgesia: a randomized, controlled, dose-ranging study after hip and knee arthroplasty. *Anesth Analg* 2003;97:1452–1457.

53 Bowrey S, Hamer J, Bowler I, et al. A comparison of 0.2 and 0.5 mg intrathecal morphine for postoperative analgesia after total knee replacement. *Anaesthesia* 2005;60:449–452.

54 Raffaeli W, Marconi G, Fanelli G, et al. Opioid-related side-effects after intrathecal morphine: a prospective, randomized, double-blind dose-response study. *Eur J Anaesthesiol* 2006;23:605–610.

55 Shapiro A, Zohar E, Zalansky R, et al. The frequency and timing of respiratory depression in 1524 postoperative patients treated with systemic or neuraxial morphine. *J Clin Anesth* 2005;17:537–542.

56 Ahn WS, Bahk JH, Lim YJ, et al. The effect of introducer gauge, design, and bevel direction on the deflection of spinal needles. *Anaesthesia* 2002;57:1007–1011.

57 Kim JT, Shim JK, Kim SH, et al. Trendelenburg position with hip flexion as a rescue strategy to increase spinal anaesthetic level after spinal block. *Br J Anaesth* 2007;98:396–400.

58 Imarengiaye CO, Song D, Prabhu AJ, et al. Spinal anesthesia: functional balance is impaired after clinical recovery. *Anesthesiology* 2003;98:511–515.

59 Horlocker TT, McGregor DG, Matsushige D, et al. Neurological complications of 603 consecutive continuous spinal anesthetics using macrocatheter and microcatheter techniques. *Anesth Analg* 1997;84:1063–1070.

60 Rigler ML, Drasner K, Krejcie TC, et al. Cauda equina syndrome after continuous spinal anesthesia. *Anesth Analg* 1991;72:275–281.

61 Salinas FV, Sueda LA, Liu SS. Physiology of spinal anesthesia and practical suggestions fort successful spinal anaesthesia. *Best Pract Res Clin Anaesthesiol* 2002;16:195–210.

62 Hartmann B, Junger A, Klasen J, et al. The incidence and risk factors for hypotension after spinal anesthesia induction: an analysis with automated data collection. *Anesth Analg* 2002;94:1521–1529.

63 Carpenter RL, Caplan RA, Brown DL, et al. Incidence and risk factors for side effects of spinal anesthesia. *Anesthesiology* 1992;76:906–916.

64 Arndt JO, Bomer W, Krauth J. Marquardt. Incidence and time course of cardiovascular effects during spinal anesthesia after prophylactic administration of intravenous fluids and vasoconstrictors. *Anesth Analg* 1998;87:347–354.

65 Mojica JL, Melendez HJ, Bautista LE. The timing of intravenous crystalloid administration and incidence of cardiovascular side effects during spinal anesthesia: the results from a randomized controlled trial. *Anesth Analg* 2002;94:432–437.

66 Lesser JB, Sanborn KV, Valskys R, et al. Severe bradycardia during spinal and epidural anesthesia recorded by an anesthesia information management system. *Anesthesiology* 2003;99:859–866.

67 Pollard JB. Cardiac arrest during spinal anesthesia: common mechanisms and strategies for prevention. *Anesth Analg* 2001;92:252–256.

68 Krismer AC, Hogan QC, Wenzel V, et al. The efficacy of epinephrine or vasopressin for resuscitation during epidural anesthesia. *Anesth Analg* 2001;93:734–742.

69 Furst SR, Reisner LS. Risk of high spinal anesthesia following failed epidural block for cesarean delivery. *J Clin Anesth* 1995;1:71–74.

70 Cullen DJ, Bogdanoiv E, Htut N. Spinal epidural hematoma occurrence in the absence of known risk factors: a case series. *J Clin Anesth* 2004;16:3786–3781.

71 Horlocker TT, Wedel DJ, Benzon HT, et al. Regional anesthesia in the anticoagulated patient: defining the risks (the second ASRA consensus conference on neuraxial anesthesia and anticoagulation). *Reg Anesth Pain Med* 2003;28:172–197.

72 Lee LA, Posner KL, Domino KB, et al. Injuries associated with regional anesthesia in the 1980s and 1990s: a closed claims analysis. *Anesthesiology* 2004;101:143–152.

73 Pollock JE. Neurotoxicity of intrathecal local anaesthetics and transient neurological symptoms. *Best Pract Res Clin Anaesthesiol* 2003;17:471–483.

74 Tong D, Wong J, Chung F, et al. Prospective study on the incidence and functional impact of transient neurological symptoms associated with 1% versus 5% hyperbaric lidocaine in short urological procedures. *Anesthesiology* 2003;98:485–494.

75 Cosar A, Yetiser S, Sizlan A, et al. Hearing impairment associated with spinal anesthesia. *Acta Otolaryngol* 2004;124:1159–1164.

76 Lybecker H, Andersen T, Helbo-Hansen HS. The effect of epidural blood patch on hearing loss in patients with severe PDPH. *J Clin Anesth* 1995;7:457–464.

77 Borgeat A, Ekatodramis G, Schenker CA. Postoperative nausea and vomiting in regional anesthesia. *Anesthesiology* 2003;98:530–547.

78 Harrington BE. Postdural puncture headache and the development of the epidural blood patch. *Reg Anesth Pain Med* 2004;29:136–163.

79 Safa-Tisseront V, Thormann F, Malasinne P, et al. Effectiveness of epidural blood patch in the management of post-dural puncture headache. *Anesthesiology* 2001;95:334–339.

7 Epidural Anesthesia

Christopher M. Bernards

I. Introduction

Compared to spinal anesthesia, epidural needle placement takes **longer**, epidural block is **slower** to set up and there is a higher likelihood that epidural block will not be **dense enough** to prevent all pain sensation during the surgical procedure. However, epidural anesthesia has distinct advantages over spinal anesthesia. Chief among these are a **lower incidence of postdural puncture headache, less hypotension** (if epinephrine is omitted), the ability to extend the extent and duration of the block if a **catheter** technique is used and the option of using the epidural catheter to provide **postoperative analgesia** (see Chapter 23).

II. Anatomy

Understanding the anatomy of the epidural space is critical for facile performance of epidural anesthesia/analgesia and for understanding the relevant pharmacology of the epidural space. Clinicians must develop a three-dimensional anatomic picture so that they can logically redirect their needle when contacting bony structures. They must also understand the relationship between spinal cord segment, spinal nerve, vertebral level and cutaneous dermatome. Finally, clinicians must recognize that the anatomy of the vertebrae and their relation to neural structures varies along the length of the spine.

A. **Bony anatomy** (Figures 7.1 and 7.2). The epidural space lies between the dura mater and the walls of the vertebral canal and extends from the foramen magnum to the sacrococcygeal ligament. The vertebrae consist of the **body** anteriorly, the **pedicles** laterally, the **lamina** and associated **transverse process** posterolaterally, and the **spinous process** in the midline posteriorly. The epidural space is accessed through the vertebral interlaminar space (Figure 7.1). Whether the interlaminar space is accessed in the midline or paramedian depends on the shape of the spinous process cephalad of the intended interspace; in the midthoracic region (T4–10) the spinous process angles caudad sufficiently that it covers the interlaminar space in the midline. Because the vertebrae increase in size as one moves caudad, the epidural space is largest at the lumbar level.

B. **Ligaments.** The anterior and posterior longitudinal ligaments run along the anterior and posterior surfaces of the vertebral bodies. The **supraspinous ligament** runs the length of the vertebral column connecting the tips of the spinous processes. The **interspinous ligament** connects the bodies of two adjacent spinous processes and the **ligamentum flavum** connects adjacent vertebral lamina.

   1. The **ligamenta flava** and interspinous ligaments are discontinuous ligaments, that is, there is an individual ligament between each adjacent vertebral pair.
   2. The ligamentum flavum consists of a distinct right- and left-sided ligament that usually, but not always, fuses in the midline (1). Failure to fuse in the midline may make it difficult to recognize the epidural space using a

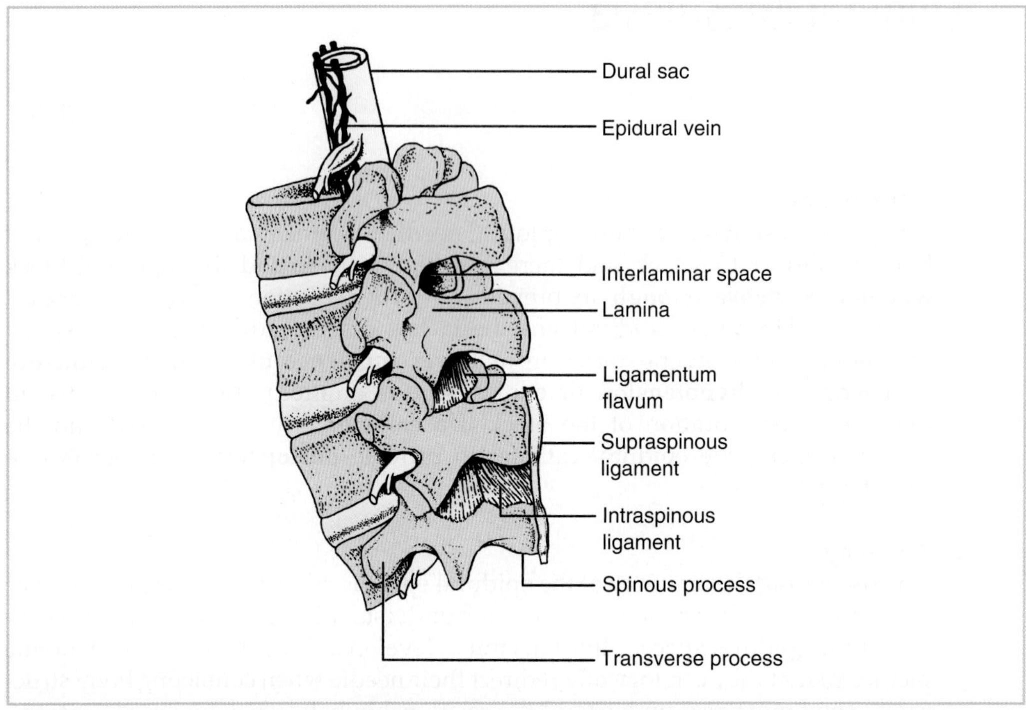

Figure 7.1. Anatomy of the bony and ligamentous components of the lumbar spine. The same structures are present at all vertebral levels although the shapes of the structures differ with vertebral level, as do the relationships between the bony components and the interlaminar space. Note also the location of the epidural veins in the anterior epidural space.

midline "loss-of-resistance" technique (see subsequent text). The ligament is 3- to 5-mm thick.

C. **Epidural fat.** Epidural fat lies between the dura mater and the vertebral canal. Although often incorrectly depicted as a continuous, uniform sheet surrounding the spinal cord, Hogan has shown that the epidural fat actually lies in discrete pockets in the posterior and anterolateral epidural space (Figure 7.3). The posterior fat compartment separates the ligamentum flavum from the dura mater, and thereby helps prevent the epidural needle from entering the subarachnoid space as it exits the ligamentum flavum.
   1. Because **hydrophobic** drugs can be extensively **sequestered** in epidural fat, it plays an important role in their pharmacokinetics (2). Whether fat acts as a reservoir that prolongs block duration or as a sink that decreases the amount of available drug (thereby slowing onset) or both is unclear.

D. **Epidural veins.** Although epidural veins are often portrayed as a reticular network surrounding the spinal cord, this view of the epidural venous plexus (Bateson plexus) is incorrect. Epidural veins are almost always confined to the anterior epidural space and only very rarely does a vein reside posterior to the intervertebral foramen through which the spinal nerves exit (3,4).

E. **Dura mater.** The dura mater, which is composed almost entirely of randomly oriented collagen fibers (5), forms the inner limit of the epidural space. The "dural sac" tapers to an end at approximately L5 where it continues through

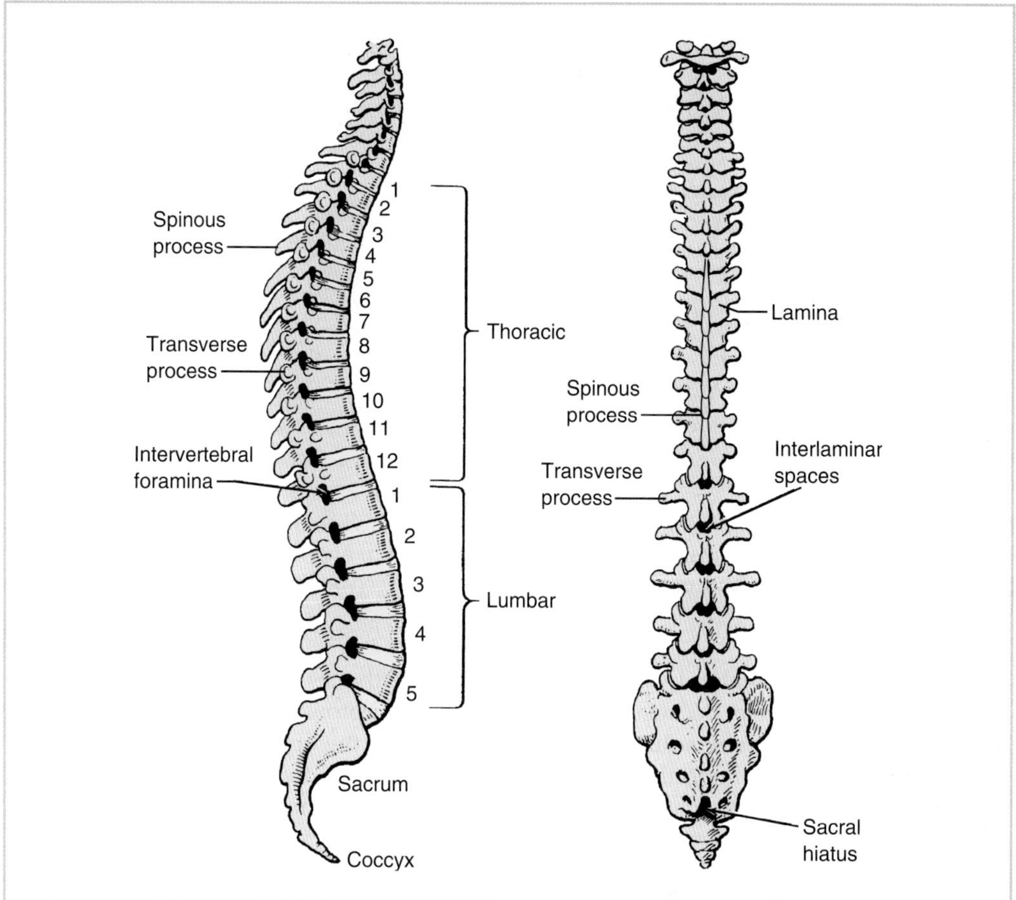

Figure 7.2. Comparative lumbar and thoracic spinal anatomy.

the sacral vertebral canal as the **filum terminale**. Consequently, the volume of the epidural space is larger below L5, a fact that likely explains the large volume of local anesthetic necessary to extend caudal epidural anesthesia to low thoracic levels. Anteriorly, the dura mater frequently fuses with the posterior longitudinal ligament thereby "obliterating" the anterior epidural space and preventing fluid spreading across the midline anteriorly.

III. Pharmacology

A. Site of action. The precise site of action of epidurally administered local anesthetics is not known. Studies in humans and animals indicate that local anesthetics penetrate the spinal meninges to reach the cerebrospinal fluid (CSF) in concentrations comparable to those produced during spinal anesthesia. However, spinal cord transmission remains intact indicating that the spinal cord itself is not the site of action. Animal studies demonstrate relatively high and comparable local anesthetic concentrations in both extradural spinal nerves traversing the epidural space and in spinal nerve rootlets within the subarachnoid space. It is not known which of these sites is the principal site of action, but is not unreasonable to assume that both play a role.

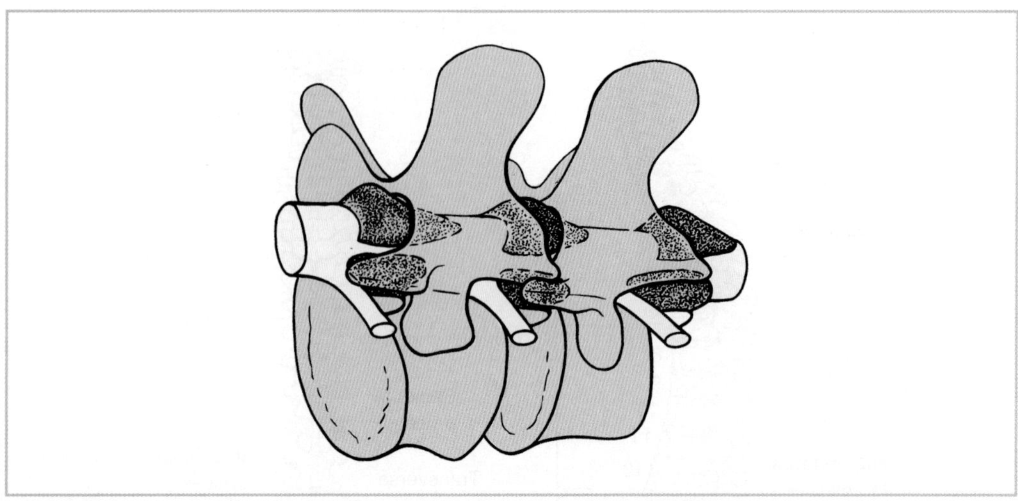

Figure 7.3. Epidural fat (*stippled area*) is discontinuously distributed within the epidural space. In areas where fat is absent, the dura mater abuts the ligamentum flavum and represents a "potential space." (Adapted from Hogan Q. Lumbar epidural anatomy: a new look by cryomicrotome section. *Anesthesiology* 1991;75:767.)

B. Local anesthetic drugs. Nearly all local anesthetics have been used for epidural anesthesia. Because of concerns about neurotoxicity only **preservative-free local anesthetic solutions** should be used in the epidural space. Local anesthetics are commonly organized in terms of their **duration of action**. However, the "duration" of any block varies depending on how "duration" is defined. For epidural anesthesia, "*two-dermatome regression*" is often used and is defined as the amount of time it takes a block to recede by two dermatomes from its maximum extent. Two-dermatome regression is a reasonable estimate of the duration of effective surgical block. **Complete resolution** is the time it takes for the patient to recover completely from sensory block and is a reasonable estimate to use for the time until outpatients may be ready for discharge. Table 7.1 lists both durations. Drugs currently used for epidural anesthesia are listed subsequently.

1. **Short duration**
   a. **Chloroprocaine** (2% or 3%) is currently available as a preservative-free solution for epidural anesthesia. Chloroprocaine produces the **fastest onset** and the **shortest duration** epidural block (Figure 7.4), although duration can be extended indefinitely by using an epidural catheter. Use of large chloroprocaine doses (more than 1,200 mg) and the presence of ethylenediamine tetraacetic acid (EDTA) have been associated with postepidural back pain more than other local anesthetics in some studies (6). Back pain has also been reported following large epidural doses of preservative-free chloroprocaine (3,000 mg over more than 7 hours) (7), whereas studies using more modest doses (900 mg) have found only mild back pain, which was not different than that experienced by subjects receiving lidocaine (8). Epidural chloroprocaine has also been associated with reduced efficacy of subsequently administered epidural morphine (9) and epidural clonidine (10) for reasons that are not known.
   b. **Procaine** is **not** a **reliable** epidural local anesthetic.

Table 7.1 Local anesthetics used for surgical epidural block

	Duration of sensory block		
Drug[a]	**Two-dermatome regression (min)**	**Complete resolution (min)**	**Prolongation by epinephrine (%)**
Chloroprocaine 3%	45–60	100–160	40–60
Lidocaine 2%	60–100	160–200	40–80
Mepivacaine 2%	60–100	160–200	40–80
Ropivacaine 0.5%–1.0%	90–180	240–420	No
Etidocaine 1%–1.5%	120–240	300–460	No
Bupivacaine 0.5%–0.75%	120–240	300–460	No

[a]These concentrations are recommended for surgical anesthesia; more dilute concentrations are appropriate for epidural analgesia.

2. **Intermediate duration.** These drugs produce a rate of block onset that is not much different than chloroprocaine, but they have a slower rate of resolution, which may result in delayed discharge of ambulatory patients.
   a. **Lidocaine** (1.5% or 2.0%) produces excellent anesthesia of 60- to 90-minute duration as a single injection, but has been associated with **tachyphylaxis** (decreasing duration with repeated injection) when

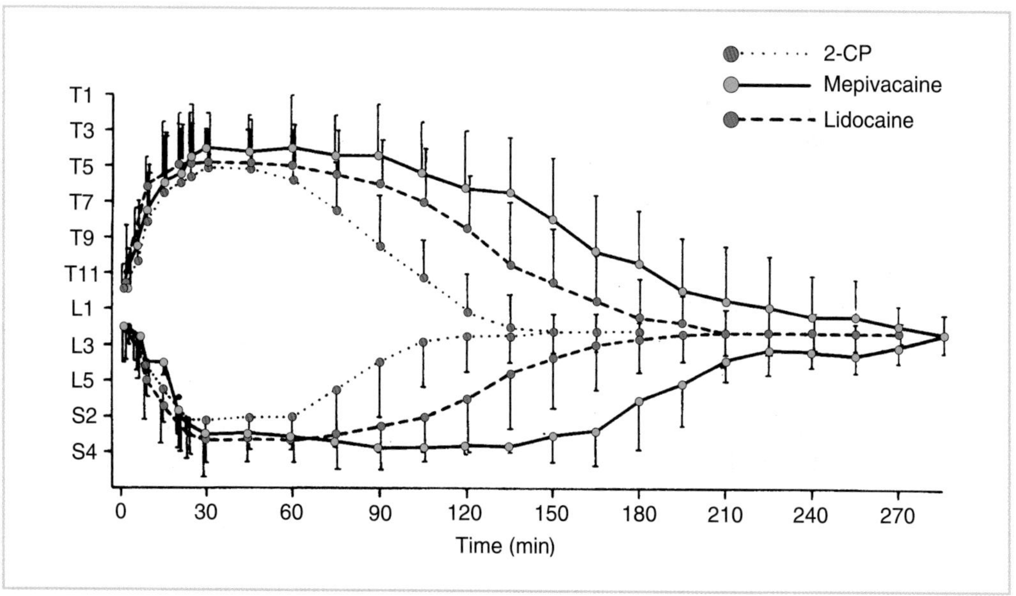

Figure 7.4. Onset and duration of epidural anesthesia. Sensory dermatomal blockade level (with standard deviations) versus time following injection of 20 mL of 3% 2-chloroprocaine (CP), 1.5% lidocaine, or 1.5% mepivacaine with 1:200,000 epinephrine at the L2 interspace. Average total durations were 133, 182, and 247 minutes, respectively. (Adapted from Kopacz DJ, Mulroy MF. Chloroprocaine and lidocaine decrease hospital stay and admission rate after outpatient epidural anesthesia. *Reg Anesth* 1990;15:19, with permission.)

repeatedly administered through an epidural catheter. The mechanism is not known but appears not to be the result of changes in drug distribution within, or elimination from, the epidural space (11).

b. **Mepivacaine** (1% or 1.5%) produces a somewhat longer average block than lidocaine.

3. **Long duration.** Given the ease with which the epidural space is catheterized, the long duration of these drugs is less of an advantage and can be a significant disadvantage for outpatient epidural anesthesia in which rapid recovery is important.

a. **Bupivacaine** (0.5% or 0.75%) is supplied as a racemic mixture of the levo- and dextrorotary optical isomers. It is reported to produce a somewhat denser sensory block compared to motor block, which has made it a favored drug for epidural **analgesia** (especially dilute concentrations). It also has slower uptake from the epidural space than the intermediate-duration local anesthetics, and therefore has less potential for systemic toxicity caused by local anesthetic absorption. Because of bupivacaine's cardiovascular toxicity (see Chapter 3) it is important to avoid high doses and avoid intravascular injection by appropriate application of a test dose use.

b. **Levobupivacaine** , the levorotary isomer of bupivacaine, is essentially indistinguishable from the racemic mixture in every way except that it is less cardiotoxic. Levobupivacaine is currently **not available** in the United States.

c. **Ropivacaine** is a single optical isomer that is approximately **40% less potent** than bupivacaine in the epidural space. If one accounts for the potency difference, it is not significantly less cardiotoxic than bupivacaine nor does it have significantly greater "motor sparing" effects than equipotent concentrations of bupivacaine. However, it is more expensive.

d. Although **etidocaine** produces effective and long-lasting epidural block, its use has largely been abandoned because of an unusual tendency to produce relatively longer duration motor block than sensory block, and it is currently **not available** in the United States.

C. **Adjuvants.** The duration of sensory and/or motor block produced by different local anesthetics can be "fine-tuned" by addition of a variety of adjuvants, including:

1. **Epinephrine**

a. **Block prolongation.** Epinephrine at a concentration 5 μg/mL (1:200,000 mg/mL) prolongs the duration of both sensory and motor block produced by short- and intermediate-duration local anesthetics, but not long-duration drugs. The mechanism(s) by which the block is prolonged is not precisely known.

(1) Evidence of a **pharmacokinetic** mechanism comes from human studies showing that addition of epinephrine **decreases peak plasma concentration**, which suggests slower drug clearance from the epidural space. This has been confirmed in animal studies (12). Contrary to what has often been taught, epinephrine does not decrease clearance by constricting the epidural venous plexus. Rather, animal studies showing that epinephrine decreases blood flow in the dura

mater (13) suggest that this is the mechanism by which epinephrine slows local anesthetic clearance.

(2) In addition to a pharmacokinetic effect, epinephrine may also have a **pharmacodynamic** effect. Specifically, because epinephrine is an α_2-adrenergic agonist it may also act within the spinal cord to decrease pain transmission. The ability of epinephrine to improve postoperative analgesia when added to dilute concentrations of epidural bupivacaine may be evidence of this mechanism.

b. **Hemodynamic effects.** Compared with plain local anesthetics, addition of epinephrine to epidural block results in a markedly **greater decrease in mean arterial pressure (MAP)** (Figure 7.5) (14). The decrease in MAP is caused by a greater fall in systemic vascular resistance (SVR), presumably because of the vasodilatory β_2-adrenergic effects of low dose epinephrine. The decrease in SVR also results in a significantly higher cardiac output

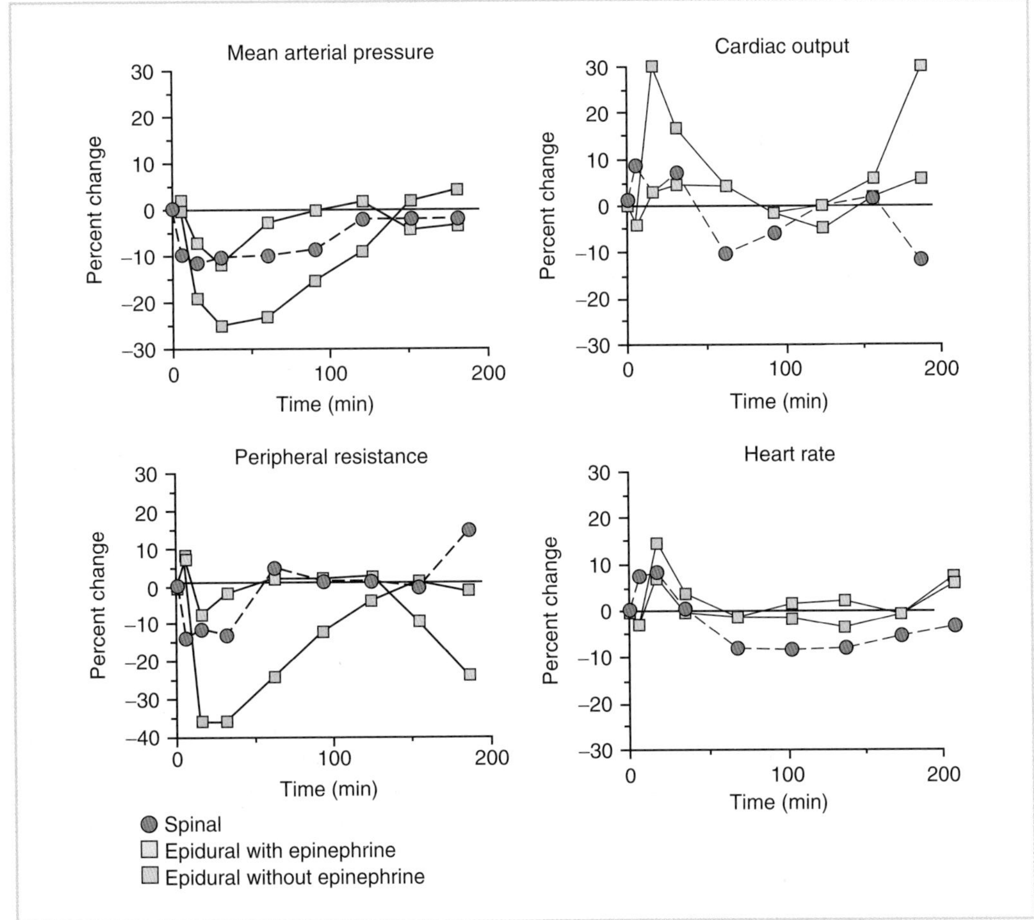

Figure 7.5. The cardiovascular effects of spinal and epidural anesthesia in volunteers with T5 blocks. The effects of spinal anesthesia and epidural anesthesia without epinephrine were generally comparable and are both qualitatively and quantitatively different from the effects of epidural anesthesia with epinephrine. (Adapted from Bonica JJ, Kennedu WF Jr, Ward RJ, et al. A comparison of the effects of high subarachnoid and epidural anesthesia. *Acta Anaesthesiol Scand Suppl* 1996;23:429.)

than occurs with epidural block without added epinephrine. Heart rate is modestly higher when epinephrine is added. Whether this is a direct effect of epinephrine or a reflexive response to decreased MAP is unknown. Animal studies indicate that the presence of epinephrine in the local anesthetic solution does not decrease the risk of cardiovascular toxicity in the event of accidental intravascular injection (15).

2. **Opioids.** Addition of opioids to epidural local anesthetics increases the **duration of sensory, but not motor block**. The magnitude and duration of the effect depends on the opioid chosen (hydrophobic opioids are significantly shorter than hydrophilic opioids) and the dose administered.
3. **Clonidine.** Epidural clonidine (150–300 μg) **prolongs sensory, but not motor block** and unlike epinephrine the effect occurs with long-acting local anesthetics (16,17). Epidural clonidine is rapidly cleared into plasma and redistribution to brain sites (locus coeruleus) causes sedation. Clonidine also causes decrease in blood pressure, likely mediated through spinal, brain and peripheral α_2-adrenergic actions. However, the effect on blood pressure is less than that of epinephrine (16). Unlike epinephrine, epidural clonidine is associated with a modest decrease in heart rate (16).
4. **Bicarbonate.** Addition of sodium bicarbonate (0.1 mEq/mL) to epidural local anesthetics has been advocated as a means to speed the onset of epidural block. However, published studies are nearly evenly split between those that found a faster onset with bicarbonate and those that found no difference. This is true for lidocaine, mepivacaine, chloroprocaine, and bupivacaine. At best, bicarbonate would seem to have an unreliable effect on block onset.

D. **Dose.** Within the epidural space, local anesthetic solutions spread cephalad and caudad from their injection site and produce a band of anesthesia that correlates reasonably well with the extent of solution spread (Figure 7.6). Unfortunately, it is impossible to look at any individual patient and predict with certainty what dose of local anesthetic is necessary to produce a given extent of epidural blockade. Consequently, clinicians must be aware of the major and minor factors that contribute to determining the spread of epidural block (Table 7.2) and use this information in conjunction with knowledge of the dermatomes that must be blocked for a particular surgical procedure to decide the local anesthetic dose necessary.

1. **Dose, volume, and concentration.** Both drug dose and volume are **independent predictors** of the spread of epidural blockade. That is, increasing drug dose while holding volume constant (increasing drug concentration) will increase the extent of epidural blockade. Conversely, increasing drug volume while holding dose constant (decreasing concentration) will also increase the extent of epidural blockade. However, the relationship is not linear; as dose is increased the *spread per milliliter injected* decreases such that the net effect is only a few dermatomes increase in spread.
2. **Technique**
   a. **Location.** Because local anesthetic spreads cephalad and caudad form the site of injection, the injection **site is a major determinant** of which dermatomes will be blocked by a given local anesthetic dose. In addition, the volume of the epidural space increases as one moves caudad; consequently to anesthetize the same number of dermatomes may take

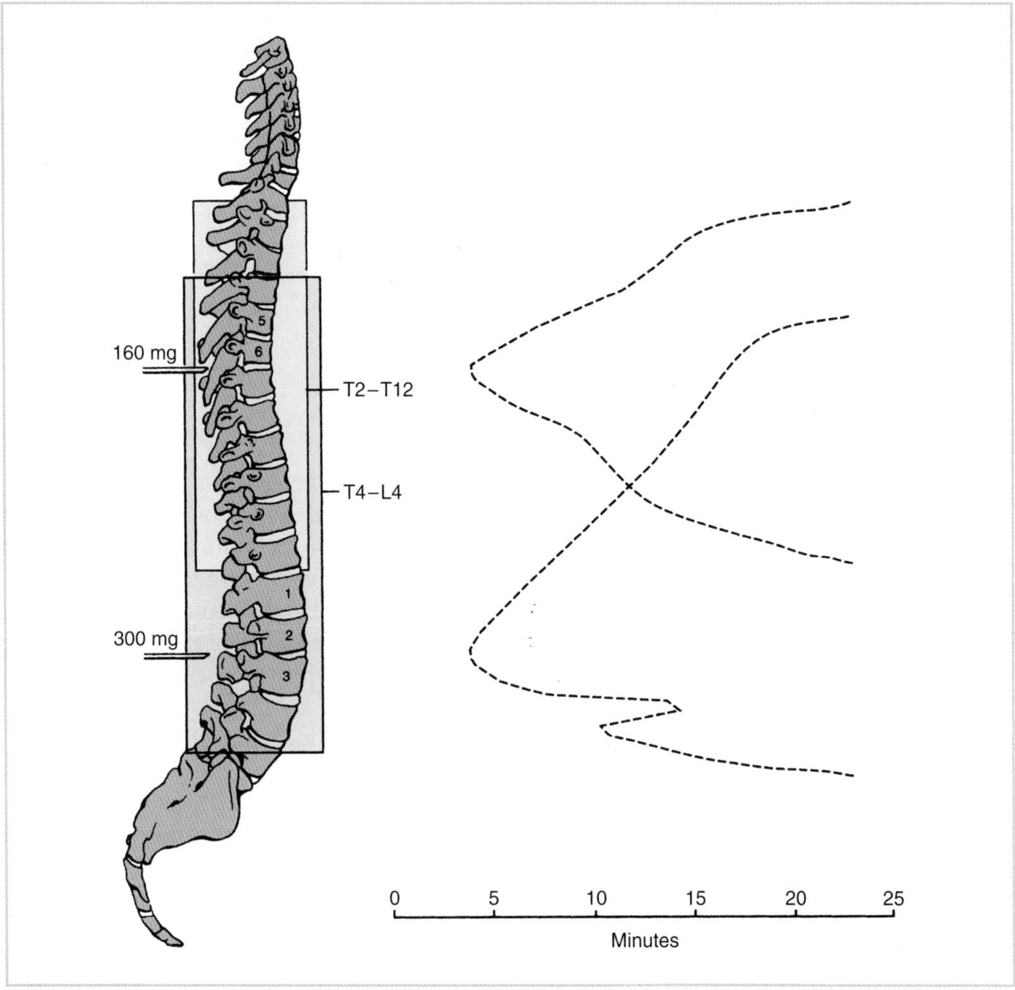

Figure 7.6. Diagram of spread of local anesthetic in the epidural space. The onset of epidural anesthesia is noted first in the segments nearest the site of injection, and spreads over the next 20 minutes both cephalad and caudad from this point.

25 mL in the caudal epidural space but only 8 mL in the thoracic epidural space.

b. **Patient position.** Gravity has no clinically important effect on the spread of local anesthetics in the epidural space.

c. **Needle angle/aperture direction.** Paramedian and midline needle insertion produce the same local anesthetic spread. Turning the needle aperture to face cephalad or caudad produces slightly greater spread in the direction the aperture faces. The magnitude of the effect is not clinically important.

d. **Injection speed.** Speed of local anesthetic injection has a very minor effect on spread of epidural block (faster = farther).

e. If the **catheter** lies in the midline, then spread should not differ significantly from that which would occur through a needle. However, catheters have an annoying tendency to deviate significantly from the

Table 7.2 Factors affecting spread of epidural block

Factors
Major factors
Site of injection
Dose
Minor factors
Age
Height
Weight
Pregnancy
Minimally relevant factors
Speed of injection
Incremental injection
Direction of needle opening

midline and if they end up traversing a vertebral foramen or lying very anterior in the epidural space then spread may be reduced and/or asymmetric (i.e., unilateral). This problem may be reduced by putting less catheter in the epidural space (3–4 cm) and using larger local anesthetic volumes. Malposition of the catheter may be particularly problematic when it is used for postoperative analgesia because of the relatively low volumes of dilute local anesthetic that are typically used.

3. **Patient factors**
   a. **Gender** is not an important determinant of local anesthetic spread.
   b. Studies of the effect of **pregnancy** are conflicting with some studies finding greater spread at all stages of pregnancy and others finding no difference. Interestingly, pregnant women have been shown to be more sensitive to the blocking effects of local anesthetics, which would be consistent with greater epidural spread.
   c. On *average*, **increasing age** results in an **increase in the spread** of epidural anesthesia, but the magnitude of the effect is not as great as once thought (18,19). The difficulty in using age as a factor in choosing a dose is that the interindividual variability is so great that it is impossible to predict *a priori* how age will affect block height in any individual patient.
   d. **Height.** On *average*, spread of epidural block is **greater in shorter people**. But, as with age, the interindividual variability is so great that it is difficult to predict how height will affect epidural block in any individual patient.
   e. **Weight.** On average, obesity increases the spread of epidural block. But, like age and height, the effect is small and **highly variable** among individuals.
4. **Choosing a dose.** As can be deduced from the preceding, the choice of local anesthetic dose is highly subjective. One approach is to consider 15 mL as an average starting dose for lumbar injections. If multiple factors suggest a reason that a larger dose may be necessary (e.g., large spread needed for planned surgery, patients who are very young and tall) then increase the dose by 5 to 10 mL. Conversely, if multiple factors suggest a reason to reduce the dose (e.g., small spread needed for planned surgery, patients who are unusually short, obese, or old) then reduce the dose by 3 to 5 mL. For thoracic epidural blocks a reasonable average starting volume would

be 6 to 8 mL. This dose might be increased by 2 to 6 mL or decreased by 1 to 2 mL for reasons outlined earlier. Importantly, it is often easier to deal with a block that is more extensive and longer lasting than necessary than it is to cover up for a block that is inadequate. Of course, use of an epidural catheter technique renders this problem moot because it permits "titration" of the epidural block.

IV. Technique

Epidural block can be performed with the patient in any position that permits access to the back (prone, lateral, sitting), although lateral is the most common and often the most comfortable for the patient. Sitting can be advantageous in the morbidly obese patient because it is easier to identify the midline. In the lumbar, low thoracic, and cervical spine, epidural blockade is similar to spinal anesthesia and is generally performed in the midline. In the high- through midthoracic spine the paramedian approach is usually necessary. As with any regional anesthesia procedure, equipment for monitoring, resuscitation, and treating side effects must be immediately available.

A. Midline. For the midline approach the following steps are taken:

1. **Prepare equipment.** Ideally, prepare the epidural "tray" before positioning the patient. Draw up local anesthetic, fill "loss-of-resistance syringe," and uncap needles, and so on. Doing this "prep-work" before positioning the patient will minimize the amount of time the the patient has to remain in a relatively uncomfortable position.
2. **Sedate patient** as deemed appropriate (see Chapter 4). Because the midline approach does not make use of intentional contact with bone/periosteum, it should not be very painful.
3. **Position patient laterally** with knees drawn up so that the legs are maximally flexed at the hips. Instruct patient to "curl up like a boiled shrimp" or similar visual metaphor. Place patient at the edge of the bed (Beware. Do not walk away from a patient thus positioned because of the risk that he or she will roll backwards onto the floor) with hips and shoulders perpendicular to the bed. This position will maximize distraction of spinous processes and minimize the need to lean over and reach for the patient.
4. **Locate desired interspace** using the iliac crest as a landmark to locate L4 (a line through the iliac crests crosses L4 $\pm$ 1 vertebral body; in obese patients the fat overlying the iliac crests may bias your estimate in a cephalad direction.) Marking the intended space with a skin pen may reduce the amount of time spent reidentifying the space throughout the procedure. Finding spinous processes can be difficult in the morbidly obese. A 90-mm (3.5-in.) spinal needle is sometimes useful as a *finder needle* to identify bony landmarks. Additionally, **ultrasonography** can sometimes be used to identify spinous processes in obese patients (Figure 7.7). Unfortunately, the limited resolution that can be achieved with the low frequencies necessary to reach greater tissue depth limit the ability to use ultrasonography in very obese subjects—the very subjects in whom it would be most useful.
5. **Prepare the skin** with appropriate antiseptic and drape as for spinal anesthesia. Use of clear plastic drapes makes it easier to reevaluate landmarks and reposition patient position if necessary.
6. **Anesthetize skin, subcutaneous tissue, and a track** along the intended path of the epidural needle. In this way the needle can be used as a "finder

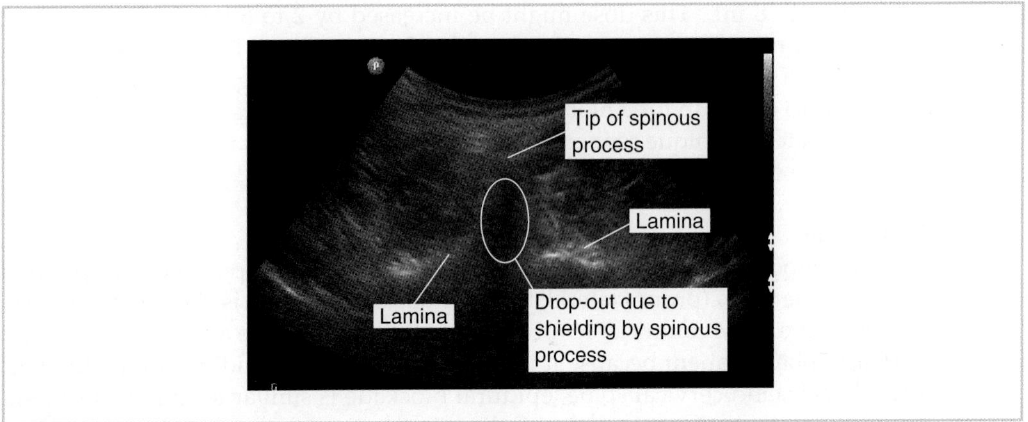

Figure 7.7. Ultrasound image of lumbar spine. The "drop-out" below the spinous process is caused by the inability of ultrasound waves to penetrate the bone. Laminas are clearly identified as bright hyperechoic areas.

needle" to delineate the path between the spinous processes. Take care not to deposit a large volume of local anesthetic in the subcutaneous tissue because the resultant "mound" may make it difficult to feel the interspace, especially in obese patients.

7. **Insert the epidural needle** through the skin with the bevel of a Tuohy or Hustead needle oriented cephalad or caudad. Orienting the bevel laterally may cause the needle to deviate from the midline. Insertion should proceed slowly and *under control* at all times (Figure 7.8). Passage through the **interspinous ligament** often results in a "gritty" sensation as if pushing the needle through a bag of tightly packed sand. Failure to appreciate this grittiness should alert one to the possibility that the needle is off midline and not within the interspinous ligament. As the needle enters the **ligamentum flavum**, resistance will increase subtly; stop at this point. The depth to the ligamentum flavum is generally between 3.5 and 5 cm in normal-sized adults, but may be significantly deeper in the obese.

   The ability to detect the increased resistance of the ligamentum flavum is an acquired skill, and it is not uncommon for the novice to have several unintentional meningeal punctures before mastering this step. Pregnant women are notorious for having "soft" ligamenta flava, and it can be particularly difficult to correctly identify the ligament in this group.

8. After identifying the ligamentum flavum, remove the stylet of the needle and attach a 5- to 10-mL saline-filled **syringe containing a clearly visible air bubble** (0.1–0.5 mL). The air bubble will act as a gauge of the amount of pressure exerted on the syringe barrel (see subsequent text). Freely moving glass syringes give a better loss of resistance than plastic syringes, although specially designed low-resistance plastic syringes intended for epidural anesthesia are also appropriate. Care must be taken to ensure that the glass syringe barrel does in fact move freely; "sticky" syringes make it very difficult, if not impossible, to detect a loss of resistance. Position the back of the nondominant hand against the patient's back and grasp the epidural needle with the thumb and forefinger (Figure 7.9). This hand is used to control needle movement and prevent accidentally plunging

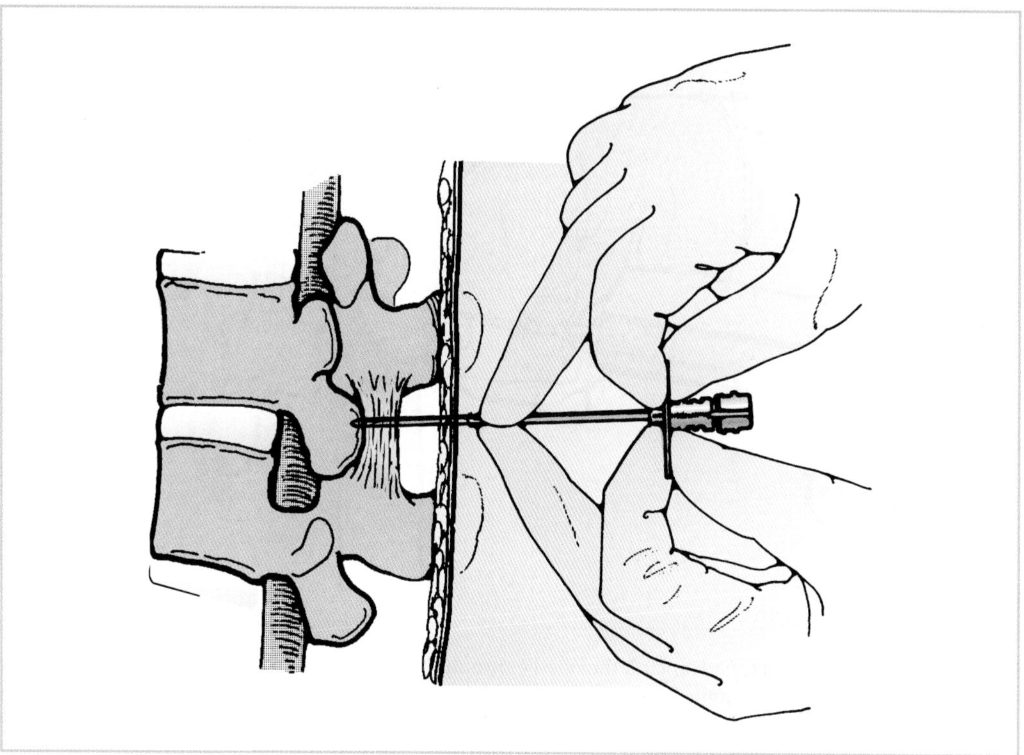

Figure 7.8. Hand position for epidural needle insertion into the ligamentum flavum. The epidural needle must be inserted under control at all times to prevent deviation from the intended path or a sudden "plunge" into the subarachnoid space or spinal cord. Multiple hand positions are appropriate, but the technique depicted here is widely employed. The thumb and forefingers hold the flanges extending from the needle hub and the tips of the middle fingers rest on the back and "grasp" the needle shaft. Resting the fingers on the back prevents the needle from being unintentionally advanced should the patient move unexpectedly. The needle is advanced using the thumbs, forefingers, and wrists—not the arms; this permits controlled advancement and appreciation of the subtle increase in resistance that heralds entry into the ligamentum flavum.

into the subarachnoid space. Apply continuous pressure on the syringe plunger with the thumb of the dominant hand. If the needle tip is in the ligamentum flavum it should be possible to exert enough pressure on the plunger to visibly compress the air bubble without injecting fluid. If it is not possible to compress the air bubble without injecting fluid then the needle tip is probably not in the ligamentum flavum. Advance the needle slightly and reattempt compression. Repeat as necessary until compression is achieved. If compression does not occur at a "reasonable depth" consider that the needle may be off the midline and reevaluate landmarks/needle angle.

9. While maintaining **constant compression** of the air bubble with the dominant hand, use the nondominant hand to slowly advance the epidural needle. Do not use the dominant hand to advance the needle because it is hard to control the advance. Warn the patients that they may feel a slight cramping sensation as the epidural needle enters the epidural space, but that **they must not move.**

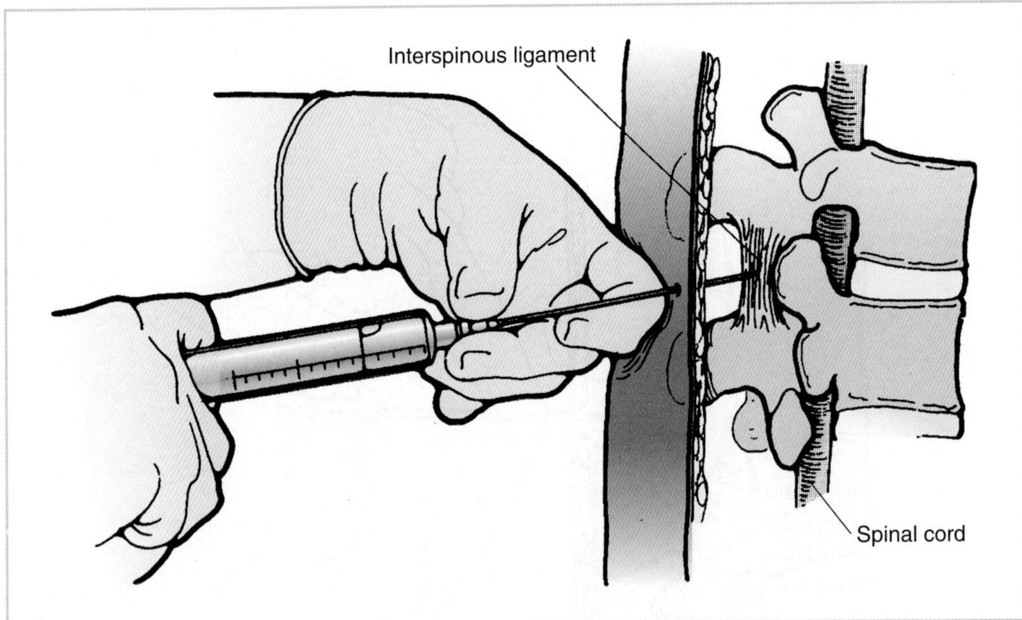

Figure 7.9. Hand position for advancing the needle through the ligamentum flavum into the space. Once the ligamentum flavum is identified, a saline-filled syringe containing a small air bubble is attached to the hub of the needle. One hand rests firmly against the back while firmly grasping the hub of the needle. This hand advances the needle and prevents a sudden plunge into the subarachnoid space. The opposite hand applies continuous pressure on the syringe plunger with sufficient force that the air bubble is compressed. Failure to compress the air bubble without injecting saline generally indicates that the needle tip is not in the ligamentum flavum. The needle is advanced by "rotating" the hand positioned against the back without using the hand compressing the plunger. Entry into the epidural space is indicated by a sudden loss of resistance and injection of the saline.

10. As the needle tip exits the ligamentum flavum and enters the epidural space there will be a dramatic **loss of resistance** as saline is suddenly injected into the epidural space. With loss of resistance, stop advancing the needle.
    a. Importantly, the tip of the needle may be against the dura mater as it enters the epidural space, especially if there is little or no epidural fat at the entry point. Maintain control of the epidural needle with the nondominant hand and carefully remove the loss-of-resistance syringe without advancing the needle.
    b. **False-positive/false-negative loss of resistance.** Not all attempts to enter the epidural space will produce the dramatic loss of resistance described in the preceding text. False positives can occur if the needle passes obliquely through the interspinous ligament and enters the paraspinous muscle; although it should not be possible to compress the air bubble if the needle tip is not in the ligamentum flavum and the loss of resistance into the paraspinous muscle is much less clear (often described as *mushy*) than is loss of resistance into the epidural space. False "negatives" may occur in pregnant women (because of their soft ligamentum flavum) or in persons whose ligament has not fused in the midline. In cases where it is not entirely clear if the needle is in the epidural space, the following additional "tests" may be tried.

(1) **Air test.** As an additional test of needle location, place a small volume (0.5–1.0 mL) of air in the loss-of-resistance syringe and very gently inject it. If the needle tip is in the epidural space air will be injected effortlessly. If not, the air will be compressed somewhat before being injected into tissue (e.g., paraspinous muscle). Omit the air test for lithotripsy because of concern that the energy of the shock wave will be dissipated at the tissue/air interface in the epidural space.

(2) **Epidural catheter test.** Sometimes trying to thread a catheter into the epidural space may be helpful. If the catheter cannot be freely threaded beyond the needle tip, then the likelihood that the needle is in the epidural space decreases. In the end, when trying to decide if the needle is in the epidural space, it is useful to remember the old teaching maxim, "if it doesn't feel right, it probably isn't" and simply repeat needle insertion.

11. **Test dose.** Once the epidural space is identified, gently aspirate the needle in an effort to detect CSF (subarachnoid placement) or blood (intravenous placement). Blood and CSF are good indicators of needle location if present, but their absence is not a foolproof indicator that the needle tip is not subarachnoid or intravenous. To more reliably detect aberrant needle location, administer a "test dose" and carefully observe the patient for evidence of intravascular or subarachnoid injection (see Chapter 3).
    a. **Test dose with a catheter.** If a catheter is inserted after the initial local anesthetic dose is administered through the aneedle, it is essential that an additional test dose be administered through the catheter to be sure it did not thread intrathecally or intravenously. If all of the local anesthetic dose is to be administered through the epidural catheter, then only a single test dose administered through the catheter is necessary. In any event, a catheter should never be used until it has been specifically tested to rule out an intrathecal or intravenous location.

12. **Drug administration**
    a. **Single-injection technique.** For a single-injection technique, administer the chosen dose in *5 mL increments* at 15- to 20-second intervals while constantly observing for evidence of subarachnoid or intravenous administration. Incremental administration provides the possibility of detecting intrathecal or intravenous injection before a catastrophically large dose is administered.
    b. **Continuous technique.** Even if using a catheter technique, administering some or all of the planned initial dose through the epidural needle may decrease the chance of the catheter threading intravenously (20). As with drug administration through the needle, local anesthetic should be administered incrementally through the catheter.

13. **Catheters**
    a. **Insertion.** As the catheter is inserted through the needle, resistance will be felt as it reaches the tip and is forced to bend to exit the needle (Tuohy or Hustead needles) or it abuts the dura mater (Crawford needle) as it exits. Steady pressure will usually overcome the resistance and the catheter will thread easily. Insert the catheter 3 to 5 cm into the epidural space. Inserting more catheter simply increases the risk that the catheter will be malpositioned (e.g., exit an intervertebral foramen). In all reported cases of catheters tying in knots within the epidural space the catheter

was inserted more than 5 cm (21,22); inserting the catheter more than 5 cm with the intention to pull it back later does not alter this risk. In addition, if the catheter is pulled back into the needle after exiting into the epidural space there is a risk that the catheter may be sheared off by the sharp edge of the epidural needle tip. If the catheter will not thread into the epidural space consider:

(1) The entire opening of the epidural needle may not have entered the epidural space. Carefully advance the needle 1 or 2 mm and reattempt catheter insertion.

(2) Contents of the epidural space (e.g., epidural fat) may be preventing catheter entry. Consider rotating the needle 90 or 180 degrees and try again.

(3) If the steps mentioned in the preceding text are unsuccessful, the needle is probably not in the epidural space.

b. Catheter position. Despite attempts to control the direction (cephalad versus caudad) that a catheter threads, 40% to 80% of the time it travels in a direction opposite the direction it was pointing as it exited the needle (23). ''Misdirection'' is more common when the needle tip points caudad. As would be expected from the fact that injection site has a major effect on epidural spread, the direction that the catheter threads has a significant effect on the local anesthetic dose required to block the targeted dermatomes (24).

c. Needle withdrawal. To prevent accidentally pulling the catheter out during needle withdrawal, push the catheter forward while slowly withdrawing the needle. Take care during this process that the catheter's free end does not flip about uncontrollably and become contaminated.

d. Secure the catheter to the patient's back. For catheters that will only be used intraoperatively, any good quality tape is probably sufficient. However, for catheters that will remain *in situ* beyond the intraoperative period, a skin adhesive (e.g., benzoin, Mastisol) and a transparent dressing (e.g., Tegaderm) work well. The transparent dressing permits daily inspection of the catheter entry site to monitor for signs of infection. To prevent the catheter from kinking when it enters the skin it is often helpful to form a loop at the entry site when securing it. Regardless of the technique used to secure the catheter, be careful that it is not dislodged as the patient is slid from the stretcher to the operating room (OR) table or hospital bed.

e. Catheter migration. Catheters do not necessarily stay where they were initially placed (25), especially in mobile patients (e.g., labor, postoperative analgesia).

(1) Outward migration is probably the most common catheter movement and has been shown to be a common cause of failed postoperative analgesia (26). Secure fastening as described earlier reduces this risk. Some have advocated subcutaneous tunneling to reduce the risk of outward migration, but the available studies fail to show a benefit (26,27).

(2) Subarachnoid and intravenous migration

(a) Intravenous migration. Entry of the catheter tip into an epidural vein may present as loss of epidural anesthetic/analgesic effect or systemic toxicity if a large enough local anesthetic bolus is administered. Consequently, an earlier negative test dose should never be construed to rule out later intravascular location of the catheter (28). Bolus local anesthetic injections through the catheter should be preceded by gentle aspiration to look for blood; why a test dose should be repeated if there is any question as to the location of the catheter and injections should be made incrementally while observing for evidence of intravascular injection.

(b) **Subarachnoid migration.** As with intravascular migration, a prior negative test dose does not rule out a later subarachnoid migration of the catheter (29). Catheters that migrate into the subarachnoid space may present as very extensive neuraxial block or even total spinal anesthesia. Detecting a subarachnoid catheter can be challenging in patients who already have an epidural block because the primary sign of subarachnoid injection (sensory/motor block) is already present. CSF aspiration is diagnostic if present but its absence can represent a false negative. If subarachnoid migration is suspected, examine the patient to determine the current extent of their sensory/motor block and administer a dose of local anesthetic that would be expected to noticeably increase the degree of block if it went subarachnoid (30). As with all injections, incremental dosing provides the possibility of detecting aberrant catheter location before serious side effects.

f. **Catheter removal.** Catheters generally slide out with minimal force. If the catheter seems to require an unusual amount of force, it is often helpful to have the patient assume the same position used when inserting the catheter. Catheter removal should not be painful. If patients experience pain, especially radicular pain, stop pulling the catheter and consider an appropriate radiologic study to identify the location of the catheter and the cause of pain. Following removal, the catheter should be inspected to make sure it was removed intact.

(1) **Retained catheter.** Catheters that are sheared off in the epidural space generally pose no risk because they are designed for implantation. They can be left in place if the patient is asymptomatic. However, the patient must be informed.

14. **Epidural block** sets up more slowly than does spinal block and onset is slower in dermatomes farther from the injection site. Some evidence of block (e.g., decreased temperature sensation) is generally detectable in dermatomes near the injection site within a few minutes; however, maximum spread may not be reached for 20 to 30 minutes depending on the drug used (Figure 7.4). In addition, onset in the L5 and S1 dermatomes is particularly slow for reasons that are not altogether clear.

B. **Paramedian approach.** A lateral (paramedian) approach can be used to access the epidural space at any level but is almost essential at mid to low thoracic levels (roughly T4–10) where the steep angle of the spinous process covers the interlaminar foramen effectively precluding the midline approach (Figure 7.2). The thoracic epidural space presents an additional anatomic challenge in that the spinal cord, which normally terminates between T12 and L2, lies beneath the dura mater and is closer to the ligamentum flavum laterally than it is in the midline. Accidental dural puncture at this level carries the very real risk of spinal cord injury.

1. **Technique.** Place the patient in the lateral or sitting position with the neck and midback flexed as much as possible. Identify the intended interspace keeping in mind the following landmarks.
   a. As you slide your hand down the back of the neck, the tip of C7 is the first prominent spinous process encountered and **T1 is the most prominent spinous process.**
   b. The **spine of the scapula** lies at approximately T4; keep in mind that the scapula is a mobile bone and its position changes as the shoulder is raised and lowered.
   c. The **tip of the scapula** lies at approximately T8; keep in mind that the scapula is a mobile bone and its position changes as the shoulder is raised and lowered.
   d. In thin patients, the **12th rib** can be palpated and followed back to its attachment to T12.
   e. The **iliac crest** can be used to identify the L4 level and the spinous processes counted upward from this point. The most common error is for the operator to feel that he or she is more cephalad than the actual level (31).
2. **Mark the intended interspace.** Keep in mind that at the midthoracic level the interlaminar foramen through which the epidural needle must pass lies 1 to 3 cm cephalad of this interspace and the tip of the cephalad spinous process lies over the lamina of the inferior vertebra. Also, the interlaminar foramen extends laterally several millimeters wider than the spinous process. It may be helpful for the beginner to draw the estimated location of the lamina and interlaminar foramen as a tool to help visualize the underlying anatomy (Figure 7.10).

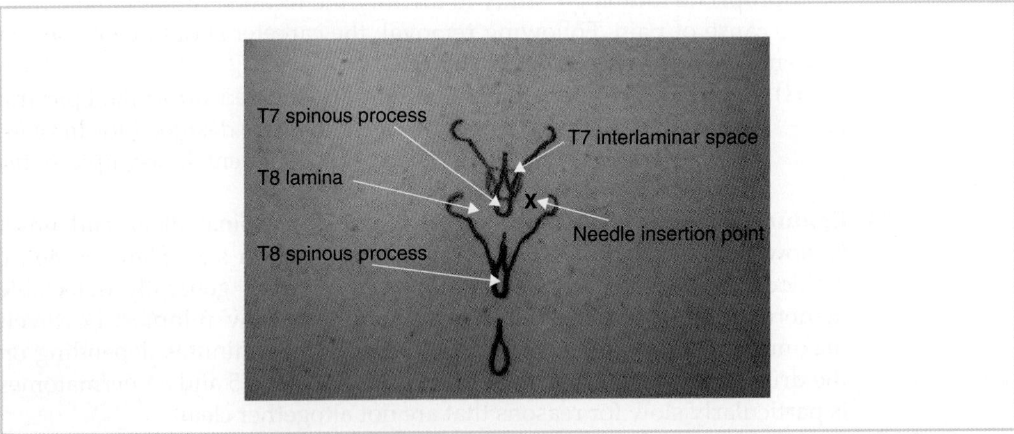

Figure 7.10. Cutaneous landmarks of palpable bony structures (spinous process tips) and underlying nonpalpable landmarks (lamina, interlaminar space) for performance of thoracic epidural block. The laminar space (*outlined in red*) lies underneath and is obscured by the elongated and downward sloping spinous process. Needle entry should occur adjacent to the spinous process overlying the targeted interlaminar space. Perpendicular needle insertion at this point will result in the needle contracting the lamina of the inferior. Drawing these landmarks will speed the performance of the block, especially for beginners, and will help the clinician develop and ability to visualize the underlying anatomy.

3. **Prepare the skin and drape** as described earlier. Anesthetize the skin and subcutaneous tissue down to the lamina and along the intended needle path.
4. **Insert the epidural needle at a point approximately 1 cm lateral to the inferior spinous process** and perpendicular to the skin in all planes. Insert until the underlying lamina is contacted (Note: If laminar contact is painful stop and inject additional local anesthetic through the needle). At this point the intent is to walk along the lamina until dropping over the edge and contacting the ligamentum flavum. Therefore, withdraw the needle sufficiently to be able to **redirect it** *slightly* **medial and slightly cephalad** and reinsert it until the lamina is contacted again. Repeat this process until the needle "firms up" in the ligamentum flavum. There are several potential "errors" that may result in missing the ligamentum flavum.
   a. Taking too big of a step as the needle is walked along the lamina may result in walking over the interlaminar foramen without dropping into it. This is easy to do, especially in obese people because what may seem like a small change in angle at the skin will result in the tip being several centimeters more cephalad by the time it reaches the depth of the lamina (Figure 7.11). This is also more likely to occur at thoracic levels where the interlaminar foramen is narrower side to side and shorter in the cephalocaudad direction than it is at lumbar levels.
   b. Angling too far medial may result in crossing the midline through the interspinous ligament. This is a potential source of a false loss of resistance as the needle firms up in the interspinous ligament and resistance decreases as it passes through and into the paraspinous muscle.
   c. Inserting the needle too far lateral, or not angling medial enough, may result in the needle walking up successive lamina where they join laterally (articular facet; Figure 7.2).

   In reality, the needle can be inserted at multiple points; one simply needs to adopt the correct medial and cephalad angulation to reach the interlaminar space from the chosen skin entry point. However, to do so requires an excellent working knowledge of vertebral anatomy so that the position of the needle tip and its relation to the interlaminar space can be accurately deduced as bone is contacted.
5. Once the needle reaches the ligamentum flavum the **loss-of-resistance technique** is applied very much as for midline insertion. One potential modification is to advance the needle with **two hands** and check for compression/loss of resistance intermittently instead of maintaining continuous pressure on the plunger. In some situations, this approach may permit greater control of the needle as it advances and reduce the risk of accidentally plunging into the epidural space and potentially the spinal cord.
6. As noted in the preceding text, because the volume of the thoracic epidural space is smaller than the lumbar epidural space local anesthetic doses are reduced 30% to 50% for segmental thoracic anesthesia/analgesia.

C. **Alternatives to the loss-of-resistance technique.** As described earlier, the air/fluid loss-of-resistance technique gives the most clear-cut identification of the epidural space and is arguably the technique of choice for most clinicians.

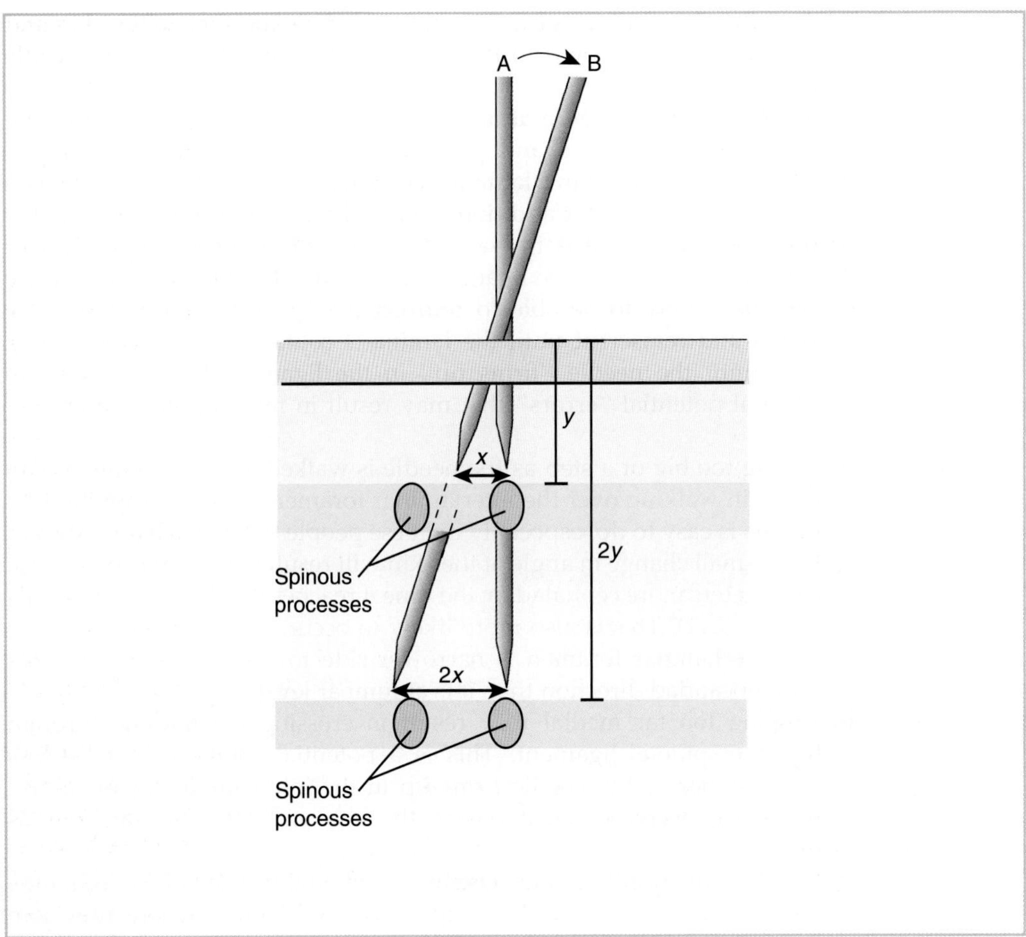

Figure 7.11. Example of the effect of tissue depth on the distance the needle tip travels. In this example, when the angle of the needle is changed from *A* to *B*, the needle tip advances distance *x* at a depth of *y*, and *x* is the correct distance to travel to put the needle between the two circles that represent the spinous processes. In a bigger person, however, that same change in needle angle at skin entry from *A* to *B* results in the tip of the needle moving cephalad a distance of 2*x* when it gets to the greater depth of the spinous processes in this patient (2*y*). In the latter case, the needle tip walks past the opening between the spinous processes.

However, other techniques have been used and may offer an advantage to some clinicians in some specific situations.

1. **Air only loss of resistance.** Because air is much easier to inject into the epidural space than into tissues, air injection can be used to identify the epidural space. When using air, the needle is advanced in small increments and the syringe plunger gently "balloted" between each motion to see if air can be easily injected. The epidural space is identified when ballottement results in air injection. The following are the difficulties of this technique.
   a. Unlike compression of an air bubble in a fluid-filled syringe, the amount of force exerted on the air is subjective, which can make for both false and failed loss of resistance.

b. Because air injection is assessed only intermittently there is an increased chance of accidentally entering the subarachnoid space before recognizing the epidural space if the needle is advanced too far between ballottements.
c. It takes longer to repeatedly stop and reassess resistance.
d. There is evidence (albeit conflicting) that air injected into the epidural space may cause "spotty" epidural block.

2. **Saline only loss of resistance.** Conflicting evidence that introducing air into the epidural space may cause "spotty" epidural blocks has caused some to omit the air bubble from the loss-of-resistance technique (although the small volume of air used has not been implicated as causing this problem). An important disadvantage of doing so is that you will lose the ability to objectively judge the amount of force being exerted on the plunger and as a result may be more likely to misidentify the ligamentum flavum. Specifically, the ligamentum flavum is dense enough that sufficient force can be exerted onto the syringe plunger to compress the air bubble without allowing fluid injection; this is not true of other tissues (e.g., interspinous ligament, paraspinous muscle). Therefore, without the air bubble as a gauge of the amount of force being applied, one may mistakenly apply too little force and misidentify other paraspinous tissues as ligamentum flavum. An additional disadvantage of omitting the air bubble is that you may not recognize a "sticky" syringe plunger, which may be misinterpreted as resistance to injection.
3. **Hanging drop technique.** If a drop of fluid is "hanging" from the hub of the epidural needle it will generally be "sucked" in as the needle enters the epidural space. Traditional teaching was that this occurred because the epidural space was under "negative" pressure relative to atmospheric pressure. Subsequent studies have shown that this is incorrect. Artificial negative pressure is created in the epidural space when the advancing epidural needle contacts the dura mater and pushes it away, causing an increase in epidural space volume. As the effective volume of the epidural space increases, pressure falls and atmospheric air rushes in to fill the void carrying the "hanging drop" with it. This technique works best in the thoracic epidural space because the epidural volume is smaller, there is less fat between the dura and the ligamentum flavum, and the dura is closer to the ligamentum flavum. Because this technique requires that the epidural needle contact the dura mater and indent it with sufficient force to displace enough CSF to artificially increase the volume of the epidural space it carries a higher risk of unintended meningeal puncture.
4. **Manometers.** Manometers have been employed as quantitative alternatives to the qualitative hanging drop technique. However, the technique is essentially the same and the same risks apply.
5. **Electrical stimulation.** Just as nerve stimulators have been used to identify peripheral nerves, they have been used to identify the epidural space, particularly in children (32). In adults, muscle contraction produced by nerve stimulators has more often been used to confirm correct epidural catheter placement (33). Experience with these techniques is still too limited to know their place in the pantheon of techniques to identify the epidural space.

V. Combined spinal–epidural technique

The combined spinal–epidural technique provides the rapid onset and dense block of a spinal anesthetic with the ability to extend the spread and duration of a block that is afforded by an epidural catheter. The technique is particularly useful in situations where sacral anesthesia is needed at the beginning of a procedure (e.g., gynecologic, lower extremity, obstetric, perineal surgery) and epidural analgesia is desired at the end. Because the subarachnoid space is entered, this technique is only appropriate at the lumbar level below the terminus of the spinal cord.

A. **Equipment.** In truth, all epidural and spinal needles are appropriate provided the chosen spinal needle fits through the epidural needle and extends at least 1 cm past the epidural needle's tip. Several manufactures market combined spinal–epidural needle kits that provide appropriately matched needles and at least one manufacturer markets a needle that has a separate lumen for the spinal needle so that it does not have to bend to exit the curved tip of the epidural needle. Small-gauge needles work best (25 and 27 gauge) both because they bend easier to exit the epidural needle tip and their smaller meningeal hole may reduce the possibility that the epidural catheter will thread into the subarachnoid space (34).

B. **The patient is positioned, prepped, draped** and the epidural needle placed using any of the approaches described in the preceding text.

C. After **identifying the epidural space**, remove the syringe and **insert the spinal needle** without its stylet. Dural puncture generally occurs within 1 cm of the epidural needle tip. If CSF is not obtained after fully inserting the spinal needle, consider.
   1. The epidural needle may not be in the epidural space.
   2. The distance from the tip of the epidural needle to the dura mater may be unusually long. If the spinal needle is fully inserted, hold the spinal needle firmly in place without its stylet and advance the spinal/epidural needle combination as a unit for an additional few millimeters. If this does not yield free-flowing CSF the needle is probably not in the epidural space.

D. Once free-flowing CSF is identified inject the subarachnoid drug and remove the spinal needle.

E. **Thread the epidural catheter,** remove the epidural needle and secure the catheter as described earlier.

F. **Test dose.** Test the epidural catheter as previously described to rule out an intravascular location. However, testing to rule out a subarachnoid location is difficult in the face of a developing spinal block. To date, no test dose that provides reliable, objective identification of a subarachnoid catheter during combined spinal–epidural anesthesia has been demonstrated. CSF aspiration is diagnostic, if present, but false-negative aspiration is always a concern. Continued vigilance is essential.

VI. Combined epidural–general anesthesia

Epidural anesthesia is often combined with a general anesthetic for cases in which an epidural catheter is placed for postoperative analgesia, but epidural anesthesia alone is not sufficient for the planned surgical procedure. For example:

A. **Indications**
   1. Surgical procedures that require tracheal intubation, for example, thoracotomy and laparoscopy
   2. Surgical procedures that are too high for the patient to remain comfortable during the procedure, for example, upper abdominal surgery
   3. Surgical procedures that are too long for the patient to remain comfortable without heavy sedation

B. **Technique.** In these settings the clinician may reasonably choose to either:
   1. Provide a surgical depth of epidural anesthesia and thereby reduce the requirement for general anesthetics (35,36). The "downside" to such an approach is that patients are more prone to develop hypotension because of the combined effects of the epidural and general anesthetics. In addition, the effectiveness of an epidural test dose containing epinephrine for identifying an intravascular epidural catheter is reduced (37).
   2. Initiate the postoperative analgesic regimen (e.g., dilute epidural local anesthetic with or without an epidural opioid) to ease the patient's transition to the postoperative period. This approach does not cause as much hypotension as a surgical depth of epidural block, but it does not provide as much "MAC-sparring" effect either.
   3. Wait until the postoperative period to initiate epidural analgesia. This approach minimizes potential hemodynamic interactions between epidural and general anesthesia, but may require some "catch up" in the recovery room to establish adequate epidural analgesia.

VII. Complications

A. **Hypotension**
   1. **Etiology.** As with spinal anesthesia, epidural anesthesia blocks sympathetic preganglionic fibers resulting in arterial **vasodilatation, decreased SVR** and a fall in MAP. Venodilatation also occurs and may result in reduced preload, especially in the hypovolemic patient.
   2. **Treatment**
      a. Restoring preload by **volume** loading may be sufficient to restore MAP in some cases, but because volume loading has no effect on SVR it is often insufficient by itself.
      b. **Ephedrine** has long been advocated as the drug of choice for treating hypotension, especially in obstetrics. However, ephedrine's primary action is to increase cardiac output by increasing contractility and heart rate. Although this approach will certainly increase MAP, it does not correct the underlying problem, namely, decreased SVR. In addition, patients on β-blockers may not respond well to ephedrine and the increase in myocardial oxygen demand may not be appropriate for patients with ischemic cardiovascular disease.
      c. **Phenylephrine,** an α_1-adrenergic agonist, is an alternative to ephedrine and one that corrects the underlying decrease in SVR instead of compensating for it by making the heart work harder. Phenylephrine is also easier to titrate than ephedrine. Therefore, phenylephrine is a reasonable choice to correct hypotension caused by epidural blockade and may be a better choice than ephedrine in some circumstances. Recent

human evidence has also shown that it may be superior to ephedrine to treat maternal hypotension during spinal or epidural anesthesia in obstetrics (38). It is also a more logical choice if tachycardia is already present, although ephedrine may be useful in increasing the heart rate if bradycardia is contributing to the hypotension.

B. Total spinal anesthesia. Total spinal is an uncommon complication resulting from anesthetic block extending to the brainstem. Patients lose the ability to breathe (C3, C4, C5 and chest wall motor block) and consciousness (block of brainstem reticular formation). Hypotension and bradycardia may be profound because all sympathetic nervous system activity is blocked at its site of origin in the brainstem. It is perhaps more likely to occur during attempted epidural anesthesia than during spinal anesthesia because of the much larger local anesthetic volumes that are used.

1. **Etiology.** During intended epidural anesthesia, total spinal can only occur if a large dose of local anesthetic is accidentally injected subarachnoid. This can occur when:
   a. The epidural needle is initially in the subarachnoid space or perhaps more likely because it is accidentally advanced into the subarachnoid space while injecting local anesthetic.
   b. A large volume of local anesthetic makes its way through the meningeal hole left by the spinal needle during a combined spinal–epidural technique or following a "wet tap" with an epidural needle. Several case reports have suggested such an etiology, and it is not unreasonable, but it has not been conclusively proved. *In vitro* studies suggest this is unlikely if the meningeal hole is made with a small-gauge spinal needle as opposed to an epidural needle (39).
   c. An epidural catheter migrates into the subarachnoid space.
   d. **Subdural injection.** Subdural (i.e., epiarachnoid) injection, *per se*, will not result in large doses of local anesthetic reaching the subarachnoid space because the arachnoid mater, not the dura mater, is the relevant anatomic barrier to drug entry into the CSF (40). In addition, the arachnoid is too delicate a tissue to confine a significant local anesthetic volume in the potential space between the dura and arachnoid. The likely scenario by which subdural injection results in a total spinal is as follows:
      (1) The epidural needle tip pierces the dura mater separating it from the arachnoid, but does not puncture the arachnoid.
      (2) Because the arachnoid is intact, CSF does not flow from the needle and dural puncture is not recognized.
      (3) A "large" volume of local anesthetic is injected, the arachnoid membrane ruptures and the local anesthetic rapidly enters the CSF. If sufficient volume is injected, total spinal may result.
2. **Treatment is entirely supportive.** With appropriate ventilation and hemodynamic support, complete recovery is to be expected. Importantly, depending on the local anesthetic used and the amount that entered the subarachnoid space, patients may need support for an hour or more.
3. **Prevention.** An appropriate test dose and **slow incremental** injection of the full local anesthetic dose with continual patient assessment are the primary means to prevent total spinal anesthesia whether local anesthetic

is injected through a needle or a catheter. In the case of an accidental wet tap with the epidural needle, consider abandoning epidural anesthesia and use the misplaced epidural needle to deliver a spinal anesthetic. If epidural anesthesia is still desired/necessary it may be prudent to move to another vertebral level in an effort to minimize drug transfer through the meningeal hole. However, whether changing vertebral levels actually reduces the risk of total spinal is unknown.

C. **Headache.** Because of its larger diameter, the risk of postdural puncture headache is much greater in the event that an epidural needle accidentally punctures the meninges, especially in young patients. Given the high risk, some have advocated immediate blood patch in young patients and have demonstrated that this approach is effective at decreasing the incidence of postdural puncture headache. The downside of course is that some patients will undergo a procedure that would not have been necessary. Postdural puncture headache is discussed in more detail in Chapter 6.

D. **Neurologic injury**

1. **Local anesthetic mediated.** As discussed in Chapter 3, all local anesthetics can produce dose-related neurotoxicity. That said, the risk of neurologic injury from local anesthetics placed in the epidural space is extremely low. The primary risk during epidural anesthesia is unintentional injection of large volumes of local anesthetic into the subarachnoid space. Multiple case reports have documented that all local anesthetics can produce permanent spinal cord injury by this mechanism. In fact, the reformulation of chloroprocaine was the result of injuries that occurred when large doses of preservative-containing (0.2% sodium bisulfite) drug intended for the epidural space were injected subarachnoid.
2. **Mechanical.** Epidural needles that contact spinal nerves or the spinal cord certainly can produce neurologic injury. However, the frequency of such injuries, especially with lumbar epidural anesthesia, is very low [Auroy et al. reported 0 cases in 35,293 epidural anesthetics (41)]. The risk with thoracic epidural anesthesia is higher, but whether that greater risk translates into more actual injuries is unknown.
3. **Nonanesthetic injuries.** Nerve injuries occur during many types of surgery and during normal vaginal delivery. When these injuries occur in the setting of epidural anesthesia/analgesia, the block is often blamed. However, in these cases careful neurologic examination will usually demonstrate that the injury was to a mixed nerve at a level well removed from the central neuraxis.

E. **Urinary retention.** Bladder contraction requires an intact parasympathetic nervous system. Blockade of parasympathetic neurons lasts longer than does blockade of sensory or motor neurons. Consequently, micturition may be inhibited well beyond the duration of sensory or motor block and may lead to retention following long duration blockade. Traditionally, many centers have required outpatients to void before discharge, which resulted in some prolonged recovery room stays in patients who were otherwise ready for discharge. Fortunately, the advent of automated bladder ultrasonographic devices, which measure bladder volume, has made management of this problem easier. Mulroy et al. showed that use of short-acting epidural blockade produced rapid return of bladder function and no greater frequency of retention than after general anesthesia (42). Patients who could not void after block resolution and who had bladder volumes less than 400 mL could be safely discharged home and would regain the ability to void without complication. This approach led to significantly shorter average discharge times compared to patients who were required to void spontaneously before discharge.

F. **Back pain.** Back pain is more common, more severe, and longer lasting following epidural anesthesia than spinal anesthesia and is cited by some patients as the reason that they would refuse subsequent epidural anesthetics (43). It is tempting to blame the larger epidural needle as the reason that pain is more of a problem with epidural anesthesia than with spinal anesthesia, but this may be too simplistic. For example, back pain may be worse following epidural anesthesia because local anesthetic exiting intervertebral foramina to reach paraspinous muscle may cause myotoxicity (see Chapter 3). Future studies are necessary to identify the cause of epidural anesthesia-related back pain before recommendations can be offered for how to prevent it. Treatment is symptomatic and patients should be encouraged to keep moving and counseled to expect resolution within 7 to 10 days in most cases.

G. **Epidural hematoma.** See Chapter 3.

H. **Epidural abscess.** See Chapter 3.

VIII. Summary

Epidural anesthesia and analgesia techniques are an essential component of modern anesthetic practice. Mastering the technique requires a thorough understanding of the relevant anatomy, the pharmacologic options (local anesthetics, opioids, adrenergic agonists, etc.) the risks unique to the technique, and the methods to reduce the risks.

REFERENCES

1 Lirk P, Kolbitsch C, Putz G, et al. Cervical and high thoracic ligamentum flavum frequently fails to fuse in the midline. *Anesthesiology* 2003;99:1387–1390.

2 Bernards CM, Shen DD, Sterling ES, et al. Epidural, cerebrospinal fluid, and plasma pharmacokinetics of epidural opioids (part 1): differences among opioids. *Anesthesiology* 2003;99:455–465.

3 Hogan QH. Lumbar epidural anatomy. A new look by cryomicrotome section. *Anesthesiology* 1991; 75:767–775.

4 Meijenhorst GC. Myelography and epidural double-catheter venography. *Br Med J* 1978;2:205–206.

5 Fink BR, Walker S. Orientation of fibers in human dorsal lumbar dura mater in relation to lumbar puncture. *Anesth Analg* 1989;69:768–772.

6 Stevens RA, Urmey WF, Urquhart BL, et al. Back pain after epidural anesthesia with chloroprocaine. *Anesthesiology* 1993;78:492–497.

7 Stevens RA, Chester WL, Artuso JD, et al. Back pain after epidural anesthesia with chloroprocaine in volunteers: preliminary report. *Reg Anesth* 1991;16:199–203.

8 Drolet P, Veillette Y. Back pain following epidural anesthesia with 2-chloroprocaine (EDTA-free) or lidocaine. *Reg Anesth* 1997;22:303–307.

9 Eisenach JC, Schlairet TJ, Dobson CE II, et al. Effect of prior anesthetic solution on epidural morphine analgesia. *Anesth Analg* 1991;73:119–123.

10 Huntoon M, Eisenach JC, Boese P. Epidural clonidine after cesarean section. Appropriate dose and effect of prior local anesthetic. *Anesthesiology* 1992;76:187–193.

11 Mogensen T, Simonsen L, Scott NB, et al. Tachyphylaxis associated with repeated epidural injections of lidocaine is not related to changes in distribution or the rate of elimination from the epidural space. *Anesth Analg* 1989;69:180–184.

12 Bernards CM, Shen DD, Sterling ES, et al. Epidural, cerebrospinal fluid, and plasma pharmacokinetics of epidural opioids (part 2): effect of epinephrine. *Anesthesiology* 2003;99:466–475.

13 Kozody R, Palahniuk RJ, Wade JG, et al. The effect of subarachnoid epinephrine and phenylephrine on spinal cord blood flow. *Can Anaesth Soc J* 1984;31:503–508.
14 Bonica JJ, Kennedy WF, Ward RJ Jr, et al. A comparison of the effects of high subarachnoid and epidural anesthesia. *Acta Anaesthesiol Scand Suppl* 1966;23:429–437.
15 Bernards CM, Carpenter RL, Kenter ME, et al. Effect of epinephrine on central nervous system and cardiovascular system toxicity of bupivacaine in pigs. *Anesthesiology* 1989;71:711–717.
16 Nishikawa T, Dohi S. Clinical evaluation of clonidine added to lidocaine solution for epidural anesthesia. *Anesthesiology* 1990;73:853–859.
17 Klimscha W, Chiari A, Krafft P, et al. Hemodynamic and analgesic effects of clonidine added repetitively to continuous epidural and spinal blocks. *Anesth Analg* 1995;80:322–327.
18 Park WY, Hagins FM, Rivat EL, et al. Age and epidural dose response in adult men. *Anesthesiology* 1982;56:318–320.
19 Park W, Massengale M, Macnamara T. Age, height, and speed of injection as factors determining caudal anesthetic level and occurence of severe hypertension. *Anesthesiology* 1979;51:81–84.
20 Cesur M, Alici HA, Erdem AF, et al. Administration of local anesthetic through the epidural needle before catheter insertion improves the quality of anesthesia and reduces catheter-related complications. *Anesth Analg* 2005;101:1501–1505.
21 Dam-Hieu P, Rodriguez V, De Cazes Y, et al. Computed tomography images of entrapped epidural catheter. *Reg Anesth Pain Med* 2002;27:517–519.
22 Renehan EM, Peterson RA, Penning JP, et al. Visualization of a looped and knotted epidural catheter with a guidewire. *Can J Anaesth* 2000;47:329–333.
23 Choi DH, Lee SM, Cho HS, et al. Relationship between the bevel of the Tuohy needle and catheter direction in thoracic epidural anesthesia. *Reg Anesth Pain Med* 2006;31:105–112.
24 Tiso RL, Thomas PS, Macadaeg K. Epidural catheter direction and local anesthetic dose. *Reg Anesth* 1993;18:308–311.
25 Hoshi T, Miyabe M, Takahashi S, et al. Evaluation of the arrow flex tip plus epidural catheter tip position and migration during continuous thoracic analgesia. *Can J Anaesth* 2003;50:202–203.
26 Motamed C, Farhat F, Remerand F, et al. An analysis of postoperative epidural analgesia failure by computed tomography epidurography. *Anesth Analg* 2006;103:1026–1032.
27 Bougher RJ, Corbett AR, Ramage DT. The effect of tunnelling on epidural catheter migration. *Anaesthesia* 1996;51:191–194.
28 Dickson MA, Doyle E. The intravascular migration of an epidural catheter. *Paediatr Anaesth* 1999;9:273–275.
29 Jaeger JM, Madsen ML. Delayed subarachnoid migration of an epidural arrow flex tip plus catheter. *Anesthesiology* 1997;87:718–719.
30 Abraham RA, Harris AP, Maxwell LG, et al. The efficacy of 1.5% lidocaine with 7.5% dextrose and epinephrine as an epidural test dose for obstetrics. *Anesthesiology* 1986;64:116–119.
31 Holmaas G, Frederiksen D, Ulvik A, et al. Identification of thoracic intervertebral spaces by means of surface anatomy: a magnetic resonance imaging study. *Acta Anaesthesiol Scand* 2006;50:368–373.
32 Tsui BC, Wagner AM, Cunningham K, et al. Can continuous low current electrical stimulation distinguish insulated needle position in the epidural and intrathecal spaces in pediatric patients? *Paediatr Anaesth* 2005;15:959–963.
33 Tsui BC, Bury J, Bouliane M, et al. Cervical epidural analgesia via a thoracic approach using nerve-stimulation guidance in adult patients undergoing total shoulder replacement surgery. *Acta Anaesthesiol Scand* 2007;51:255–260.
34 Holmstrom B, Rawal N, Axelsson K, et al. Risk of catheter migration during combined spinal epidural block: percutaneous epiduroscopy study. *Anesth Analg* 1995;80:747–753.
35 Hodgson PS, Liu SS. Epidural lidocaine decreases sevoflurane requirement for adequate depth of anesthesia as measured by the Bispectral Index monitor. *Anesthesiology* 2001;94:799–803.
36 Hodgson PS, Liu SS, Gras TW. Does epidural anesthesia have general anesthetic effects? A prospective, randomized, double-blind, placebo-controlled trial. *Anesthesiology* 1999;91:1687–1692.
37 Liu SS, Carpenter RL. Hemodynamic responses to intravascular injection of epinephrine-containing epidural test doses in adults during general anesthesia. *Anesthesiology* 1996;84:81–87.
38 Ngan Kee WD, Khaw KS. Vasopressors in obstetrics: what should we be using? *Curr Opin Anaesthesiol* 2006;19:238–243.
39 Bernards CM, Kopacz DJ, Michel MZ. Effect of needle puncture on morphine and lidocaine flux through the spinal meninges of the monkey *in vitro*. Implications for combined spinal-epidural anesthesia. *Anesthesiology* 1994;80:853–858.
40 Bernards CM, Hill HF. Morphine and alfentanil permeability through the spinal dura, arachnoid, and pia mater of dogs and monkeys. *Anesthesiology* 1990;73:1214–1219.

41 Auroy Y, Benhamou D, Bargues L, et al. Major complications of regional anesthesia in France: the SOS Regional Anesthesia Hotline Service. *Anesthesiology* 2002;97:1274–1280.
42 Mulroy MF, Salinas FV, Larkin KL, et al. Ambulatory surgery patients may be discharged before voiding after short-acting spinal and epidural anesthesia. *Anesthesiology* 2002;97:315–319.
43 Seeberger MD, Lang ML, Drewe J, et al. Comparison of spinal and epidural anesthesia for patients younger than 50 years of age. *Anesth Analg* 1994;78:667–673.

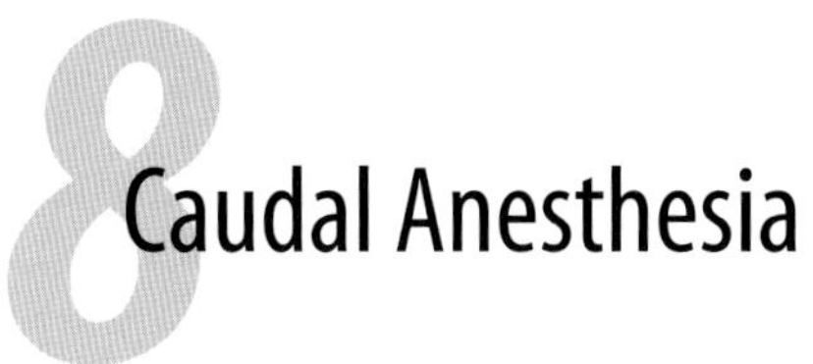

8 Caudal Anesthesia

Michael F. Mulroy

An alternative approach to the peridural space is through the base of the spine at the sacral hiatus. Injection into the sacral canal produces an epidural block but requires a higher volume of solution to reach abdominal levels. The caudal approach is handicapped by a greater **variability of the anatomy** and a higher potential for venous injection, and is used primarily in pediatric practice.

I. Anatomy

A. The caudal canal is the lowermost extension of the spinal canal. The dorsal roof is the fused posterior laminae of the sacral vertebral bodies. The only direct opening into the canal normally occurs at the level of the fifth sacral vertebra, where the failure of development of the spinous process and the laminae leaves a hiatus in the bony roof of the canal. This opening is bounded laterally by the prominent cornu (the incompletely developed articular processes) and covered by the thick sacral–coccygeal ligament. Along the lateral border of the canal itself are openings both anterior and posterior in the sacral bone at the levels of S1 through S4. The sacral nerve roots emerge both posteriorly and anteriorly through these modified intervertebral foramina.

B. The canal is concave anteriorly but basically flat at the point of entry from the sacral hiatus (Figure 8.1). The angle of the canal to the skin surface varies with sex and race. In whites, the canal is angled approximately 35 degrees to the skin surface, whereas in blacks, the angle may be 45 degrees. In women of each race, the angle is slightly less steep than in their male counterparts. The degree of fusion of the bones is variable; the canal may be absent in 5% to 10% of the population (1,2).

C. A helpful **relationship is the distance between the posterior superior iliac spines and the sacral hiatus.** This distance is consistently equal to the distance between the two spines themselves, forming an equilateral triangle (Figure 8.2) **(2)**. This relationship can be helpful if the sacral cornu are difficult to palpate.

D. Within the canal, the dural sac can normally be expected to terminate above the level of the **second sacral vertebra**. It may extend into the sacral portion of the canal and be as close as 3.5 cm (1.4 in.) from the hiatus. Areolar tissue, nerve roots, and a generous venous plexus are the other occupants of the space.

II. Indications

A. Local anesthetics injected into the sacral canal produce dense sacral root anesthesia. This is an ideal technique for **perineal and perianal surgery**, such as hemorrhoidectomy or rectal tumor fulguration. With adequate lumbar levels of block, **foot or leg procedures** are possible. If larger volumes are used, anesthesia to the lower thoracic dermatomes can be obtained, and **transurethral prostatectomy or vaginal hysterectomy** is possible. The advantages of a continuous technique can be obtained by inserting a catheter in the canal.

B. Caudal anesthesia offers an advantage over lumbar epidural anesthesia in that anesthesia for lower-extremity surgery is **limited to lumbar and sacral** roots.

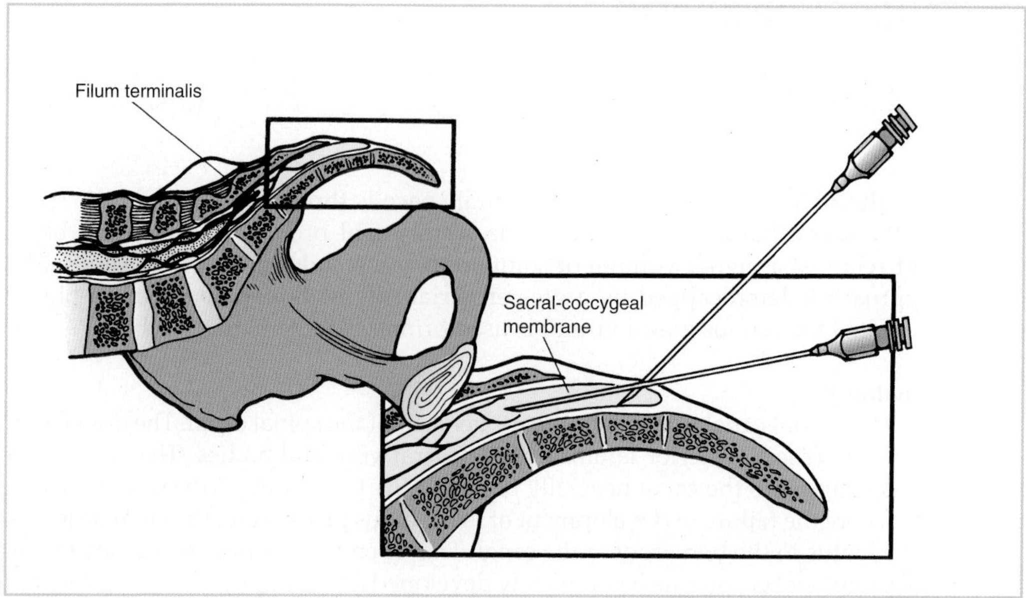

Figure 8.1. Sacral anatomy, lateral view. A needle directed through the sacral–coccygeal membrane at a 45-degree angle will usually "pop" through the ligament and contact the anterior bone of the sacral canal. The needle needs to be rotated so that the bevel does not scrape the periosteum of this layer, and the angle of advancement changed to allow passage directly 2 to 3 cm up the canal without contacting bone again. This space is generously endowed with blood vessels, and the terminal point of the dural sac extends a variable distance into the sacral canal, but usually lies at the S2 level.

When compared to spinal anesthesia, caudal anesthesia offers less chance of postdural puncture headache than spinal anesthesia, but this complication is still possible. With the lower incidence of headache with rounded-bevel spinal needles, this advantage is less significant. These potential comparative advantages must be weighed against the **slower-onset, higher drug dose, and anatomic difficulties** of caudals.

C. The major application of the caudal approach is in **pediatric anesthesia**, where the anatomy is more superficial and reliable, and excellent postoperative analgesia can be offered. Obstetric practice has seen a decline in the use of continuous caudals, related to the high volume of anesthetic solution required and the greater interference with the "pushing" reflex. Caudal anesthesia is available for the rare patient who cannot be offered the advantages of lumbar epidural anesthesia, such as the mother with a previous Harrington rod spinal fusion.

III. Drugs

A. The drugs used for caudal anesthesia are the same as those used for lumbar epidural anesthesia. The same considerations apply when choosing desired density (motor versus sensory) and duration of anesthesia.

B. Because of leakage through the lateral sacral foramina and the greater space in the canal, the **volume of solution required is greater** for caudal than for epidural anesthesia. A dose of 15 mL of solution may produce only sacral (perineal) anesthesia, whereas 25 mL is required to obtain a T10-12 level of

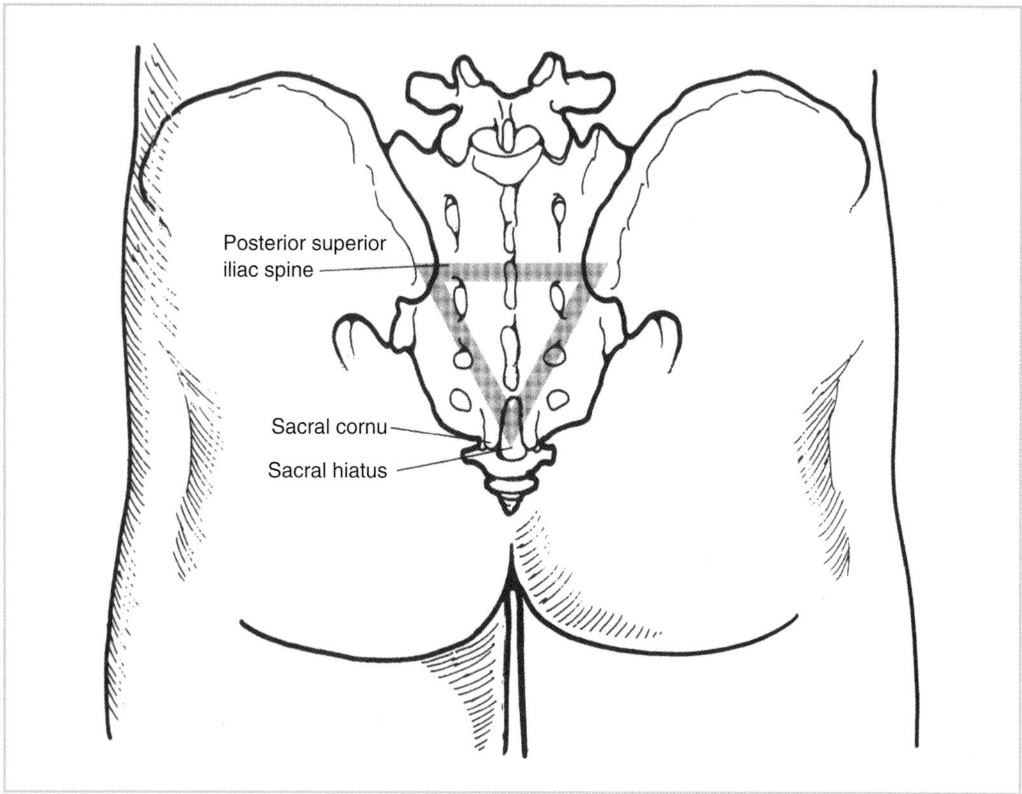

Figure 8.2. Sacral anatomy, posterior view. The sacral hiatus is covered by a thick ligament that lies between and slightly inferior to the two prominent sacral cornua. A triangle drawn between the posterior superior iliac spines and this foramen is usually equilateral in shape.

block. This is an average of 2 to 3 mL per segment, in contrast to the requirement for half this amount with lumbar injections.

C. **Age and weight are not predictable** determinants of extent of anesthesia, as they are in adult lumbar epidural anesthesia. The dose requirement does appear to be slightly reduced in pregnancy; 16 to 18 mL will give a T10 level of block.

D. The same additives can be used as in epidural injection. Epinephrine prolongs duration. Clonidine and opioids will enhance degree and duration of analgesia (3,4).

IV. Technique

A. **Position.** Caudal anesthesia may be performed with the patient in the prone, lateral, or knee-chest position.

1. The **knee-chest** position is preferred in obstetrics, where the uterus makes lying prone unsuitable. For that position, the patient is instructed to turn prone but with the knees brought up into a kneeling position. It is the least "glamorous" position, but it is the most effective in causing the gluteal muscles to "fall away" from the sacral hiatus.
2. In the **lateral** position, the upper leg is flexed at the hip and knee, again to help spread the gluteal muscles away from the hiatus.

3. In the **prone** patient, a pillow is placed under the hips to flex the hip joint and spread the muscles, and the patient is also asked to spread the legs and internally rotate the feet.

B. **Standard technique**

1. Once the patient is in the appropriate position, the landmarks are identified. The **sacral cornu** may be easily palpated on the thin patient, lying just above the intergluteal crease. The **sacral coccygeal membrane** forms a soft valley between and just below these peaks. The position is confirmed by drawing the **triangle** formed by the hiatus and the posterior superior iliac spines; it should be equilateral. The membrane should also be 4 to 5 cm (1.8 to 2 in.) above the palpable tip of the coccyx. The sacral foramina may also be drawn (Figure 8.2).
2. Before skin preparation in the prone position, a small sponge is placed in the gluteal skin crease to prevent solution dripping into the perineal area. Following aseptic preparation and draping, a small **skin wheal** is raised with a small-gauge needle over the membrane. Generous infiltration will obscure the landmarks.
3. **Deeper infiltration** is done with a 22-gauge needle, again avoiding excessive distortion of the tissues. If a catheter is not used, the entire single-injection block can be performed with the 22-gauge needle, keeping in mind that the loss of resistance in the peridural space will be harder to appreciate with the smaller needle than with the traditional 17- to 19-gauge needle. Even when a large needle is used, the preliminary approach with the 22-gauge needle helps identify the membrane and canal so that the larger needle can be placed in a single attempt.
4. The needle is introduced through the anesthetized tissue to the membrane at approximately a **70-degree angle** to the skin (perpendicular to the membrane [Figure 8.1]). Firm pressure will allow the needle to penetrate the fibrous band and "drop" into the caudal canal. The canal here is shallow, however, and vigorous advancement will produce a painful laceration of the periosteum of the anterior wall of the canal. If multiple attempts do not produce a penetration of the membrane within a few minutes, the landmarks are reassessed. Six percent to 10% of patients will have a fusion of the structures that prevents entry (1,2), and alternative techniques may have to be considered.
5. Once in the canal, the hub of the needle is **dropped downward** toward the gluteal crease so the tip now advances no more than 4 cm (1.8 in.) up the center of the canal, almost parallel to the axis of the back itself. The bevel should be rotated in the appropriate direction to reduce the chance of the sharp point lacerating the tender periosteum as it advances. The **angle of the canal can normally be expected to be almost flat** in relation to the skin in females, but somewhat steeper in males or blacks (the hub will drop less from the perpendicular). If the angle is 50 degrees or greater, intraosseous or transsacral placement should be suspected. The path of advancement should be directly up the caudal canal following the midline course of the spine; if lateral deviation occurs, the needle is withdrawn and the landmarks are reassessed.
6. With 2 to 4 cm (0.8–1.8 in.) of needle within the canal, a **small syringe** with 1.5 mL of air is attached to the hub, and **gentle aspiration** is performed. If no blood or cerebrospinal fluid (CSF) is obtained, the air is injected

forcefully to gauge the resistance. There should be **no resistance** to injection other than the caliber of the needle itself, just as in the epidural space. Sharp pain on injection indicates subperiosteal placement and requires reinsertion.

7. If injection of this volume of **air is undesirable** (as in pediatric patients), other tests are available. Ultrasound guidance is becoming more common (5). Listening over the sacrum with a stethoscope for a "whoosh" sound associated with local anesthetic injection is also helpful (6). An alternative confirmation of proper entry is the use of the nerve stimulator, which will produce perirectal contractions if the needle is in the caudal canal (7).
8. If **no pain or resistance** is felt, an additional 5 mL **of air is injected forcefully** while the fingers rest lightly on the area of skin over the tip of the needle. If crepitus is felt, the needle is probably in the subcutaneous tissue and needs to be reinserted. Air may emerge laterally through the sacral foramina (Figure 8.2); this is acceptable. The patient may confirm proper needle placement by describing cramping discomfort in the posterior thighs with injection.
9. If a **catheter** is used, it is inserted after these confirmatory tests. A longer length of insertion (12 to 13 cm [5 in.]) into the canal may be required here than in the lumbar area, especially if lower abdominal (thoracic root) anesthesia is desired.
10. A **test dose** of 3 mL of local anesthetic with 1:200,000 epinephrine is injected through the catheter or needle (single-injection technique), and the heart rate or blood pressure is monitored appropriately.
11. If no intravascular or subarachnoid injection is demonstrated, the anesthetic dose may be injected and the catheter secured. **Twenty minutes** is usually required before adequate surgical anesthesia is obtained.
12. As with all continuous techniques, the **test dose** is repeated before each injection.

V. Complications

A. **Intravascular injection is the most common serious problem,** and is more likely here than with epidural anesthesia (8). The canal is **highly vascular**, but the veins have a low pressure that frustrates detection of vascular entry by aspiration of blood. Careful test doses are mandatory, along with frequent monitoring of the patient's mental status. Incremental injection is appropriate.

B. **Periosteal damage** is infrequent but may be a painful disability for the patient for several weeks. Vigorous treatment with heat and anti-inflammatory drugs, along with concerned support, is needed.

C. **Dural puncture is rare and carries the same risks of total spinal anesthesia** and postspinal headache as epidural anesthesia.

D. **Intraosseous injection** is rare, but it **can produce systemic toxicity** similar to that of intravenous injection. Aspiration of the thick marrow is usually not possible, and absorption is slow enough that a test dose may not clearly reveal improper needle placement. Systemic symptoms may not occur for several minutes following injection of a therapeutic dose.

E. **Presacral injection** is also rare, but rectal injection and injection into the fetal scalp have occurred. Careful attention to landmarks and angles will reduce this possibility, and the needle need not be advanced its entire length into the tissues. Some authors suggest that obstetric caudal anesthesia is contraindicated once the fetal head has descended into the pelvis (and lies just anterior to the sacrum).

F. **Hypertension** has also been described on **rapid injection**. This may be due to a response to compression of the cord or spinal nerves. It is usually transient and can be avoided with slow injection.

REFERENCES

1 Crighton IM, Barry BP, Hobbs GJ. A study of the anatomy of the caudal space using magnetic resonance imaging. *Br J Anaesth* 1997;78:391.

2 **Senoglu N, Senoglu M, Oksuz H, et al. Landmarks of the sacral hiatus for caudal epidural block: an anatomical study. *Br J Anaesth* 2005;95:692–695.**

3 Constant I, Gall O, Gouyet L, et al. Addition of clonidine or fentanyl to local anaesthetics prolongs the duration of surgical analgesia after single shot caudal block in children. *Br J Anaesth* 1998;80:294.

4 Van Elstraete AC, Pastureau F, Lebrun T, et al. Caudal clonidine for postoperative analgesia in adults. *Br J Anaesth* 2000;84:401.

5 Roberts SA, Galvez I. Ultrasound assessment of caudal catheter position in infants. *Paediatr Anaesth* 2005;15:429–432.

6 Orme RM, Berg SJ. The 'swoosh' test—an evaluation of a modified 'whoosh' test in children. *Br J Anaesth* 2003;90:62–65.

7 Tsui BC, Tarkkila P, Gupta S, et al. Confirmation of caudal needle placement using nerve stimulation. *Anesthesiology* 1999;91:374.

8 Brown DL, Ransom DM, Hall JA, et al. Regional anesthesia and local anesthetic-induced systemic toxicity: seizure frequency and accompanying cardiovascular changes. *Anesth Analg* 1995;81:321.

9 Intercostal and Terminal Nerve Anesthesia of the Trunk

Michael F. Mulroy

Intercostal nerve block, like the paravertebral approach, provides an alternative to spinal or epidural anesthesia for superficial anesthesia for abdominal and chest-wall procedures. This technique provides intraoperative and postoperative analgesia for up to 12 hours without the price of the sympathectomy associated with the axial blocks, and is a useful alternative if neuraxial blockade is contraindicated. It is more tedious because multiple injections must be made and one missed nerve can reduce the analgesia provided. More distal blockade of the terminal branches of the thoracic and upper lumbar nerves at the rectus sheath or in the groin can also provide extensive postoperative analgesia for small midline or groin incisions.

I. Anatomy

A. The peripheral somatic nerves of the thorax depart the spinal column and immediately form a small dorsal and a major ventral branch. These ventral somatic branches travel laterally under their respective ribs. The interior lower edge of each rib provides a channel for the nerve and its companion artery and vein, thereby leaving an overhanging external edge that protects these fellow travelers from direct external assault. This intercostal groove is further enclosed by the fascia of the internal and external intercostal muscles. Beneath the internal intercostal muscle lies the parietal pleura.

B. Near the **midaxillary line** the groove becomes less well defined, and the nerve migrates away from the rib and gives off a **lateral cutaneous branch** as it moves anteriorly. Because of these two factors, reliable anesthesia is more difficult beyond the anterior axillary line. The main trunk continues anteriorly to provide sensory and motor innervation to the muscles and skin of the anterior chest (T2-6) and abdomen (T7-11). The terminal branches of these nerves pierce the sheath of the rectus abdominis muscle as they approach the midline, and are once again enclosed in a well-defined fascial plane in that sheath along the midline.

C. The **12th intercostal nerve** is unique in that it is **not closely associated with its rib**. Branches from the 12th nerve depart early to join the ilioinguinal nerve, and the standard subcostal injection is less likely to produce anesthesia of this nerve.

D. The ilioinguinal nerve is a branch of the first lumbar root, which travels alongside its companion branch, the iliohypogastric nerve, as they extend into the groin. These two nerves pierce successively the transversalis muscle and the internal and external oblique muscles of the abdomen near the level of the anterior superior iliac spine as they eventually emerge to provide sensation to the hypogastric and upper inner thigh areas.

E. The first and second intercostal nerves also differ in that their primary branches join with the lower nerves of the brachial plexus or extend onto the arm itself as the intercostobrachial nerve to provide sensation to the medial aspect of the upper arm.

F. The ribs themselves vary. In the posterior midline, all of them are well protected medially by the thick paravertebral muscle. The **lower six are easily palpated**

lateral to this muscle and are broad, flat, and relatively superficial. The **upper ribs are more protected** by the scapula and its associated muscles, appear narrower and deeper, and are technically more difficult to reach, making the **paravertebral approach more practical in this region**.

II. Indications

A. Bilateral blockade of the 6th through 12th intercostal nerves provides sensory anesthesia of the **abdominal wall in these respective dermatomes, that is, from the xiphoid to the pubis**. The abdominal muscles in this distribution are also relaxed. There is **no anesthesia of the visceral peritoneum**. Anesthesia of these nerves will therefore produce sufficient analgesia and relaxation for an anterior abdominal incision. Bilateral blockade is needed for any midline incision because there is lateral overlap of innervation such that sensory dermatomes for each side cross over the midline.

B. Supplemental anesthesia of the **celiac plexus** or general anesthesia is necessary for intra-abdominal procedures. This combined technique is ideally suited for upper abdominal surgery, such as cholecystectomy, splenectomy, or gastrectomy. Even with visceral anesthesia, endotracheal intubation, controlled ventilation, and light supplemental general anesthesia are usually required in all but the more debilitated patients. For midabdominal surgery (abdominal aortic aneurysm repair, colectomy, etc.), this technique can be further supplemented with **paravertebral block of the first and second lumbar nerve** roots.

C. Unilateral blockade of the intercostal nerves is also useful in reducing the anesthetic requirement during thoracotomy (1). It will reduce postoperative analgesia requirements, although not as successfully as for abdominal surgery. A paravertebral approach may be needed for the upper ribs (see Chapter 10). Intercostals can rarely be useful as the sole anesthetic for superficial operations of the chest wall. They are applicable, however, for insertion of chest tubes or for providing analgesia for percutaneous biliary drainage. Unilateral blockade of three or more ribs is useful in relieving the **pain of fractured ribs**. The segments above and below the injury also must be blocked because of sensory dermatome overlap. This technique is also useful for acute **post-thoracotomy pain** or for subcostal incisional pain, as well as midline abdominal pain. Intercostal block in this setting has been shown to improve ventilatory function and reduce narcotic requirements in healthy patients. The relief is not as effective as with epidural infusions, and the intercostal blocks **need to be repeated** frequently to preserve the gains.

D. Blockade of the terminal branches of the 9th through 11th nerves in the rectus sheath provides approximately 10 hours of postoperative analgesia for umbilical hernia repair or gynecologic umbilical laparoscopic incisions (2).

E. Blockade of the ilioinguinal and iliohypogastric nerves near the anterior superior iliac spine similarly provides analgesia for hernia or groin operations (3), and a combination blockade of the rectus sheath and these two nerves can provide analgesia for lower midline incisions, such as for cesarean delivery (4).

III. Drugs

Prolonged duration is usually a primary goal of this technique, and the longer-acting amino amides are ideal.

A. **Bupivacaine** or levobupivacaine 0.5% with 1:200,000 epinephrine in a dose of 3 to 5 mL per rib for intercostal blocks will give 9 to 14 hours of analgesia as well as adequate intraoperative muscle relaxation for a shorter time. Similar analgesia is produced with the rectus sheath and groin injections of the terminal nerves.
B. **Ropivacaine** is equally effective, but the duration is shorter by a third (5).
C. The **lower concentration** of 0.25% is more appropriate for postoperative analgesia when motor relaxation is not needed. The total dose is therefore reduced. This is an important consideration because the highly vascular area of injection produces the highest blood levels of any of the peripheral nerve injections.

IV. Technique

A. **Intercostal nerve block, posterior approach.** This classical approach can be performed with the patient in the traditional **prone position** (Figure 9.1) or in the **sitting or lateral positions** for patients with abdominal pain or tenderness. The lateral position allows the greatest lateral displacement of the scapula, but it allows only one side to be blocked at a time. The major risk of the prone position is respiratory depression or airway obstruction from the sedation that is normally required for the patient to tolerate 14 injections. Close monitoring is needed.
   1. The patient is positioned prone with the arms hanging over the sides of the stretcher or bed so that the scapulae fall laterally away from the midline. A pillow placed under the abdomen helps to arch the back and facilitate palpation of the ribs. The head is turned to one side, and an **adequate airway** is ensured.
   2. The **landmarks** are drawn. The spinous processes are marked, and then a mark is drawn on the lower border of the 12th rib at a point 7 cm from the midline (Figure 9.1). This usually marks the point of the sharpest posterior angulation of the rib. The sixth or seventh rib is then marked where it can be most easily felt between the scapula and the paraspinous muscles, usually 4 to 5 cm from the midline. A line is drawn on each side joining these two initial rib markings. The lower borders of the rest of the ribs from the 6th to the 11th are marked along these lines on each side. These lines should fall along the prominent posterior angle of each rib. The distance between the 11th and 12th rib will be greater than that between the other ribs. If a celiac plexus block is to be performed also, skin markings are made at this time (see Chapter 11).
   3. While preparation of the back and equipment is proceeding, an assistant continues **monitoring and begins intravenous sedation**. A combination of analgesic and amnestic drugs is most appropriate.
   4. After **skin preparation and draping**, a **skin wheal** is made at each mark with a small needle. The patient's reaction to these 14 injections will usually indicate whether sedation is adequate.
   5. Starting at the lowest rib, the intercostal nerves are blocked. The 12th nerve may be skipped because its variable course makes anesthesia unreliable. The anesthesiologist stands at the patient's side with the syringe in his or her caudad hand (right hand if he or she is on the patient's left). The index finger of the cephalad hand is placed on the skin just above the lowest skin mark and should lie on the body of the rib. The skin wheal is retracted cephalad so that it lies over the midpoint of the rib. The **22-gauge needle is**

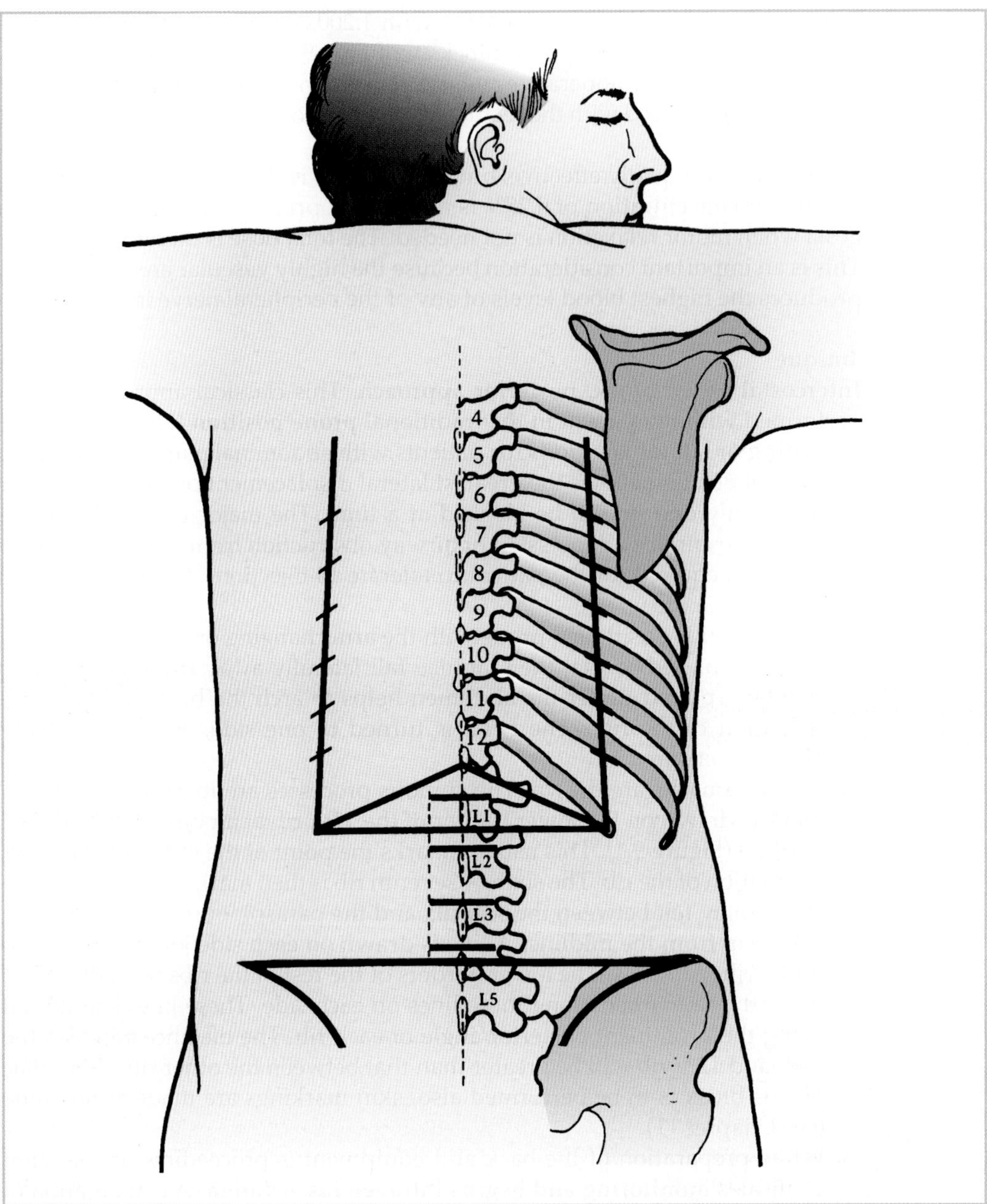

Figure 9.1. Landmarks for intercostal block. The inferior borders of the ribs are identified at their most prominent point on the back. The marks usually lie along a line that angles slightly medially from the 12th to the 6th rib. The marks for the 12th rib usually lie approximately 7 cm from the midline. For a celiac plexus block (see Chapter 11), a triangle is drawn between the 12th rib marks and the inferior border of the 12th spinous process, with the base formed by joining the two rib marks with a straight line. For lumbar somatic (see Chapter 10) or lumbar sympathetic blocks (see Chapter 11), the transverse processes of the lumbar vertebrae are identified by drawing a line across the superior border of the lumbar spinous processes; the transverse process for each vertebra usually lies along this line in the lumbar area.

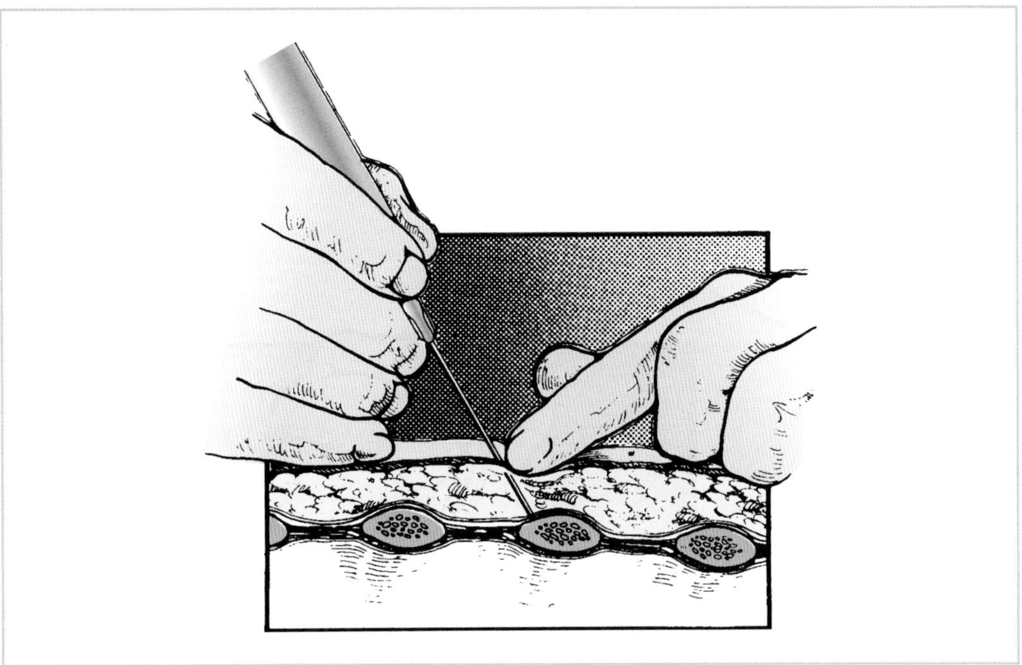

Figure 9.2. Hand and needle position for intercostal block; needle on rib. The index finger of the cephalad hand identifies the lower margin of the rib and the needle is gently inserted onto the bone. The cephalad hand is then used to grasp the hub of the needle and control the movement of the syringe.

inserted through the wheal to rest on the rib (Figure 9.2). The periosteum is contacted gently, both to avoid patient discomfort and to avoid barbing the point of the needle.

6. With the **needle resting safely on the rib**, the cephalad hand now assumes control of the needle and syringe. The hub of the needle is grasped between the thumb and forefinger while the middle finger rests along the needle shaft (Figure 9.3). The ulnar border of the palm rests on the back and steadies the hand to prevent unintentional changes in depth. The fingers of the caudad hand now move to the rings of the syringe and prepare for injection. While maintaining a 20-degree cephalad angulation of the needle and syringe, the **needle tip is raised slightly off the periosteum and "walked" inferiorly** until it passes under the inferior border of the rib. The natural traction of the skin (previously pulled upward to move the skin wheal over the rib) helps move the needle to the correct position. The **syringe and needle must always remain parallel to their original cephalad angulation** with each "step" toward the rib margin. The most frequent cause of inadequate analgesia is allowing the syringe to pivot to a caudad angle.
7. Once the needle is under the rib, the cephalad angulation is maintained and the **needle is advanced 2 to 3 mm** to lie in the intercostal groove. While the cephalad hand continues to control the syringe, 3 to 4 mL of anesthetic solution is injected. Intravascular injection should be prevented by careful aspiration. A deliberate infinitesimal "jiggling" of the needle tip may help prevent intravenous injection. If the needle lies within a vessel, the jiggling makes the intravascular presence temporary. Paresthesias are not necessary

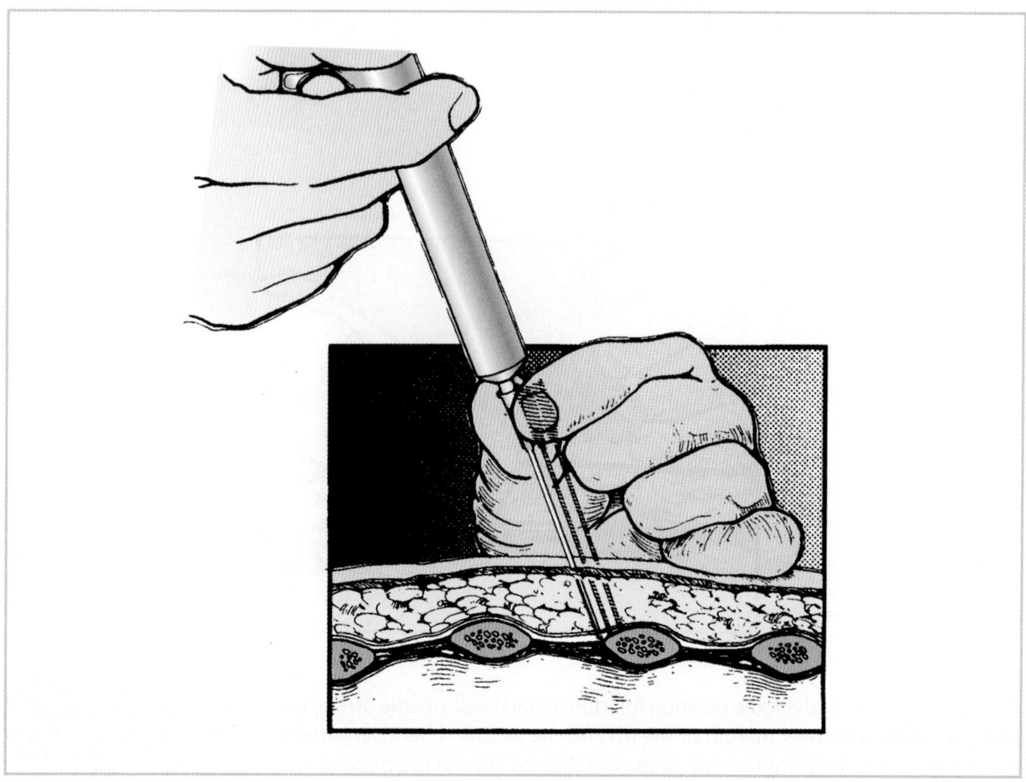

Figure 9.3. Hand and needle position for intercostal block; needle under rib. The depth of the needle is controlled by the hand resting on the back. The other hand injects solution when the needle is under the rib, but this is the only function performed while the needle is near the pleura.

unless a neurolytic block is sought. During the injection, the upper hand rests on the chest wall, providing **firm control of the syringe**. The fingers of the caudad hand are used only to inject, not to advance the syringe or needle.

8. **After injection, the needle and syringe are immediately moved back** to the safe dorsal surface of the rib. The fingers of the caudad hand are removed from the rings of the syringe, and the barrel is cradled between the thumb and forefinger to allow control of the syringe. Now the upper hand relinquishes control to the caudad hand and is again employed to seek the next rib while the needle remains "parked" on the rib just blocked.
9. By alternating control of the syringe between the hands, the syringe and needle are moved from one rib to the next. If the syringe is to be refilled, it is detached from the needle, and the needle is left in the skin as a marker of the last nerve injected.
10. The ribs of the **opposite side** may be injected by reaching across the midline or by moving to the opposite side of the stretcher. If the anesthesiologist moves to the opposite side, the syringe is best held in the caudad hand again. This is now an opposite arrangement, and appears awkward to the beginner when the nondominant hand is caudad. If a right-handed anesthesiologist attempts to block the patient's right side with the syringe in his or her right hand, it is difficult to maintain the necessary cephalad angle. The needle

often pivots and points caudad when "walked off" the rib, and the local anesthetic (LA) solution is injected away from rather than toward the nerve.

11. If a **celiac plexus or lumbar somatic** block is to be added, it is performed at this point.
12. After completion of the block, the stretcher can be taken to the operating room and the patient simply rolled over onto the operating table, where the block can be tested and further anesthesia and surgery can begin.

B. Intercostal nerve block, **midaxillary approach.** When the patient's abdomen is distended or pain prevents the prone or lateral approach, the intercostal nerves can be reached in the mid- or posterior axillary line while the patient lies supine. This is also a good approach for postoperative pain relief at the conclusion of surgery if intercostal blocks were not performed at the beginning of the procedure. It is more awkward, but it is not difficult technically.

1. With the patient in the supine position, the patient's arms are extended laterally on armrests. The ribs are palpated and marked as far posteriorly as practical, usually in the posterior axillary line.
2. Skin preparation and draping are done on both sides, and skin wheals are raised if the patient is alert. (This can be performed at the start or end of a general anesthetic with no need for local anesthesia.)
3. The anesthesiologist may stand either at the head of the bed or at the side. The technique of injection is the same as that in the prone position, with the syringe held in the caudad hand and control alternating between the upper and lower hands as the needle is "walked off" the rib, injection is made, and the syringe is advanced to the next rib.

C. Continuous intercostal block technique. A **continuous technique** has also been described, using insertion of a standard epidural catheter in the intercostal space by means of a Tuohy needle. This may produce anesthesia of several levels because of medial spread of injected solutions to the peridural or paravertebral levels. This usually provides **anesthesia for three or four segments**. This technique of intrapleural injection may be useful for postoperative analgesia (see Chapter 10).

D. Rectus sheath block. Bilateral blockade is necessary for midline analgesia.

1. The original approach is a tactile one. A 4-cm (1.5-in.) 22-gauge needle is inserted on each side just medial to the lateral border of the rectus muscle at the level of the umbilicus. The needles are advanced until the anterior sheath of the rectus is identified by an increased resistance, or the firm fascial plane is identified by moving the needle back and forth until a "scratching" sensation is appreciated. The anterior sheath is entered, and then the posterior sheath sought in a similar manner. LA (10–20 mL) is then injected on each side after aspiration and a suitable test to avoid intravascular injection. If the fascial planes cannot be identified easily, the technique should be abandoned to avoid the risk of peritoneal entry and perforation of a viscus.
2. This block is easier to perform with **ultrasound guidance**, which allows easy identification of the fascial planes, and can reduce the chance of intravascular or intraperitoneal injection by direct visualization of the needle tip (Figure 9.4). The planes are identified by placing the probe lateral to the umbilicus, and an in-plane injection made with the same needle as above, depositing the LA just above the posterior sheath.

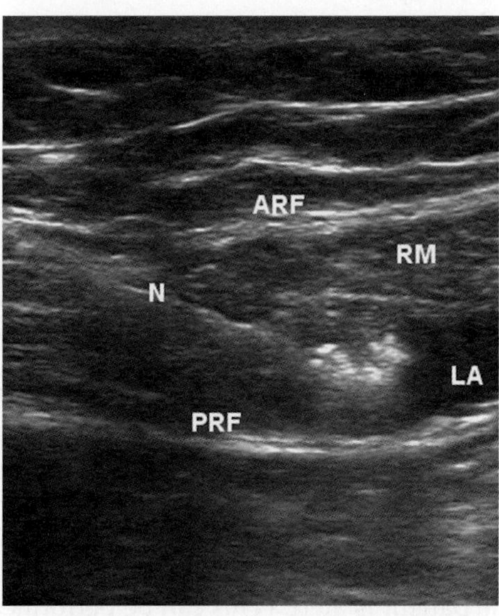

Figure 9.4. Rectus sheath block. The terminal branches of the intercostal nerves of the abdomen lie between the posterior rectus sheath and the muscle. The needle (*N*) can be advanced in-plane from the lateral border of the rectus muscle (*RM*) to pierce the anterior fascia of the rectus sheath (*ARF*) and stop on the anterior surface of the posterior sheath (*PRF*). Local anesthetic (*LA*) injected in this plane will produce anesthesia of several of the terminal branches, usually T9-11. Blockade needs to be performed bilaterally to produce anesthesia for periumbilical procedures.

E. Ilioinguinal-iliohypogastric blockade This technique is most commonly done in children, and is described in Chapter 21, but is also suitable (and desirable!) for hernia repairs in adults.

1. For adults, a 4 cm (1.5 in.) 22-gauge needle is inserted perpendicularly through the skin 2 cm (1 in.) medial to the anterior superior iliac spine. The fascial planes of the external oblique, internal oblique, and the transversalis muscle can be appreciated. Several fan-wise injections of 5 mL of LA are injected as the needle is withdrawn from the level of the transversalis to create a "wall" of solution between the iliac crest and the umbilicus, along the paths of the nerves. Care is taken not to advance the needle through the transversalis into the abdominal contents.
2. Ultrasound guidance, again, allows a more precise identification of the nerves, which may lie at varying levels in the fascial planes at this point. The probe is placed over the skin just medial to the anterior superior iliac spine, perpendicular to the path of the nerves (Figure 9.5). The nerves are identified as hypoechoic areas between the fascial layers, commonly between the internal and external obliques, but they may be in variable positions. A 4 cm (1.5 in.) needle is introduced in-plane and 5 mL of LA injected directly on each nerve under direct visualization.

V. Complications

A. Pneumothorax is the most commonly feared complication of intercostal block, but it is **rare in experienced hands**. The key to prevention is **rigid control of**

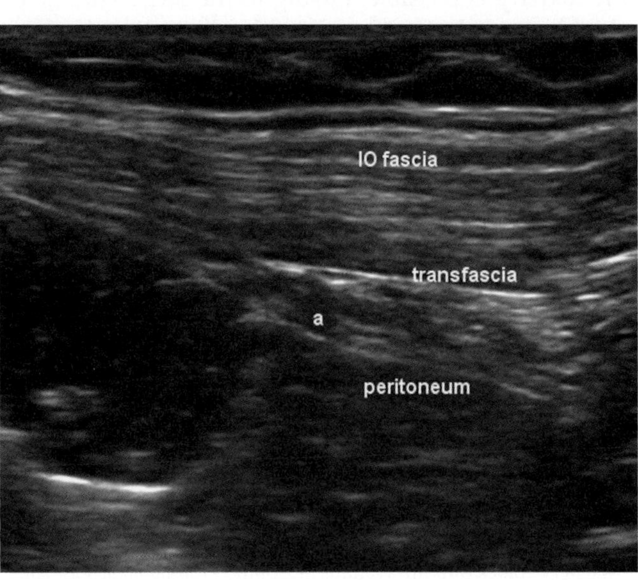

Figure 9.5. Ultrasound guidance for ilioinguinal block. The linear probe is placed over the inguinal area medial and caudad to the anterior superior iliac spine. The internal oblique muscle and fascia (*IO fascia*) and the transversalis muscle and fascia (*transfascia*) are readily identified. The ilioinguinal and iliohypogastric nerves pierce the transversalis at a variable point, and lie between the transversalis and the internal oblique. The ideal technique is to advance the needle in-plane under ultrasound vision to the plane of the nerves, where a small volume of local anesthetic is effective. The peritoneum and abdominal cavity lie just beneath, and small branches of the femoral artery (*a*) can also be seen.

the depth of penetration of the needle by the upper hand resting solidly on the back during the time of injection. In addition, the needle remains safely on top of the rib for every part of the block except the injection itself. The lower hand, which exerts poorer control because of its lack of fixation and longer "lever arm," does nothing except inject while the needle is below the rib. The fingers of this hand are not moved in and out of the rings except when the needle is "parked" on the top of the rib. With these precautions, the technique is quite safe and pneumothorax will occur in less than 1% of patients. It should be suspected if the patient experiences coughing or chest pain during injection or if localization of the ribs is difficult and associated with frequent, deep, and blind probings (an undesirable variant of the technique). If pneumothorax is suspected clinically, **a chest x-ray** should be ordered and the air leak treated appropriately if confirmed.

B. **Airway obstruction and respiratory depression** are the **more frequent complications** of intercostal blockade, related to generous sedation in the prone position during performance of the block. **Ventilation and resuscitation equipment, including naloxone, should be available**. Supplemental nasal oxygen and pulse oximetry are indicated.

C. **Respiratory inadequacy** can occur after intercostal block if **motor blockade of the intercostal** and upper abdominal muscles is produced in a patient whose diaphragm is ineffective and who depends on intercostal muscles for tidal ventilation.

D. **Systemic toxicity** is possible. Owing to the large volume of solution injected into a highly vascular space, systemic absorption is significant. Even with epinephrine added to 0.5% bupivacaine, blood levels of bupivacaine may reach 2 mg/mL, the highest for any of the peripheral nerve blocks. A **lower concentration** of either bupivacaine or ropivacaine (0.25%) will reduce the blood levels to approximately 1 mg/mL (5). Similar considerations are appropriate when using large volumes for rectus sheath blockade to attempt to provide wider spread.

E. **Hypotension** occurs rarely and may be the result of subarachnoid injection into a dural sleeve if the injection is made too far medially. More commonly, it is produced by epidural or paravertebral spread of LA to the sympathetic chain. Drugs injected in the intercostal space can easily track medially and spread to several dermatomes above and below the injection.

REFERENCES

1 Concha M, Dagnino J, Cariaga M, et al. Analgesia after thoracotomy: epidural fentanyl/bupivacaine compared with intercostal nerve block plus intravenous morphine. *J Cardiothorac Vasc Anesth* 2004;18:322–326.

2 Willschke H, Bosenberg A, Marhofer P, et al. Ultrasonography-guided rectus sheath block in paediatric anaesthesia—a new approach to an old technique. *Br J Anaesth* 2006;97:244–249.

3 Willschke H, Bosenberg A, Marhofer P, et al. Ultrasonographic-guided ilioinguinal/iliohypogastric nerve block in pediatric anesthesia: what is the optimal volume? *Anesth Analg* 2006;102:1680–1684.

4 Templeton T. Rectus block for postoperative pain relief. *Reg Anesth* 1993;18:258–260.

5 Kopacz DJ, Emanuelsson BM, Thompson GE, et al. Pharmacokinetics of ropivacaine and bupivacaine for bilateral intercostal blockade in healthy male volunteers. *Anesthesiology* 1994;81:1139.

10 Paravertebral Block

Christopher M. Bernards

I. Introduction

Paravertebral block refers to blockade of spinal nerves as they exit the intervertebral foramen. Intercostal block is often preferred over paravertebral block in areas where the rib is easily identified because it requires less local anesthetic per nerve blocked and is often technically easier. However, at spinal levels lacking a rib (lumbar) or where the rib may be difficult to locate posteriorly (e.g., upper and lower thoracic), paravertebral block can be used to block spinal nerves. Unlike peripheral nerve blocks, paravertebral block produces anesthesia with a strictly dermatomal distribution.

II. Anatomy

A. The spinal nerves exit the spinal canal through the intervertebral foramina. The foramina are formed by a "notch" in adjacent vertebral pedicles (Figure 10.1).

B. The foramina lie anterior to and approximately midway between the transverse processes of adjacent vertebrae. The transverse process is the critical bony landmark for paravertebral block (see the following text). Importantly, the anatomic description that follows is of the "average" patient. Individuals may differ from this for multiple reasons (e.g., normal human variability, compression fractures, kyphoscoliosis). As with all regional techniques, clinicians must keep this in mind so that they can adjust their technique as necessary when encountering an individual whose landmarks seem to differ from the "mean."

1. The **transverse processes** cannot be palpated but must be located in relation to the more readily identified spinous process. The relationship of the transverse process to the spinous process varies along the length of the spine because the angle of the spinous process varies as a function of vertebral level.
   a. In **lumbar vertebrae**, the spinous processes are elongate and the cephalad edge of the spinous process is at the level of the transverse process of the same vertebra.
   b. In thoracic vertebrae, the spinous processes have a bulbous tip. This tip lies at the level of the transverse process of the vertebra ***below*** it.
   c. The 11th and 12th thoracic vertebra represent a transition between the more cephalad thoracic vertebrae and the lumbar vertebrae. The spinous process of these vertebrae are elongate like the lumbar vertebrae but the cephalad edge does not quite extend to the lower edge of its own transverse process.
2. In the thoracic and lumbar regions, the spinal nerves (and associated dermatome) are named for the vertebrae that forms the **cephalad** half of the intervertebral foramen through which they pass. For example, the L4 spinal nerve exits between the L4 and L5 vertebrae.

C. In the **thoracic area**, the vertebral body, spinous process, and pleura form a triangular area through which the spinal nerve courses (Figure 10.2). This area is important because the spinal nerve gives rise to a posterior branch here, which courses posteriorly to innervate the skin of the back. This posterior

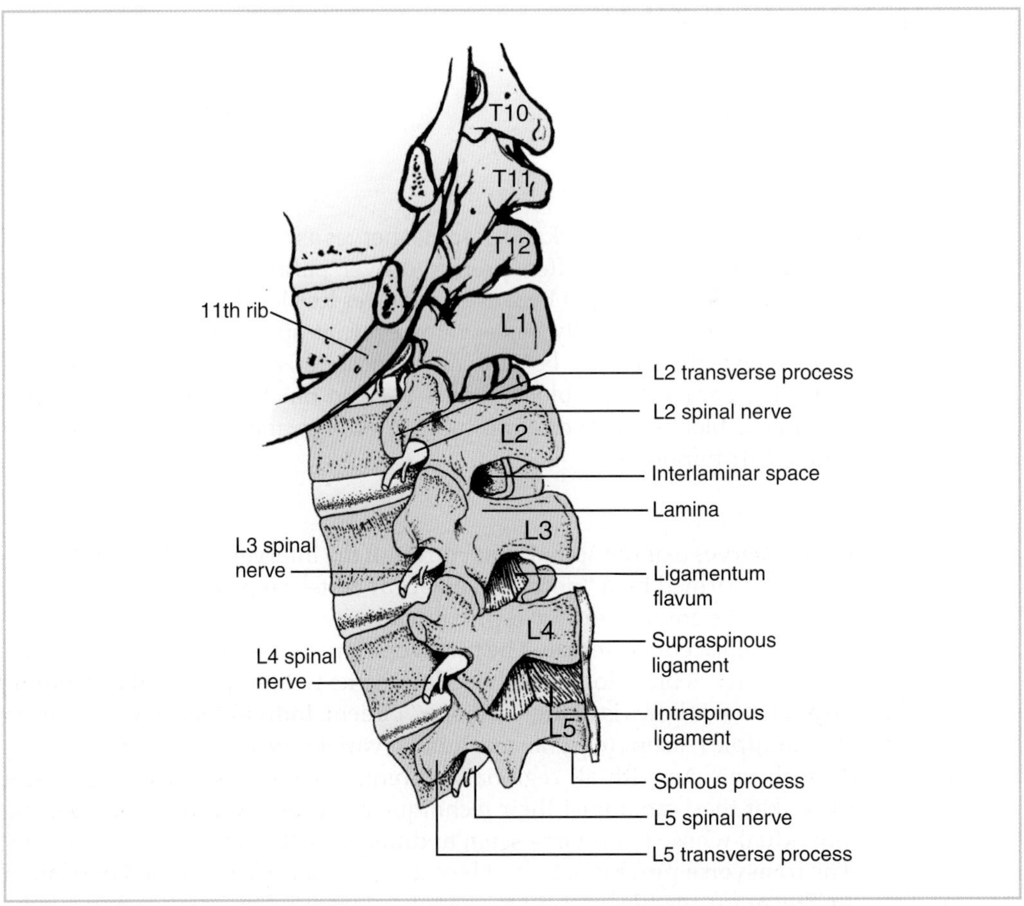

Figure 10.1. Relationship between the spinous processes, transverse processes, and spinal nerves in the lumbar and thoracic spine. The lumbar spinal nerves course caudad to the transverse process of the vertebrae for which they are named.

branch can be missed during intercostal block if local anesthetic is placed too far laterally. Paravertebral block obviates this potential problem.

III. Indications

A. Paravertebral block is indicated any time a **dermatomal** block distribution is desired. It is particularly useful when a strictly unilateral block is desired.

1. Caveat. Because innervation overlaps across the midline, areas near the midline may not be adequately blocked by unilateral paravertebral (or intercostal) block. Similarly, there is overlap between adjacent dermatomes on the same side so that it is almost always necessary to place blocks one dermatomal level above and below the desired level(s) to assure complete block of the targeted dermatome(s).

B. Outpatient surgery. Paravertebral block is well suited to outpatient surgery because it generally does not impair the sympathetic nervous system as extensively as does epidural/spinal anesthesia and can produce analgesia lasting 10 hours or more with long-acting local anesthetics. Also, unlike central neuraxial block, paravertebral block is unlikely to affect micturition or to

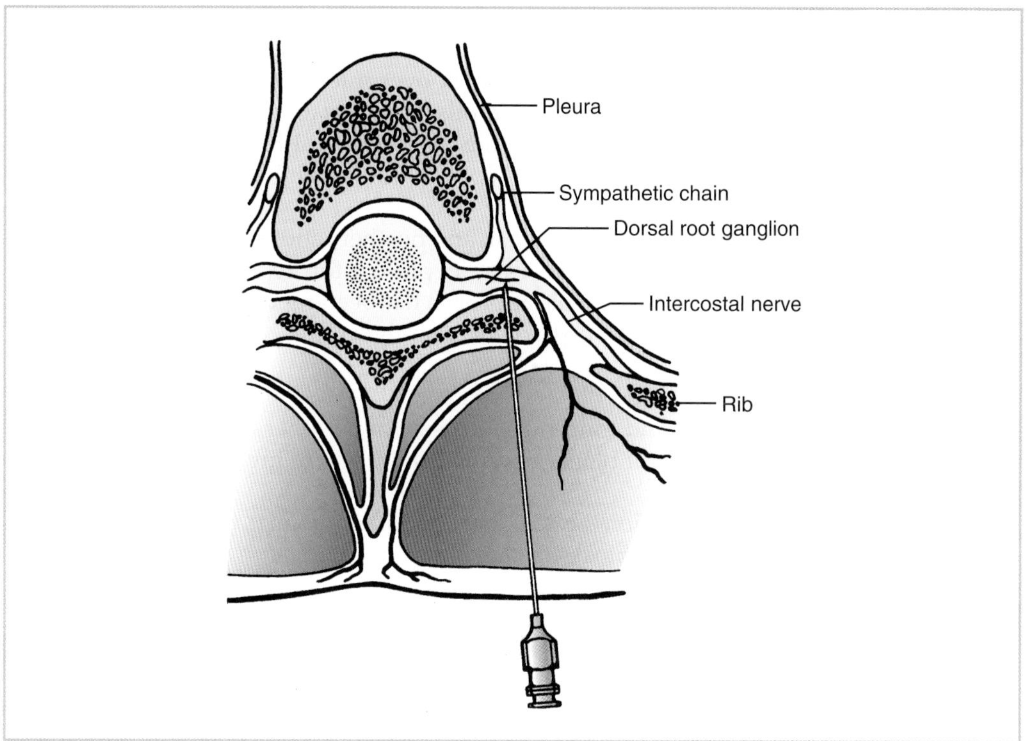

Figure 10.2. Thoracic paravertebral block. The thoracic spinal nerves exit the intervertebral foramen and enter a small triangular space formed by the vertebral body, the pleura, and the plane of the transverse process. The needle is advanced off the superior border of the transverse process and into this triangle. The depth from the transverse process to the nerve is approximately 2 cm. Some medial angulation is important to reduce the chance of entering the pleura and causing a pneumothorax.

significantly impair lower extremity motor function (above L2), which should speed discharge.

C. **Specific uses.** There are numerous potential uses of paravertebral block, either as a "stand-alone" regional anesthesia technique or in combination with other blocks (e.g., intercostal). Given in the subsequent text are a few common examples.

1. **Breast surgery.** Thoracic paravertebral block has been shown to be superior to general anesthesia in terms of postoperative pain, nausea/vomiting incidence, and ambulatory discharge time (1).
2. **Inguinal hernia.** As with breast surgery, paravertebral block has been shown to be superior to general anesthesia (less postoperative pain, nausea/vomiting, and faster discharge) for inguinal hernia repair (2, **3**).
3. **Postsurgical analgesia: thoracotomy/thoracoscopy.** Thoracic paravertebral block provides excellent analgesia for thoracic surgery and has been shown to be superior to thoracic epidural analgesia (lower pain scores, less hypotension, less nausea/vomiting, better pulmonary function). The ability to place a catheter for continuous local anesthetic infusion is an important advantage of paravertebral block over intercostal block (**4**, 5).
4. **Other pain therapy.** Both single-injection and continuous techniques can be useful with longer-term pain problems.

a. **Rib fracture.** Rib fractures are readily treated by paravertebral block (6). The ability to place a catheter for continuous infusion is a significant advantage of paravertebral block over intercostal block and a reduced effect on the sympathetic nervous system is an advantage over thoracic epidural analgesia. Continuous paravertebral block also has potential advantages over epidural block in the setting of concomitant spinal trauma.

b. **Herpes zoster** (acute outbreak and postherpetic neuralgia). Unlike intercostal block, a catheter can be placed for repetitive or continuous paravertebral block. This approach has been reported to be successful in treating refractory postherpetic neuralgia (7).

IV. **Local anesthetics**

A. Any local anesthetic and concentration used for peripheral nerve block is appropriate for paravertebral block. Specific examples are given in the subsequent text.

1. Intermediate-duration amide local anesthetics (e.g., **lidocaine, mepivacaine**) will produce blocks lasting 3 to 5 hours.
2. Long-duration amide local anesthetics (e.g., **bupivacaine, levobupivacaine, ropivacaine**) will produce blocks lasting 8 to 14 hours.
3. As with other blocks, more dilute solutions (lower doses) produce less motor block and shorter-duration sensory blocks.

B. The local anesthetic volume required per nerve blocked is significantly higher with paravertebral blocks than with intercostal blocks; therefore, fewer dermatomes can be safely blocked than would be the case with intercostal block.

V. **Lumbar technique**

A. **Position.** The block can be performed with the patient in any position, although prone (with an abdominal pillow to flex the spine) and sitting are probably easier (especially for bilateral blocks) than lateral.

B. **Mark injection sites.** Identify the spinous processes associated with the nerves to be blocked and mark them along their entire length. Draw transverse lines through the spinous processes of the vertebrae for the targeted nerves. Three to four centimeters lateral to the spinous processes, draw vertical lines connecting the transverse lines (Figure 10.3). The lines should intersect over the inferior edge of the vertebra's transverse process.

1. In the lumbar region, the superior border of the spinous process is at the same level as the caudad edge of its own transverse process (Figure 10.1). Also, because the spinal nerve is named for the vertebra forming the cephalad half of the intervertebral foramen, the spinal nerve exits **inferior** to the transverse process of the vertebra for which it is named.

C. Aseptically prepare and drape the skin and raise local anesthetic skin wheals at each intersection of the transverse and vertical lines.

D. **Needle placement**

1. **Fixed-depth technique.** Insert a 6- to 8-cm (2.5–3.5 in.) 22-gauge or larger needle through the skin wheal at a 10- to 30-degree cephalad angle (Figure 10.4).

a. Depending on the girth of the patient, the transverse process should be contacted at a depth of 2.5 to 5 cm (1–2 in.). If the transverse process is not contacted at the expected depth, gently probe cephalad and caudad parallel to the neuraxis.

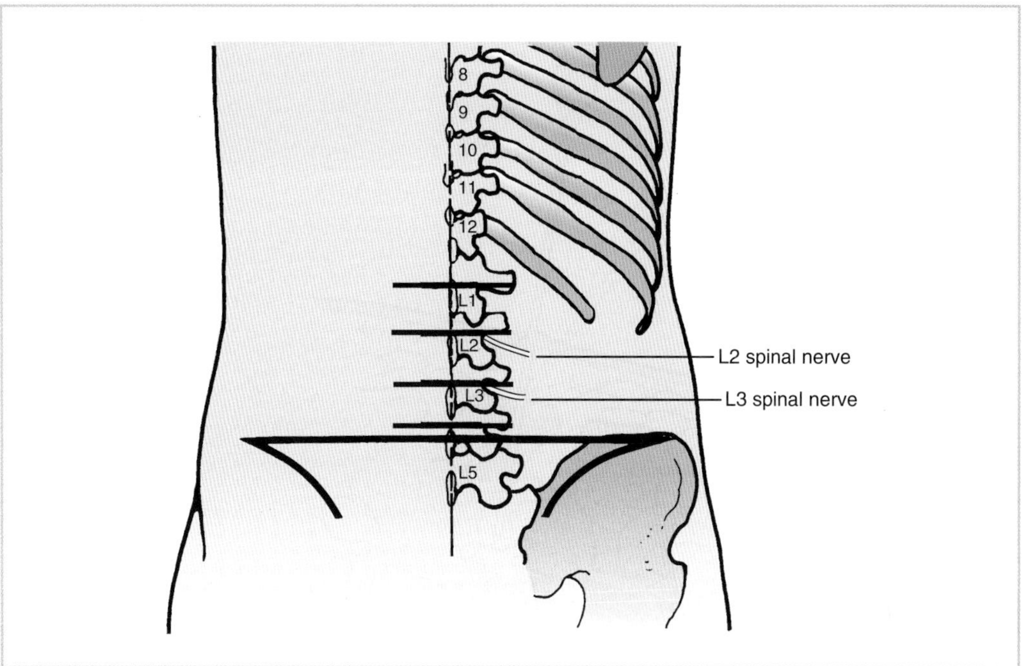

Figure 10.3. Cutaneous landmarks for lumbar paravertebral block. The entire spinous process is outlined, and the horizontal lines pass through the cephalad edge of the process. The intersection of the horizontal and vertical lines should lie above the caudad edge of the transverse process, and the needle should be inserted at this point with a slight (10- to 30-degree) cephalad angle to contact the transverse process.

b. Once the transverse process is contacted, mark the depth. The depth is important because the nerve will lie approximately 2 cm deeper than the posterior surface of the transverse process.

c. Withdraw the needle to the skin and redirect caudally (i.e., more perpendicular to the skin) and slightly medially to a depth approximately 2 cm deeper than the inferior edge of the transverse process.

(1) If bone is contacted at roughly the same depth at which the transverse process was originally contacted, then the needle was probably not directed caudally enough and the transverse process has been hit again (Figure 10.4). Withdraw the needle and direct slightly more caudally until the needle passes beyond the transverse process.

(2) If bone is contacted deeper than the transverse process, this is probably the vertebral body. Withdraw the needle and contact the transverse process. Reinsert the needle with slightly less medial angulation to a depth 2 cm beyond the transverse process.

2. Ultrasonographic technique. Because the hyperechoic transverse process causes the image to drop out below it, ultrasonography cannot generally be used to visualize the spinal nerve. However, ultrasonography can be used to identify the transverse process and to determine the depth from the skin to the process (8). This measurement makes it easier to place the needle at the correct depth.

3. Nerve stimulator technique. As with peripheral nerve blocks, nerve stimulation can aid in identifying the spinal nerve during paravertebral block.

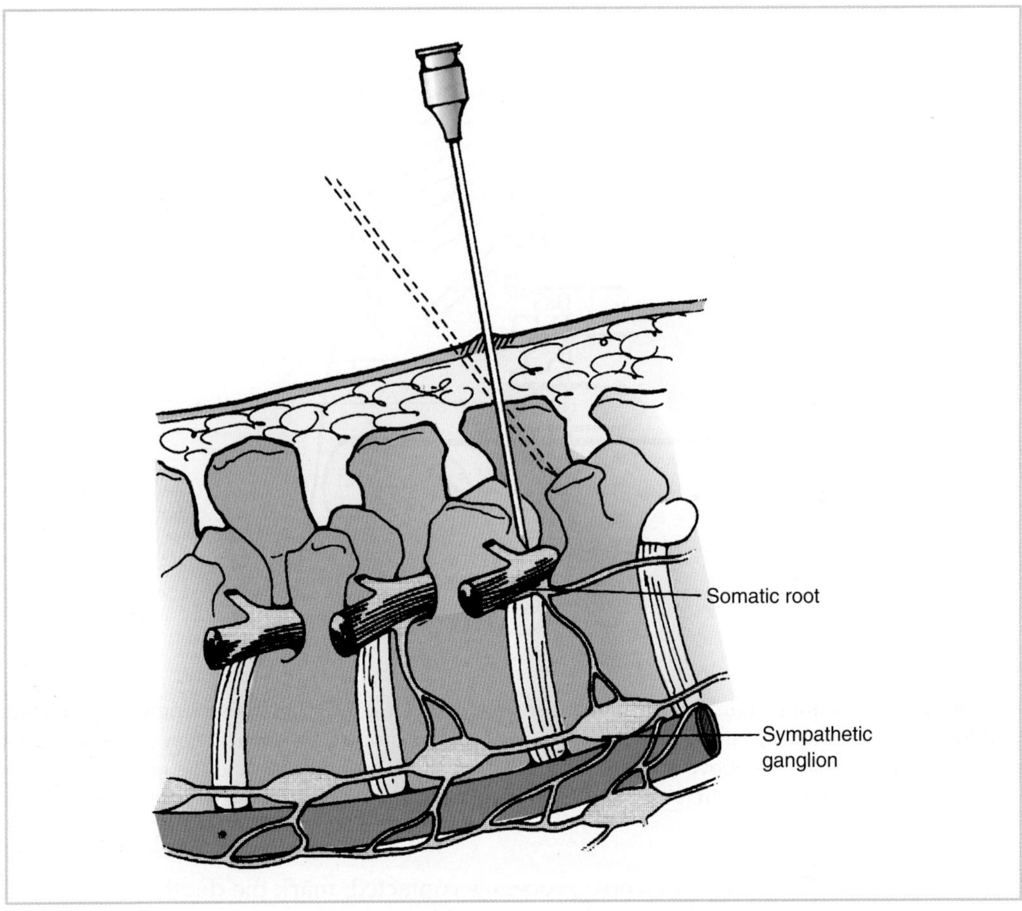

Figure 10.4. Lumbar paravertebral block, lateral view. The needle is introduced at the lower border of the transverse process (Figure 10.3) and angled slightly cephalad to contact the transverse process. The needle is then walked caudad off the transverse process and advanced 2 cm beyond the depth at which the process was contacted. Paresthesias are not necessary, and injection of 10 mL of anesthetic will block the nerve.

Segmental muscle contraction corresponding to the targeted nerve at a current of 0.4 to 0.6 mA has been reported to yield a 100% successful block rate for thoracic paravertebral block in 60 women undergoing breast surgery (1).

E. **Drug injection.** With the needle fixed in position, aspirate to detect intravascular (blood) or subarachnoid (cerebrospinal fluid [CSF]) location and incrementally inject 4 to 8 mL local anesthetic.

VI. Thoracic technique

A. **Position.** As with the lumbar paravertebral block, prone, lateral, or sitting positions are appropriate.

B. **Marking injection sites.** The skin is marked much as described for lumbar paravertebral block except that the vertical lines are placed only 3 cm lateral to the midline because the vertebrae are narrower in the thoracic region.

1. Importantly, because thoracic transverse processes slope caudally, the tip of the spinous process is at the level of the **caudad** vertebrae's transverse

process, not its own. Therefore, when blocking thoracic spinal nerves the needle is walked off the **cephalad** edge of the transverse process to reach the spinal nerve corresponding to the palpated spinous process.

C. Aseptic **skin preparation** and local anesthetic skin wheals are as for the lumbar paravertebral block.

D. **Needle placement.** The same techniques (fixed depth, nerve stimulator, ultrasonography) used to place the needle for lumbar paravertebral block can be applied to thoracic paravertebral block. Differences are as follows:

   1. The depth from the skin to the transverse process is less (2–4 cm).
   2. The needle may contact the rib (which connects to the spine at the transverse process) if it is inserted too far lateral.
   3. After contacting the transverse process, the needle is redirected **cephalad** (instead of caudad) and walked over the edge (see Section VI.B.1).

E. **Loss-of-resistance technique.** Although not as clear as the loss of resistance used to identify the epidural space, there is a **subtle** loss of resistance as the tip of the block needle exits the superior costotransverse ligament to lie in the thoracic paravertebral space (8). This technique is not applicable to the lumbar paravertebral space because there is no costotransverse ligament equivalent.

   1. To use the loss-of-resistance technique, an air-filled loss-of-resistance syringe is attached to the block needle and **gentle** pressure exerted as the needle is advanced beyond the transverse process. Loss of resistance indicates entry into the paravertebral space. This is a technique that can be used by anybody even when using fixed depth, ultrasonography, or nerve stimulation as the primary technique. However, use of the loss-of-resistance technique as the sole means of identifying the thoracic paravertebral technique should probably be left to those with significant experience.
   2. A dramatic loss of resistance should make one concerned that the needle is in the thorax.

F. **Paravertebral catheterization.** The thoracic paravertebral space is amenable to catheterization. Catheters are generally placed with **Tuohy needles**. Unlike the epidural space, catheter advancement will be met with significant resistance because the paravertebral space is not a "space" in the same sense as the epidural space. This problem can be overcome by injecting 5 to 10 mL of solution to create a space to accommodate the catheter.

   1. If the catheter threads easily, one should be concerned that the needle is in the thorax.

G. **Drug injection.** As with lumbar paravertebral block, aspirate in an effort to detect intravascular or subarachnoid needle placement. Incrementally inject 3 to 7 mL local anesthetic.

   1. Unlike the lumbar paravertebral block, drug injected into the thoracic paravertebral space can spread cephalad and caudad to reach spinal nerves one or more levels beyond the targeted nerve. Consequently, if multiple contiguous nerves are to be blocked a somewhat smaller volume of local anesthetic can be used at each site. In fact, this approach is preferable to injecting a large volume at a single level (9). There is no such communication between different levels in the lumbar paravertebral block.

VII. Complications

Paravertebral blocks are subject to the same types of complications associated with other nerve blocks.

A. **Failed block.** Reported failure rates range from 0% to 10%. The largest single study to date reported a failure rate of 6.1% in adults ($n = 620$) and zero in children ($n = 42$) using a nerve stimulator technique (10).
B. **Intravascular needle placement.** When defined as positive blood aspiration, Naja et al. reported the rate of intravascular needle placement to be 6.8% in adults and zero in children (10). Not surprisingly, the risk in any individual patient increased as the number of injections increased.
C. **Hematoma.** Naja et al. reported that hematomas occurred in 2.4% of patients (10). All hematomas were superficial and successfully treated with local pressure.
D. **Pneumothorax.** Naja et al. reported a 0.5% incidence of pneumothorax (10). The risk of pneumothorax increased with increasing number of injections.
E. **Central neuraxial block.** Naja et al. reported that signs of epidural or intrathecal injection occurred in 1% of patients (11). Spinal block may occur if the needle enters the "dural sleeve," where it extends beyond the intervertebral foramen and may result in "total spinal" if the dose is sufficient (especially at high thoracic levels) (10). Epidural block may occur if local anesthetic tracks back along the spinal nerve to reach the epidural space.
F. **Hypotension.** The risk of hypotension would be expected to be very low with paravertebral block and in fact Naja et al. reported an incidence of just 4%. There are multiple potential mechanisms by which paravertebral block might cause hypotension. Block of the spinal nerve will cause a dermatomal sympathetic block, which would not be expected to cause hypotension unless a large number of nerves are blocked bilaterally. The sympathetic chain ganglia lie along the vertebral body slightly anterior and medial to the site for paravertebral block. A misplaced needle could cause hypotension by blocking the sympathetic chain. Unintentional epidural and spinal blocks could also cause hypotension for obvious reasons.
G. **Systemic toxicity.** Because of the relatively large local anesthetic doses required and the rapid absorption (12) of local anesthetic following paravertebral block, the risk of central nervous system toxicity is probably greater than with central neuraxial or peripheral nerve blocks.

VIII. Summary

Although less commonly performed than central neuraxial and peripheral nerve blocks, there are clinical situations in which the paravertebral block may be nearly ideal. Mastering the technique will significantly increase the regional anesthesiologist's versatility.

REFERENCES

1 Naja MZ, Ziade MF, Lonnqvist PA. Nerve-stimulator guided paravertebral blockade *vs.* general anaesthesia for breast surgery: a prospective randomized trial. *Eur J Anaesthesiol* 2003;20(11):897–903.
2 Naja Z, Ziade MF, Lonnqvist PA. Bilateral paravertebral somatic nerve block for ventral hernia repair. *Eur J Anaesthesiol* 2002;19(3):197–202.
3 **Hadzic A, Kerimoglu B, Loreio D, et al. Paravertebral blocks provide superior same-day recovery over general anesthesia for patients undergoing inguinal hernia repair. *Anesth Analg* 2006;102(4):1076–1081.**
4 **Davies RG, Myles PS, Graham JM. A comparison of the analgesic efficacy and side-effects of paravertebral *vs.* epidural blockade for thoracotomy—a systematic review and meta-analysis of randomized trials. *Br J Anaesth* 2006;96(4):418–426.**

5 Richardson J, Sabanathan S, Jones J, et al. A prospective, randomized comparison of preoperative and continuous balanced epidural or paravertebral bupivacaine on post-thoracotomy pain, pulmonary function and stress responses. *Br J Anaesth* 1999;83(3):387–392.
6 Karmakar MK, Critchley LA, Ho AM, et al. Continuous thoracic paravertebral infusion of bupivacaine for pain management in patients with multiple fractured ribs. *Chest* 2003;123(2):424–431.
7 Naja ZM, Maaliki H, Al-Tannir MA, et al. Repetitive paravertebral nerve block using a catheter technique for pain relief in post-herpetic neuralgia. *Br J Anaesth* 2006;96(3):381–383.
8 Pusch F, Wildling E, Klimscha W, et al. Sonographic measurement of needle insertion depth in paravertebral blocks in women. *Br J Anaesth* 2000;85(6):841–843.
9 Naja MZ, Ziade MF, El Rajab M, et al. Varying anatomical injection points within the thoracic paravertebral space: effect on spread of solution and nerve blockade. *Anaesthesia* 2004;59(5):459–463.
10 Naja Z, Lonnqvist PA. Somatic paravertebral nerve blockade. Incidence of failed block and complications. *Anaesthesia* 2001;56(12):1184–1188.
11 Lekhak B, Bartley C, Conacher ID, et al. Total spinal anaesthesia in association with insertion of a paravertebral catheter. *Br J Anaesth* 2001;86(2):280–282.
12 Karmakar MK, Ho AM, Law BK, et al. Arterial and venous pharmacokinetics of ropivacaine with and without epinephrine after thoracic paravertebral block. *Anesthesiology* 2005;103(4):704–711.

11 Sympathetic Blockade

Christopher M. Bernards

I. Introduction

The sympathetic nervous system is a **purely efferent** system involved in a wide range of homeostatic functions including vasomotor tone, myocardial contractility, heart rate, bronchial tone, perspiration, gastrointestinal secretions, genitourinary function, pupil diameter, and so on. Sympathetic blocks can be used both **diagnostically** and **therapeutically** to block these functions (e.g., perspiration in hyperhydrosis or vasomotor tone in vascular insufficiency). Also, there are pathological pain states involving the sympathetic nervous system (e.g., sympathetically maintained pain) that can benefit from sympathetic block.

In addition, there are afferent sensory nerves, particularly from the viscera, that travel with the efferent sympathetic fibers. Blockade of these sensory afferents can relieve pain either as an adjunct to surgical anesthesia or to treat both malignant and nonmalignant chronic pain.

Sympathetic blockade can be performed based solely on the **anatomic landmarks** described in the subsequent text and this degree of accuracy is generally sufficient when using these blocks as an adjunct to surgical anesthesia (e.g., celiac plexus block as part of a general anesthetic for cholecystectomy). However, when used for diagnostic or neurolytic block use of **radiographic** (e.g., computed tomography [CT], fluoroscopy) or **ultrasound** guidance is recommended because of the greater accuracy these techniques provide.

II. Anatomy

A. The cell bodies of sympathetic **preganglionic neurons** arise in the intermediolateral gray matter of spinal segments from T1 to L2. These cell bodies receive input from both local spinal interneurons as part of sympathetic reflex arcs and descending control from brainstem centers (Figure 11.1).

B. Sympathetic preganglionic neurons from each spinal cord segment course within the **corresponding spinal nerve** as it traverses the intrathecal and epidural spaces. After exiting the spinal canal, the sympathetic neurons leave the spinal nerve as the white **rami communicantes** to enter one of the sympathetic chain ganglia where they then take one of three paths (Figure 11.1):

1. The preganglionic neuron may synapse with the **second order** (postganglionic) neuron within the nearest paravertebral (sympathetic chain) ganglion.
   - **a.** The sympathetic chain or "paravertebral" ganglia are generally paired ganglia on the right and left anterolateral aspect of the T1 to L2 vertebral bodies.
2. The preganglionic neuron may pass through the paravertebral ganglion and travel rostral or caudal to synapse with a postganglionic neuron in another local or distant paravertebral ganglion.
   - **a.** The postganglionic neurons originating in the paravertebral ganglia pass through the gray rami communicantes to rejoin the adjacent spinal nerve and travel with it to provide sympathetic innervation to the tissues innervated by that nerve.

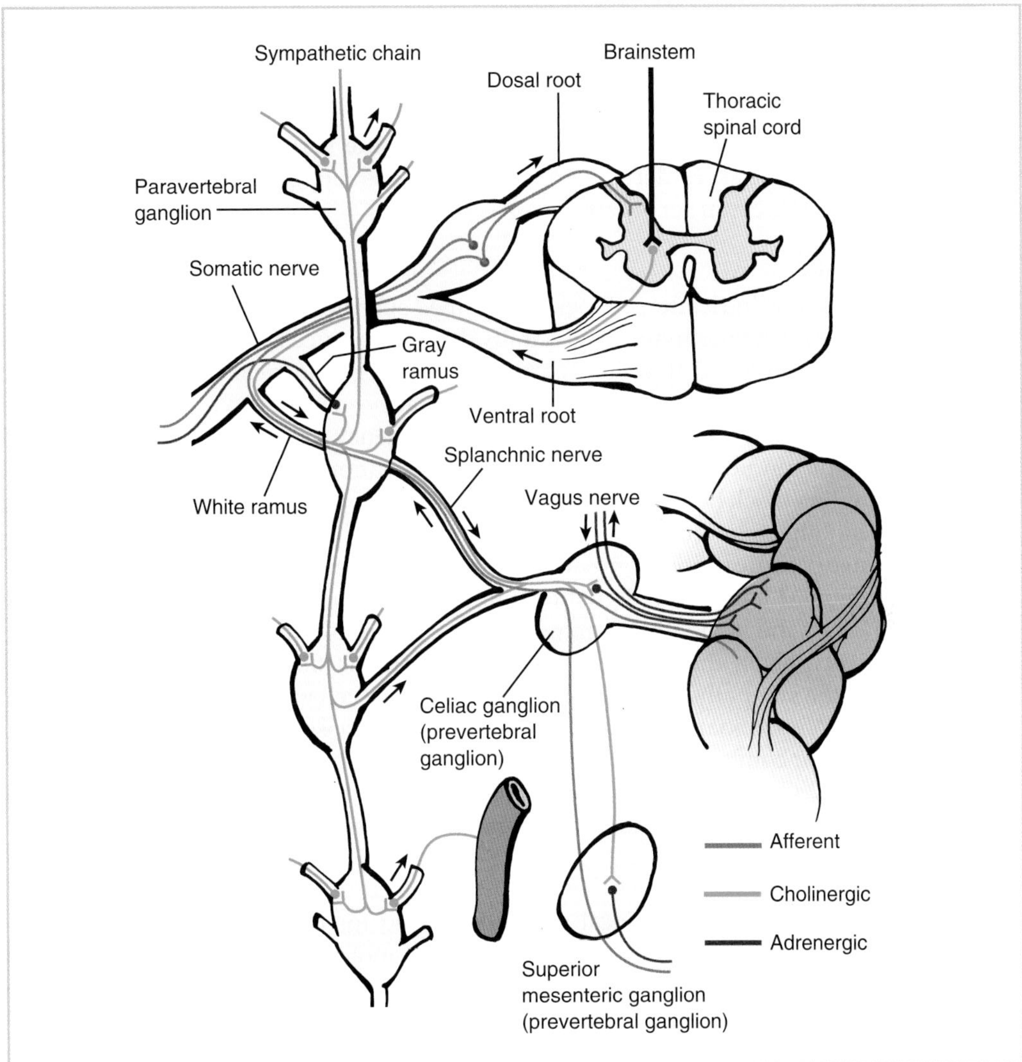

Figure 11.1. Sympathetic nervous system pathways. Sympathetic preganglionic cell bodies reside in the intermediolateral gray matter of the spinal cord (T1-L2) and receive input from neurons descending from the brainstem and from local interneurons. Preganglionic sympathetic fibers (cholinergic) exit the spinal cord within the corresponding spinal nerve and enter the sympathetic chain ganglia through the white rami communicantes where they may (i) synapse with a postganglionic sympathetic neurons (adrenergic), (ii) pass through the sympathetic chain ganglion without synapsing and reenter the spinal nerve of origin through the gray rami communicantes and synapse with a postganglionic neuron in one of the distant prevertebral ganglia, or (iii) travel along the sympathetic chain to synapse with a postganglionic neuron in a different ganglion in the sympathetic chain.

b. There is a great deal of **overlap** in sympathetic innervation so that a single spinal nerve may carry sympathetic activity arising in multiple spinal cord segments.

3. The **preganglionic neuron** may pass through the paravertebral ganglion to synapse with the postganglionic neuron in a prevertebral ganglion (e.g., superior cervical, superior mesenteric) or the adrenal gland.

C. **Plexuses.** Aggregations of sympathetic nerves and prevertebral ganglia in the thoracic, abdominal, and pelvic cavities are termed *plexuses*. There are four generally recognized plexuses: **cardiac, pulmonary, celiac, and hypogastric,** which innervate the heart, lungs, abdominal viscera, and pelvic organs, respectively.

1. Plexuses lie along the **anterior aspect of the vertebral bodies** or the aorta and the nerves derived from them course along nearby blood vessels to reach their target organs.

III. Indications

A. **Autonomic indications.** Blocks performed specifically to interrupt sympathetic nervous system activity are generally done to produce vasodilatation in an effort to improve blood flow in a particular area (1) or to treat hyperhydrosis. For example, block of the sympathetic chain has been used successfully to increase blood flow in the setting of vascular insufficiency, particularly in patients who are not candidates for surgical revascularization (2). More recently, stellate ganglion block has been shown to be effective in producing long-lasting (weeks to months) relief from severe "hot flashes" associated with menopause (3).

B. **Sensory indications.** Sympathetic blocks are probably most often used to treat malignant and nonmalignant pain. In this context, they are employed not to block the sympathetic ganglia *per se*; rather the intent is to block afferent sensory fibers that travel with the sympathetic fibers and pass through or near the sympathetic ganglion. Blockade of the celiac plexus to treat malignant and nonmalignant intra-abdominal pain is a classic example. Celiac plexus blockade combined with intercostal blocks can be used for upper abdominal surgery. Ganglionic blockade has also been used to supplement surgical general anesthesia and to provide postoperative analgesia.

IV. Drugs

A. **Local anesthetics.** All local anesthetics used for peripheral nerve blocks are appropriate for ganglionic blocks. Because motor block is not an issue when performing ganglionic blocks (there are no somatic motor fibers present), **dilute local anesthetic solutions** can be used if desired (e.g., 0.25% bupivacaine, 0.5% lidocaine). Shorter-acting agents might be useful for diagnostic blocks or for efficacy trials before surgical extirpation or neurolytic block.

B. **Neurolytic agents.** Both **alcohol** and **phenol** have been used successfully to produce neurolytic block of ganglia. Alcohol is often preferred for use around great vessels (e.g., celiac block) because it is thought to be less likely to damage them. Both agents can cause unintended damage to nearby neural structures, for example, spinal nerves or spinal cord.

V. Specific blocks

A. Stellate ganglion block

1. **Anatomy.** The stellate ganglia are formed by a variable fusion of the first (sometimes second, third, and even fourth) thoracic ganglion and the lower two cervical segmental ganglia, which is why it is sometimes called the *cervicothoracic ganglion*. Position is somewhat variable but "on average" the ganglion lies just anterior to the lateral edge of the C7 and T1 vertebral bodies. At this level, a good portion of the ganglion is behind the vertebral and subclavian arteries and medial to the cupola of the lung (Figure 11.2).

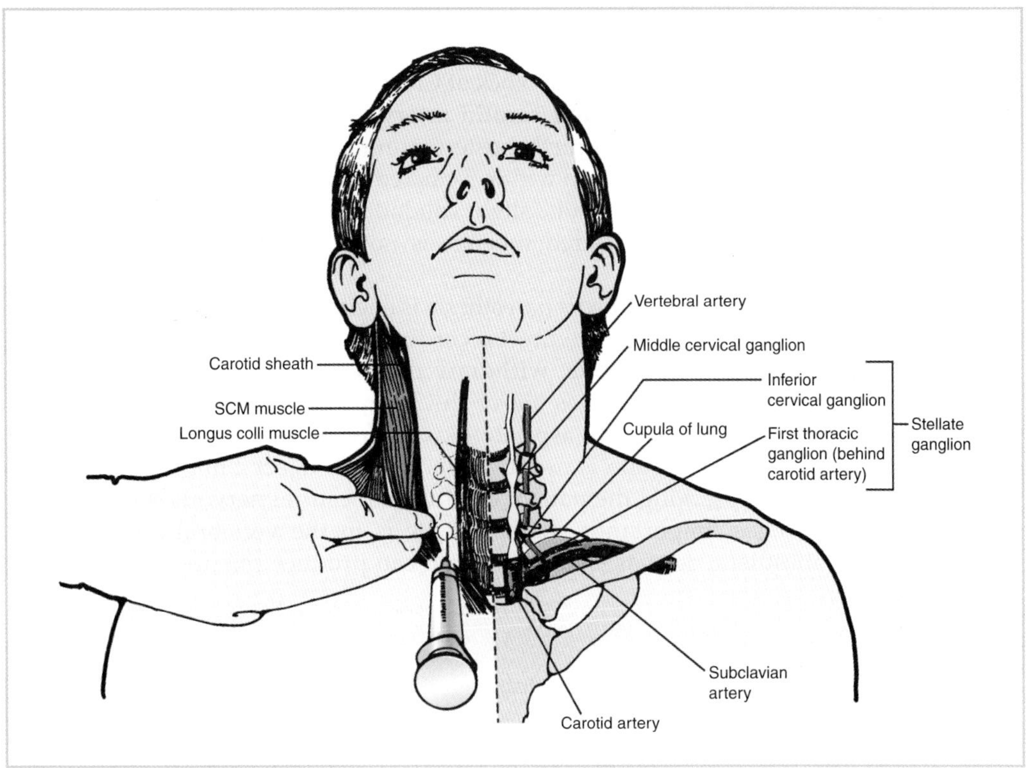

Figure 11.2. Stellate ganglion block. The stellate ganglion is formed by a variable fusion of the first thoracic (sometimes second, third, and fourth as well) and inferior cervical ganglia (sometimes middle cervical ganglion also). The ganglion generally lies along the lateral border of C7 and T1 vertebrae sometimes extending to the inferior edge of C6 or as low as T4. The bulk of the ganglion lies posterior to the carotid and vertebral arteries and posteromedial to the cupula of the lung. Because of the proximity of multiple "high-risk" structures the block is usually performed at the level of the C6 or C7 transverse processes and sufficient volume (7–10 mL) is used to assure sufficient inferior spread. SCM, sternocleidomastoid.

a. Because of the proximity of multiple "high-risk" structures, the stellate ganglion is generally not blocked directly. Rather the block is made at the C6 or C7 transverse process and ganglionic blockade relies on administration of a sufficient local anesthetic volume to spread caudally to reach the ganglion. Direct block of the ganglion, as would be needed for neurolytic drugs, is probably best accomplished under CT guidance.

2. Technique

a. Position the patient supine with the neck in slight extension.

b. Skin **landmarks**. Mark the cricoid cartilage and the medial border of the sternocleidomastoid muscle on the side to be blocked. Approximately 2 cm lateral to the edge of the cricoid cartilage, palpate the tubercle of the C6 vertebral process (**Chassaignac tubercle**). This is usually the most prominent transverse process in the neck. Mark the skin overlying the tubercle. If the block is to be made at C7, place a second mark approximately 2 cm directly caudad of the mark overlying the C6 tubercle. This second mark will lie over the C7 transverse process.

c. After aseptic preparation, raise a skin wheal at the mark to be used for the block.

d. Whether performing the block at C6 or C7, gently retract the **sternocleidomastoid** muscle and **carotid artery** laterally and insert a 22- or 25-gauge 6-cm needle directly posterior until bone is contacted (Figure 11.3). If bone is not contacted within 5 cm, redirect the needle slightly medially and reinsert. If this fails, slight caudad or cephalad angulation may be required. If the desired tubercle is not easily contacted, reassess the landmarks.

   (1) If a brachial plexus paresthesia is elicited, the needle is too far lateral and posterior—redirect accordingly.

e. After contacting bone, **withdraw** the needle approximately 2 mm so that the needle tip lies above the longus colli muscle in the plane of the ganglion. Gently **aspirate** looking for blood or cerebrospinal fluid (CSF). If aspiration is negative, very slowly inject 2 mL local anesthetic while observing the patient carefully for central nervous system (CNS) changes. Importantly, if the needle is in the vertebral artery a local anesthetic dose as small as 0.5 mL can produce seizures (4). If the test

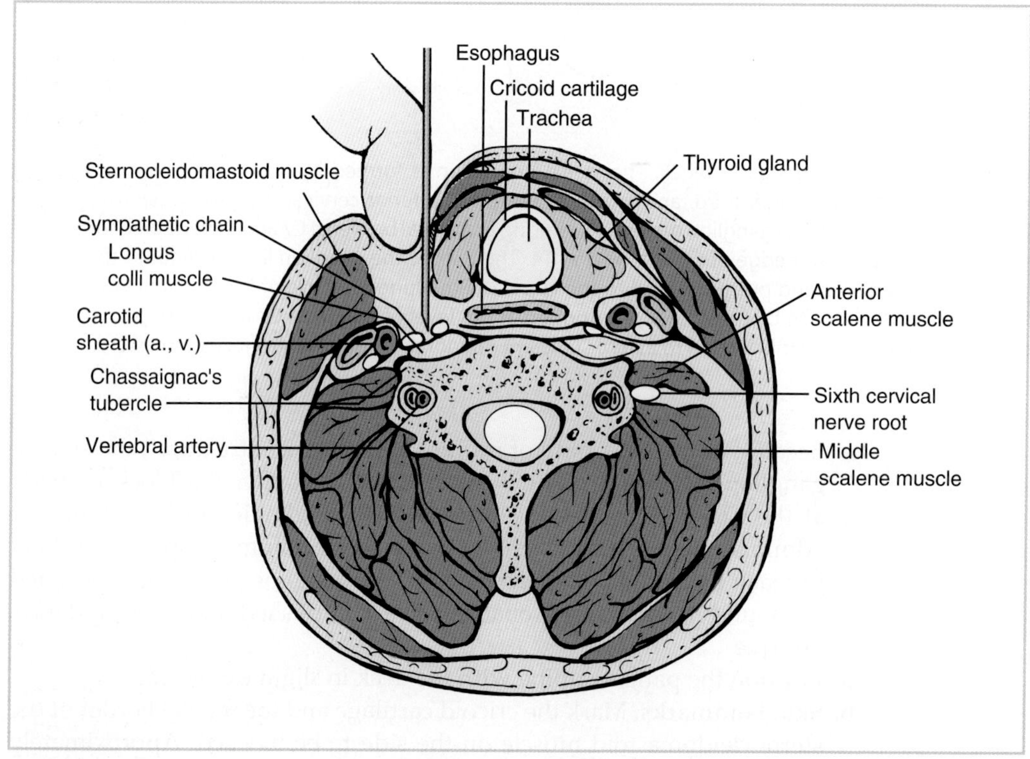

Figure 11.3. Cross-section of stellate ganglion block. Palpate the tubercle of C6 and retract the sternocleidomastoid muscle and carotid sheath laterally. Insert the needle onto the tubercle. Once bone is contacted, withdraw the needle approximately 2 mm so that the needle tip lies above the longus colli muscle. The stellate ganglion lies caudad to the C6 vertebral body and block results from caudal spread of local anesthetic. At this level, only fibers of the sympathetic chain running between the stellate ganglion and the middle cervical ganglion are present. The block is performed similarly at C7 (see text).

dose is negative, incrementally inject an additional 5 to 10 mL local anesthetic with frequent aspiration and constant assessment of mental status.

3. **Signs/symptoms of block.** Stellate ganglion block will result in **Horner syndrome** (ptosis, miosis, facial anhidrosis, enophthalmos, and injected sclera) within 10 minutes. Also, nasal congestion and varying degrees of vasodilatation of the arm will likely occur.
4. **C6 versus C7 approach.** The C6 approach offers the potential benefit of a lower risk of pneumothorax and intravascular injection. However, sympathetic block of the upper extremity is more complete when the block is performed at C7.
5. **Complications.** Complications of stellate ganglion block include the following:
   a. **Hematoma/hemorrhage**
   b. **Pneumothorax**
   c. **Intravascular injection/systemic toxicity**
   d. **Epidural/intrathecal injection**
   e. **Spinal cord trauma**
   f. **Unintended nerve blocks.** Vagus, phrenic, recurrent laryngeal, and other nerves can be blocked either by inaccurate needle placement or by excessive local anesthetic spread.
   g. **Physiological effects.** Stellate ganglion block can both shorten (left-sided block) and prolong (right-sided block) QTc; therefore, care should be exercised in patients with preexisting prolonged QTc (5). Stellate ganglion block also decreases cerebrovascular resistance on the ipsilateral side resulting in increased blood flow to that side and a simultaneous decrease on the contralateral side. Whether this poses a risk to patients with cerebrovascular or carotid vascular disease is unknown.

B. Celiac plexus block

1. **Anatomy** (Figure 11.4)
   a. **Location.** The celiac plexus is a **variable collection** of ganglia and autonomic nerves (both sympathetic and parasympathetic) located anterior to the aorta at the level of the T12 to L1 vertebral bodies (lower on the left than the right).
   b. **Ganglia.** The number of ganglia present in the celiac plexus has been found to range from 2 to 10 with an average of 5.5 (6).
   c. **Innervation.** The celiac plexus receives sympathetic preganglionic fibers from the **greater, lesser, and least splanchnic nerves**. The greater and lesser splanchnics course from their spinal segments of origin through the mediastinum to pierce the diaphragmatic crura to reach the celiac plexus. The splanchnic or retrocrural approach to the celiac plexus block aims to block these nerves as opposed to the plexus *per se*. The least splanchnic nerve is derived from the lumbar sympathetic chain ganglia.

      Parasympathetic nerves from the vagus also pass through the celiac plexus as do afferent sensory fibers originating in the abdominal organs. It is these afferent sensory fibers that are generally being targeted by celiac plexus block.

      Sympathetic postganglionic fibers are distributed to most of the organs of the upper abdomen including liver, spleen, stomach, pancreas, kidneys, small bowel, and large bowel to the splenic flexure.

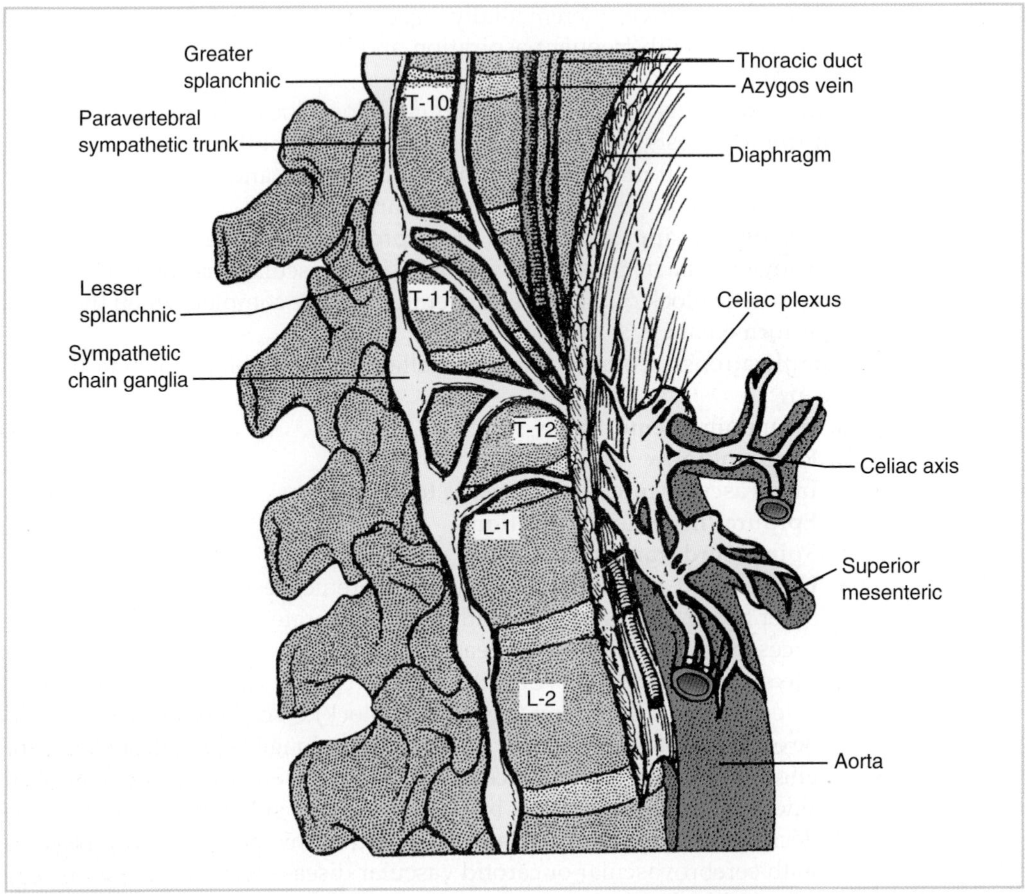

Figure 11.4. Celiac plexus anatomy: The celiac plexus comprises a variable number of sympathetic ganglia and associated nerves straddling the aorta near the takeoff of the celiac and superior mesenteric arteries. Sympathetic afferents reach the plexus through the greater, lesser, and least splanchnic nerves and sympathetic efferent nerves course along the arterial branches arising from the aorta to supply blood to abdominal organs and viscera. Parasympathetic fibers from the vagus and afferent sensory fibers from the abdomen also travel through the celiac plexus.

   d. **Surrounding structures.** The celiac plexus is distributed along the anterior and lateral surface of the **aorta** between the origin of the celiac and superior mesenteric arteries. The **adrenal glands** lie lateral to the plexus and the stomach and pancreas are anterior.

2. **Technique**
   a. Position the patient **prone** with a pillow under the hips to minimize lumbar lordosis.
   b. Identify and mark the caudad edge of **the 12th thoracic and 1st lumbar spinous processes**. Mark the inferior edge of the 12th rib at a point 7 to 8 cm lateral to the midline. Connect the marks over the rib margins with the mark over the T12 spinous process. This will result in a **shallow triangle,** the sides of which will provide guides for the direction of the block needles (Figure 11.5).

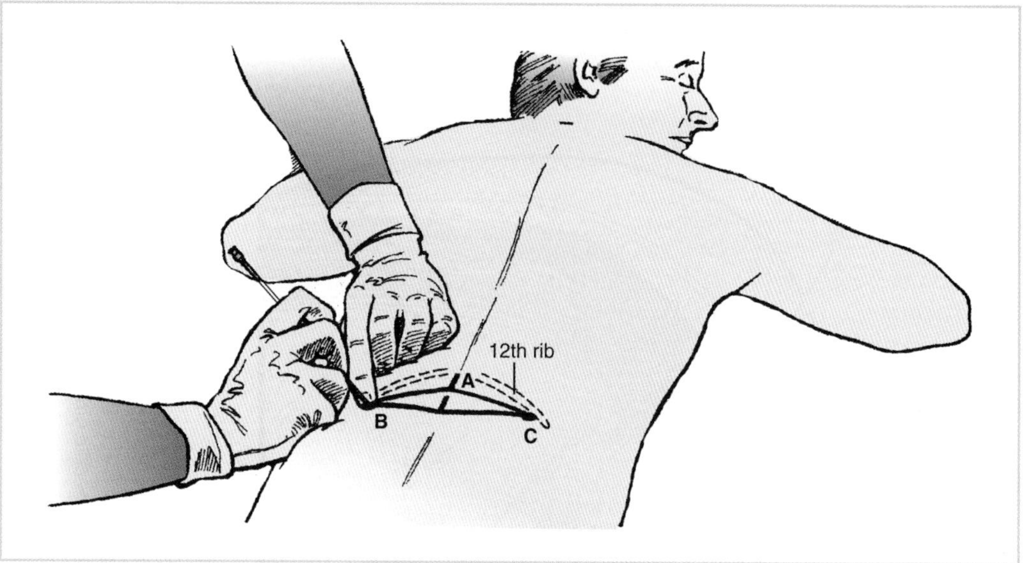

Figure 11.5. Celiac plexus block: cutaneous landmarks. Mark the inferior edge of the T12 (point *A*) and L1 spinous processes and the inferior edge of the 12th rib at a point 7 to 8 cm lateral of the midline (points *B* and *C*). Connect points *A*, *B*, and *C* to form a triangle, the base of which should pass over the inferior edge of the L1 spinous process.

c. Aseptically prepare the skin and raise skin wheals at the marks over the ribs. Infiltrate local anesthetic 4 to 6 cm deeper toward the L1 vertebral body in the direction of the T12 spinous process.

d. Bilaterally, insert 10- to 15-cm (depending on the patient's size) 20-gauge needles at a 45-degree angle (relative to a sagittal plane running through the spine) beginning at the marks over the 12th rib and directed along the lines connecting the rib with the T12 spinous process. Insert the left-sided needle first because it will serve to indicate the depth for the right-sided needle.

e. The needles should contact the **L1 vertebral body** at a depth of 7 to 10 cm. More superficial bony contact is likely the L1 transverse process (Figure 11.6). It is important to correctly distinguish the superficial transverse process from the deeper vertebral body so that drug injection is not made too superficially where it could produce extensive epidural, spinal, or psoas compartment blocks.

f. After identifying the L1 vertebral body, withdraw the needle sufficiently to be able to redirect it at a slightly less steep angle (again, relative to a sagittal plane running through the spine) so that the needle tip just slides off the lateral side of the vertebral body. **Multiple redirections** may be necessary.

g. After clearing the edge of the vertebral body, slowly advance the left needle constantly feeling for the transmitted pulsations of the aorta. When **aortic pulsations** are felt, stop advancing the needle. On the right side, slowly advance the needle to a depth approximately 1 cm farther than the aorta was encountered on the left. A lateral radiograph should confirm that the needle tips project just ahead of the vertebral body (Figure 11.6).

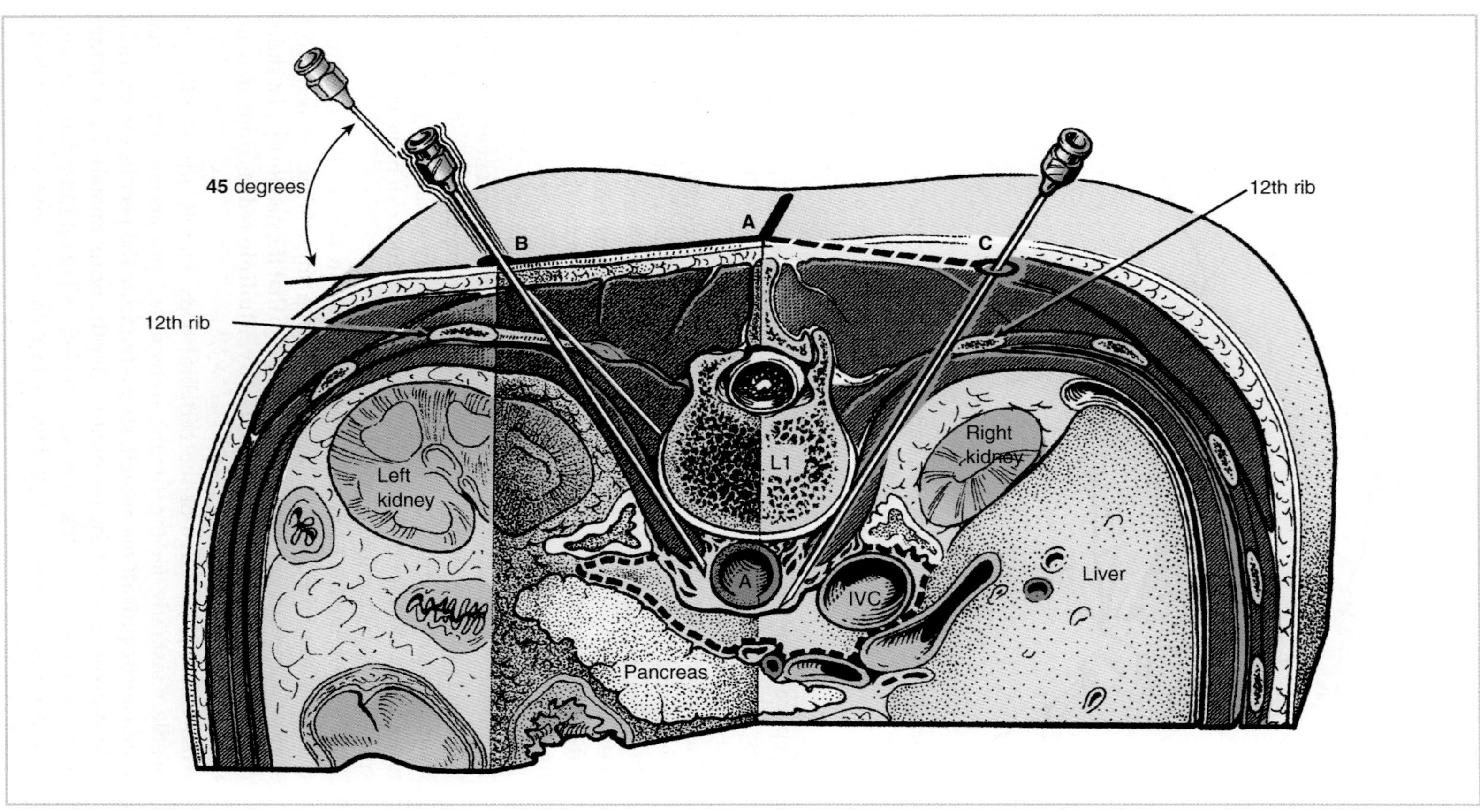

Figure 11.6. Celiac plexus block: needle insertion. Advance the first needle at a 45-degree angle along line *BA* (*left side*). The L1 vertebral body should be contacted at a 7 to 10 cm depth. After contacting the vertebral body, partially withdraw the needle and reinsert it at a slightly more vertical angle so as to walk off the lateral edge of the vertebral body. Insert the needle until aortic pulsations are felt. Insert the right-sided needle (line *CA*) similarly but advance 1 cm deeper than the needle on the left. See text for full details.

h. Carefully **aspirate** while slowly rotating the needles to identify intravascular, intrarenal, or subarachnoid location of the needle tip. If negative, inject 3 mL of an epinephrine-containing local anesthetic test dose and observe for signs of intravascular, epidural, or subarachnoid location.

i. Following a negative **test dose**, incrementally inject 20 to 25 mL local anesthetic through each needle. This relatively large volume is necessary because of the diffuse localization of the components of the plexus and the fact that the needles are located behind the aorta and vena cava and local anesthetic solution must spread anteriorly to reach the plexus.

   Injection should meet little resistance if made through a 20-gauge needle and some authors prefer this diameter needle because the low resistance to injection helps confirm correct needle location in the loose tissue of the retroperitoneal space. Other authors prefer the smaller-diameter 22-gauge needle because it makes a smaller hole if the aorta, hollow viscus, or solid organs are accidentally pierced. However, this needle requires significant force to overcome the higher resistance to injection and therefore provides no "feedback" as to the location of the needle.

j. **Radiographic guidance.** Celiac plexus block can and for many years has been performed solely based on the landmarks discussed earlier. However, for diagnostic and therapeutic neurolytic blocks the greater precision/confidence afforded by radiographic visualization (e.g., fluoroscopy, CT scan) is highly desirable.

3. **Signs/symptoms of block.** One of the earliest signs of celiac plexus block is significant **hypotension** because of widespread vasodilatation. Patients may also experience an urge to defecate (and in fact may have uncontrolled defecation) because sympathetic block results in unopposed parasympathetic stimulation of the bowel. This seems to be especially true of patients who have been on high-dose opioids for pain.

4. **Other approaches**
   a. **Paramedian.** Singler has described a paramedian approach in which needles are inserted caudad to the T12 spinous process at a point 3 cm lateral to the midline in a plane perpendicular to the skin (7). This technique decreases the risk of hitting the kidney but makes identifying the correct depth difficult without radiographic guidance.
   b. **Anterior.** The plexus can be approached through the anterior abdominal wall using either fluoroscopic or ultrasound guidance with a reportedly low incidence of complications (8).
   c. **Endoscopic.** More recently, the gastroenterology literature has described an endoscopic ultrasound-guided approach to the celiac plexus block (9, 10).

5. **Complications.** Celiac plexus block is associated with many of the same types of complications inherent in all regional anesthesia procedures:
   a. **Hematoma/hemorrhage**
   b. Damage to **adjacent structures** (e.g., kidney, bowel, and adrenal) either because of needle contact or because injected drug (especially neurolytic drugs) causes tissue damage.
   c. **Pneumothorax**
   d. **Infection** (especially if the bowel is punctured)

e. **Bowel, bladder, and sexual dysfunction** if local anesthetic/neurolytic spread is excessive and reaches the lumbar plexus or the spinal cord.

C. **Deep splanchnic block is an alternative approach** to blocking the nerves traveling to and from the celiac plexus and some have referred to this as the *retrocrural approach* to the celiac plexus. However, it will miss the sympathetic nerves that reach the plexus from below the diaphragm (e.g., least splanchnic nerve) and any sensory fibers traveling with it. It is generally used for diagnosis/treatment of abdominal pain and not for surgical anesthesia/analgesia.

1. **Anatomy** is described in the preceding text for the celiac plexus (Figure 11.7).
2. **Technique.** The same equipment is used and the patient is positioned and landmarks identified and marked as for celiac plexus block. The needles are directed slightly more cephalad than for celiac plexus block so that the tips end up anterior to the body of the **12th thoracic vertebra** just posterior to the crura of the diaphragm. Contrast injection (1–2 mL) should result in linear spread along the vertebral bodies **above the diaphragm**. Once appropriate spread is confirmed, 4 to 5 mL local anesthetic solution or neurolytic agent is usually sufficient.
3. **Splanchnic or celiac block?** Splanchnic block offers the potential advantage of a much **smaller volume** of local anesthetic/neurolytic solution; a lower risk of damage to subdiaphragmatic structures; and much lower risk of bladder, bowel, or sexual dysfunction. However, not as many pathways that might be contributing to abdominal pain will be blocked by deep splanchnic block as by celiac plexus block.
4. **Complications.** Similar to celiac plexus block except that the risk of **pneumothorax** is higher and the risk of damage to nerves controlling bowel, bladder, and sexual function is less. Because the thoracic duct traverses the left side of the retrocrural space, injury is possible resulting in chylothorax or lymphedema. Hypotension is less than with celiac plexus block.

D. **Lumbar sympathetic block**

1. **Anatomy.** Sympathetic innervation to the lower extremities can be blocked at the **lowermost of the paired parasympathetic chain ganglia**. Most of the sympathetic innervation to the lower extremities passes through these **"gateway" ganglia**, which lie along the anterolateral aspect of the vertebral bodies. Human cadaver studies suggest that the best places to block these ganglia are the caudal third of the L2 vertebral body or the cephalad third of the L3 vertebral body (11). For local anesthetic blocks, a single injection of a large volume (20–25 mL) will generally spread sufficiently cephalad and caudad to block multiple paravertebral ganglia. For **neurolytic** blocks where excessive spread increases the risk of unintended damage to nearby structures (e.g., somatic nerves), it may be advisable to perform blocks at several levels with small volumes.
2. **Technique**
   a. Position the patient prone with a pillow under the lower abdomen if necessary to remove the lumbar lordosis.
   b. Mark the L2 spinous process. Draw a line perpendicular to the spine through the middle of the L2 spinous process and mark an "X" along this line 5 cm lateral of the midline. This line should overlie the L2 transverse process (Figure 11.8).

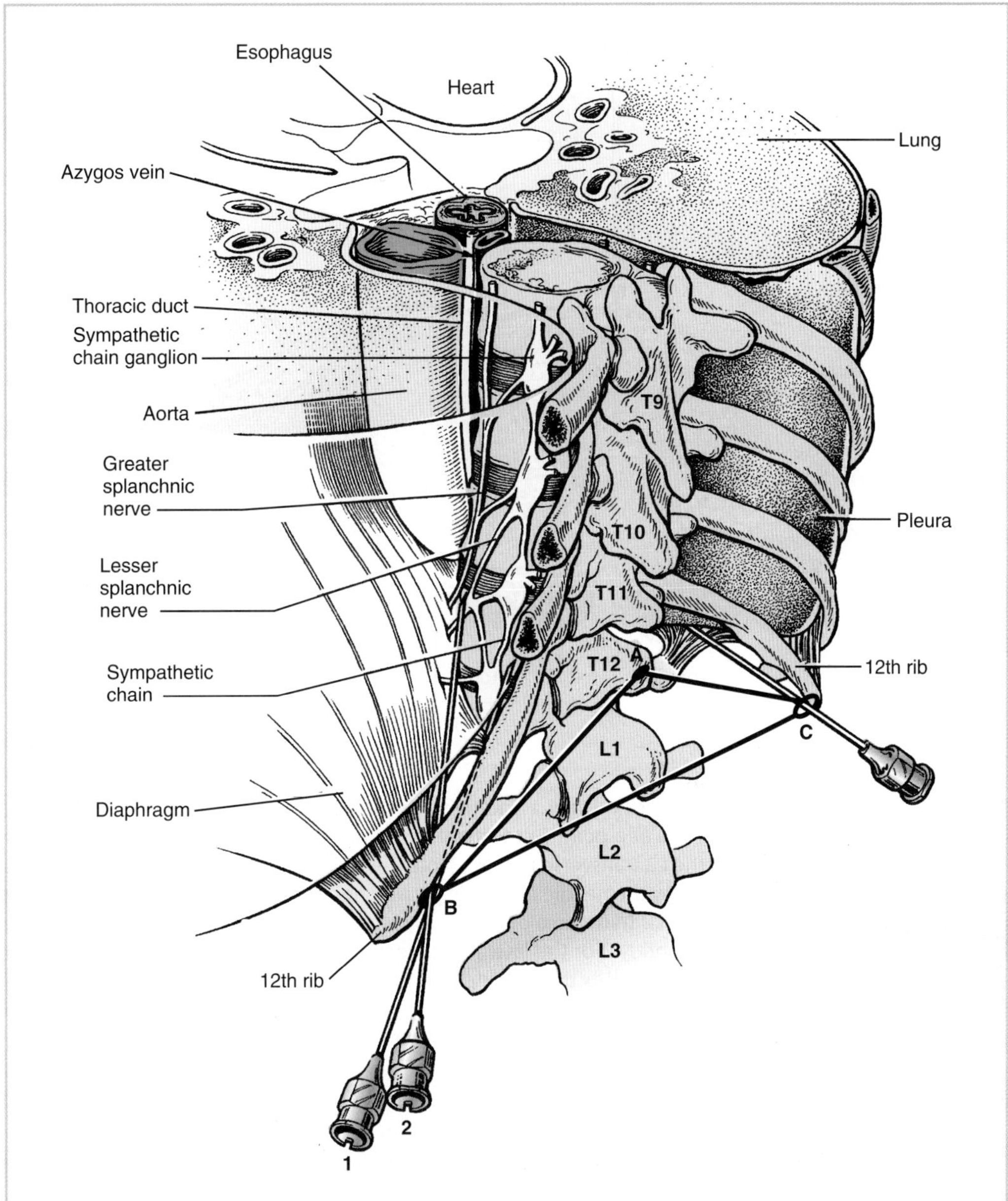

Figure 11.7. Deep splanchnic block. Skin markings are similar as for celiac plexus block except that point *A* is made at the superior edge of T12. The needles are advanced along lines *BA* and *CA* so that the tips end up anterior to the T12 vertebral body just posterior to the diaphragm.

c. Aseptically prepare the skin and raise a skin wheal at each X. Insert a 10 cm long 20- or 22-gauge needle through the skin wheel at a 45-degree cephalad angle. Slowly advance the needle until it contacts the **L2 transverse process** (Figure 11.8). Note the depth.
d. Withdraw the needle sufficiently to allow it to be redirected perpendicular to the skin in the cephalocaudad plane and slightly medially.

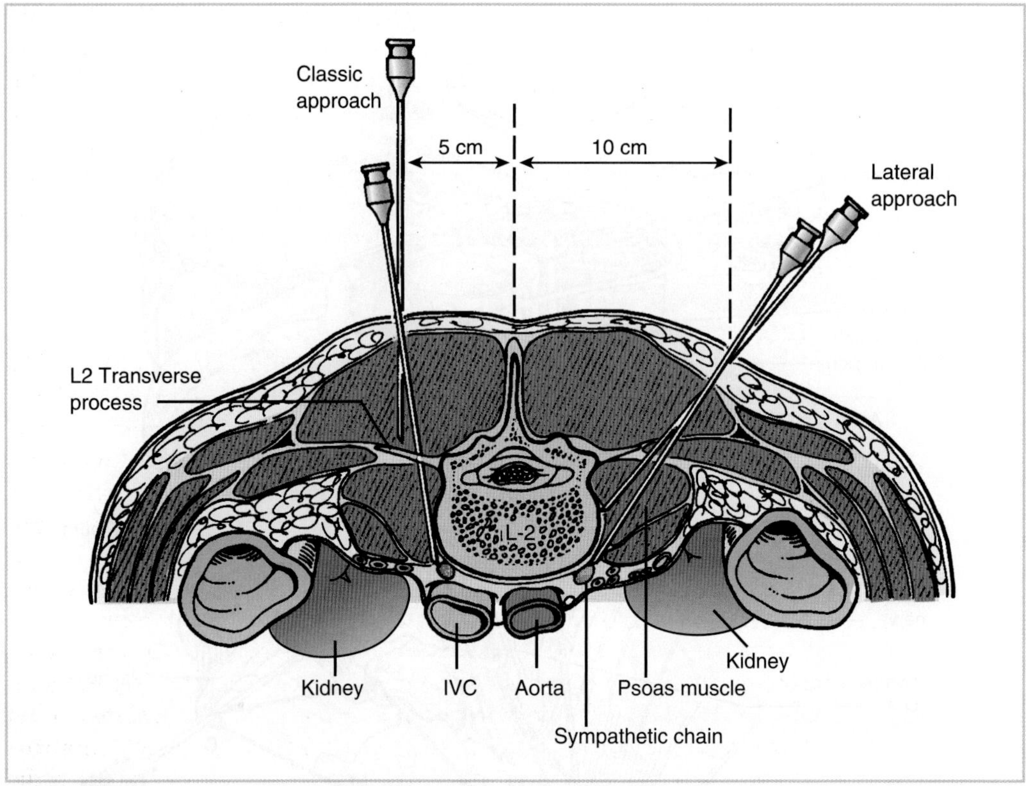

Figure 11.8. Lumbar sympathetic block. Draw a line through the midpoint of the L2 spinous process. The needle is inserted along this line at a point 5 cm lateral to the midline and is directed approximately 45 degrees cephalad to contact the L2 transverse process. Note the depth at which the transverse process was contacted and partially withdraw the needle redirecting it perpendicular to the skin. Insert to a depth 5 cm deeper than that at which the L2 transverse process was contacted. The needle tip should lie at the anterolateral edge of the vertebral body. For the lateral approach, the same landmarks are used except that the needle is inserted 10 cm lateral to the midline and directed medially toward the midpoint of the vertebral body. After contacting the vertebral body, partially withdraw the needle and reinsert it at a steeper angle until it pierces the psoas fascia. IVC, inferior vena cava.

Insert the needle approximately 5 cm deeper than the depth at which the transverse process was contacted. The needle will pass between the transverse processes to lie at the anterolateral edge of the vertebral body. If the vertebral body is contacted before advancing 5 cm, redirect slightly less medially and "walk off" the vertebral body to the desired depth (Figure 11.8).

e. Carefully **aspirate** looking for blood, CSF, or urine. If aspiration is negative, inject an epinephrine-containing test dose while observing for evidence of intravascular, epidural, or intrathecal injection. If negative, inject 5 to 10 mL on each side. Do not inject local anesthetic as the needle is withdrawn because the corresponding spinal nerve lies superficial to the targeted ganglia. Block of the somatic spinal nerve may confuse diagnostic sympathetic blocks or incapacitate the patient because of motor block.

3. **Signs/symptoms of block.** The block should produce **vasodilatation** and increased **skin temperature** after 5 to 10 minutes. This can easily be evaluated by placing a skin temperature sensor on the foot and looking for a 3°C temperature increase. Complete block may require 20 minutes or more. Sensory block of the lateral thigh indicates block of the L2 nerve root and suggests either that the local anesthetic was deposited too superficially or that local anesthetic spread from the sympathetic ganglia onto the L2 nerve root. The absence of a skin temperature change suggests the former.
4. **Alternative approaches**
   a. **"Lateral"** approach. The ganglia can also be reached using a more lateral needle insertion point. From a point **10 cm lateral to the middle of the L2 spinous process,** insert a 15-cm 20-gauge needle directed medially toward the midpoint of the vertebral body. After contacting the vertebral body, withdraw and redirect the needle more anterior so as to "walk off" the side of the vertebral body to reach its anterolateral edge (Figure 11.8). After a negative aspiration and a negative epinephrine-containing test dose incrementally inject 5 to 10 mL local anesthetic.
   b. **Bryce-Smith** approach (12). The gray rami communicantes, which carry preganglionic sympathetic nerves, leave the spinal nerve where it exits the spinal canal and form a reticular network as they wrap around the side of the vertebral body to reach the paravertebral ganglia. To block the ganglia at this point, the needle is inserted **5 cm lateral to the midline of the L2 spinous process** at an angle of approximately **70 degrees** until it contacts the vertebral body. With the needle against the vertebral body, inject 15 to 20 mL local anesthetic solution. The local anesthetic will track anteriorly to reach the paravertebral ganglia and **may track posteriorly to reach the L2 somatic root.** Consequently, this approach is not appropriate for diagnostic or neurolytic blocks.
5. **Complications**
   a. **Hematoma/hemorrhage**
   b. **Subarachnoid/epidural injection.** Needles directed too shallow can enter the intervertebral foramen.
   c. **Spinal nerve injury.** Needle contact injury or chemical injury can occur because the spinal nerves course near the path of the block needle (Figure 11.8). Pain, dysesthesia, or motor impairment in the area innervated by the spinal nerve indicates spinal nerve injury. It is most likely to occur with large volumes of neurolytic solutions.
   d. **Spinal cord injury.** Needles directed too shallow can enter the intervertebral foramen to pierce the spinal cord.
   e. **Renal injury.** Needles angled too steep or introduced too far lateral of the midline can pierce the kidney.
   f. Perforation of intervertebral disk.

E. **Superior hypogastric plexus block.** Block of the superior hypogastric plexus is used primarily to treat pelvic pain, especially from cancer. It was first described by Plancarte et al. for this purpose (13).
   1. **Anatomy.** The superior hypogastric plexus lies in the retroperitoneal space just anterior to the caudad third of L5 and the cephalad third of S1 just distal to the bifurcation of the common iliac vessels (Figure 11.9).

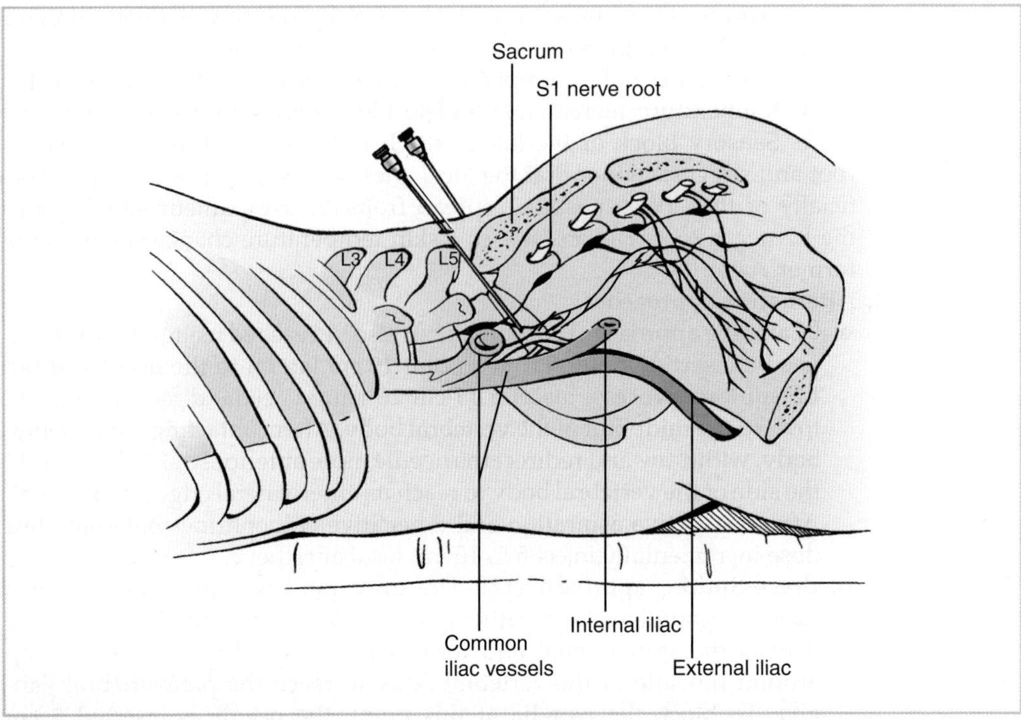

Figure 11.9. Superior hypogastric block. In the prone position, 15- to 20-cm needles are inserted on the right and left side approximately 6 cm from the midline at the middle of the L4-5 interspace. The needles are advanced 45 degrees medial and 30 degrees caudal to contact the L5 vertebral body. The needles are partially withdrawn and redirected to "walk off" the lateral edge of the vertebral body. Advance the needles approximately 1 cm past the anterior edge of the L5 vertebral body until a distinct "pop" is felt as the needle advances through the anterior psoas fascia to lie in the retroperitoneal space at the L5-S1 junction.

2. **Technique**
   a. Position the patient supine with a pillow under the lower abdomen to straighten the lumbar lordosis.
   b. Identify the **L4-5 interspace** and draw a line through the center of it. Place bilateral marks along this line approximately **6 cm from the midline** (Figure 11.9).
   c. Aseptically prepare the skin and raise skin wheals at the marks. Insert 15-cm long 20- or 22-gauge needles at the skin wheals at an angle **30 degrees caudad and 45 degrees medial**. If the spinous process of L5 is contacted, redirect the needle slightly more caudad and reinsert the needle until the body of L5 is contacted.
   d. Withdraw the needle sufficiently to redirect it slightly less medial and "walk off" the lateral edge of the vertebral body. Carefully advance the needle approximately 1 cm past the vertebral body at which point a distinct "pop" may be felt as the needle pierces the fascia on the anterior surface of the psoas muscle to lie in the retroperitoneal space at the L5 through S1 junction.
   e. After careful **aspiration** and a negative epinephrine-containing test dose, incrementally inject 6 to 8 mL local anesthetic through both needles.

3. **Alternative approaches.** Both anterior (14) and posterior transdiscal (15) approaches have been described.
4. **Complications**
   a. **Hematoma/hemorrhage.** Iliac as well as other vessels can be injured.
   b. **Subarachnoid/epidural injection.** Needles directed too shallow can enter the intervertebral foramen.
   c. **Spinal nerve injury.** Needle contact injury or chemical injury can occur because the L5 spinal nerves course near the path of the block needles. Pain dysesthesia or motor impairment in the area innervated by L5 could result.
   d. Because the block is performed below the termination of the spinal cord, needle stick injury to the cord is not a risk; however, **intrathecal injection** can occur and neurolytic agents can injure the spinal cord.
   e. Bowel, bladder, and sexual dysfunction have not been reported in the large series published to date.

REFERENCES

1 Pieri S, Agresti P, Ialongo P, et al. Lumbar sympathectomy under CT guidance: therapeutic option in critical limb ischaemia. *Radiol Med (Torino)* 2005;109(4):430–437.
2 Holiday FA, Barendregt WB, Slappendel R, et al. Lumbar sympathectomy in critical limb ischaemia: surgical, chemical or not at all? *Cardiovasc Surg* 1999;7(2):200–202.
3 Lipov E, Lipov S, Stark JT. Stellate ganglion blockade provides relief from menopausal hot flashes: a case report series. *J Womens Health (Larchmt)* 2005;14(8):737–741.
4 Kozody R, Ready LB, Barsa JE, et al. Dose requirement of local anaesthetic to produce grand mal seizure during stellate ganglion block. *Can Anaesth Soc J* 1982;29(5):489–491.
5 Egawa H, Okuda Y, Kitajima T, et al. Assessment of QT interval and QT dispersion following stellate ganglion block using computerized measurements. *Reg Anesth Pain Med* 2001;26(6):539–544.
6 Ward EM, Rorie DK, Nauss LA, et al. The celiac ganglia in man: normal anatomic variations. *Anesth Analg* 1979;58(6):461–465.
7 Singler RC. An improved technique for alcohol neurolysis of the celiac plexus. *Anesthesiology* 1982;56(2): 137–141.
8 Romanelli DF, Beckmann CF, Heiss FW. Celiac plexus block: efficacy and safety of the anterior approach. *AJR Am J Roentgenol* 1993;160(3):497–500.
9 Michaels AJ, Draganov PV. Endoscopic ultrasonography guided celiac plexus neurolysis and celiac plexus block in the management of pain due to pancreatic cancer and chronic pancreatitis. *World J Gastroenterol* 2007;13(26):3575–3580.
10 Tran QN, Urayama S, Meyers FJ. Endoscopic ultrasound-guided celiac plexus neurolysis for pancreatic cancer pain: a single-institution experience and review of the literature. *J Support Oncol* 2006;4(9):460–462, 464; discussion 463–4.
11 Umeda S, Arai T, Hatano Y, et al. Cadaver anatomic analysis of the best site for chemical lumbar sympathectomy. *Anesth Analg* 1987;66(7):643–646.
12 Bryce-Smith R. Injection of the lumbar sympathetic chain. *Anaesthesia* 1951;6(3):150–153.
13 Plancarte R, Amescua C, Patt RB, et al. Superior hypogastric plexus block for pelvic cancer pain. *Anesthesiology* 1990;73(2):236–239.
14 Kanazi GE, Perkins FM, Thakur R, et al. New technique for superior hypogastric plexus block. *Reg Anesth Pain Med* 1999;24(5):473–476.
15 Gamal G, Helaly M, Labib YM. Superior hypogastric block: transdiscal versus classic posterior approach in pelvic cancer pain. *Clin J Pain* 2006;22(6):544–547.

12 Brachial Plexus Blocks

Susan B. McDonald

The brachial plexus is conveniently arranged to allow regional nerve blockade. There are several anatomic locations to provide operative anesthesia or postoperative analgesia of the entire upper extremity from the shoulder to the hand with minimal patient cooperation. Many approaches have been published; this chapter will describe several of the common approaches that have proved useful.

I. Anatomy

The brachial plexus comprises roots, trunks, divisions, cords, and terminal nerves (Figure 12.1).

A. **Roots.** The ventral nerve roots of C5 through T1 intertwine to form a closely approximated bundle known as the *brachial plexus.* At their origin in the neck, all the roots exit the spinal column in a trough between the anterior and posterior tubercle of the transverse process of the vertebral body. The roots pass laterally in a long narrow compartment between the posterior fascia of the anterior scalene (AS) muscle and the anterior fascia of the middle scalene (MS) muscle. **Interscalene block is performed at this level.** Anesthesia of the roots produces a pattern that follows the dermatomal distribution, typically C4 through C7.

B. **Trunks.** As the nerve roots course further distally, the C5 and C6 roots typically form the upper trunk, the C8 through T1 roots form the lower trunk, and C7 becomes the middle trunk. The **trunks** are compactly arranged in a vertical manner between the AS and MS muscles in the lower part of the interscalene space. The trunks pass over the first rib behind the insertion of the AS, where they may already be dividing into anterior and posterior **divisions**. The subclavian artery (SA) rises from the thorax and also crosses the first rib immediately behind the AS insertion, lying just anterior to the nerve bundle. **Supraclavicular blocks are performed at this level.**

C. **Divisions.** Each trunk divides into an **anterior** and **posterior division**. Ultrasonography has demonstrated that the six divisions are still compactly arranged and are typically located superior and posterior to the SA, as the artery passes over the first rib. The plexus closely surrounds the artery from this level before departing on their unique courses distal to the axilla.

D. **Cords.** Three cords arise from the divisions at the level of the coracoid process and are named for their relationship to the axillary artery. **Infraclavicular block is performed at the level of the cords.**

1. **Lateral cord.** Sends off a major branch that combines with a branch from the medial cord to form the median nerve (MN) before continuing on as the **musculocutaneous** (MC) nerve
2. **Medial cord.** Sends off a major branch that combines with a branch from the lateral cord to form the **MN** before continuing on as the **ulnar** nerve. Sensory branches of the **medial brachial cutaneous** nerve and the **medial antebrachial cutaneous** nerves branch off early.
3. **Posterior cord.** The axillary nerve branches off early; the cord continues on as the **radial nerve** (RN).

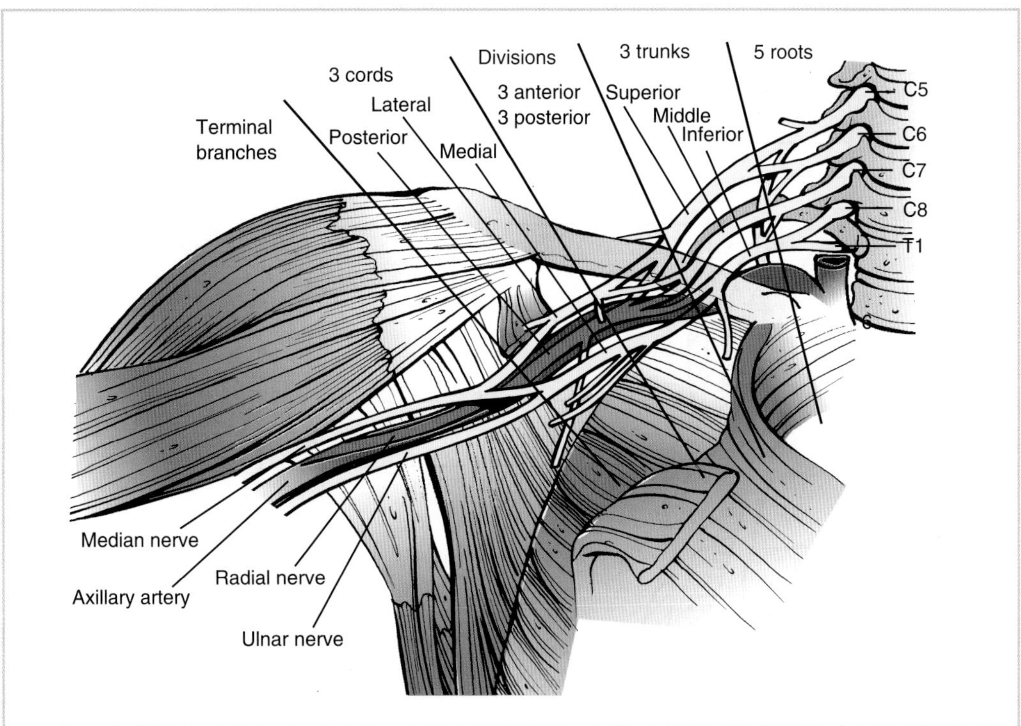

Figure 12.1. Brachial plexus overview: The ventral roots of the fifth cervical through the first thoracic spinal nerves form the brachial plexus. The upper and lower pairs of roots merge, creating three trunks, which join the subclavian artery as it crosses the first rib. The trunks then divide and recombine to form three cords and then divide into the four terminal nerves of the forearm, which surround the axillary artery—the radial, median, ulnar, and musculocutaneous.

E. **Terminal nerves.** Axillary block is performed at the level of the terminal nerves, where there is greater variability of anatomy (1).
   1. The three main terminal nerves to the hand remain closely approximated to the axillary artery, with the median generally superior to the vessel and the others inferior and posterior, but with considerable variability in location.
   2. Sensory branches to the forearm have already departed the neurovascular bundle at this level and travel in the coracobrachialis muscle (**musculocutaneous**) or in the subcutaneous tissues **(medial brachial cutaneous, medial antebrachial cutaneous).**

F. Although knowledge of these derivations is helpful, the approach to brachial plexus anesthesia is **based on the reproducible landmarks of the neck**—the vertebral **tubercles**, the first **rib**, the **coracoid** process, or the axillary **artery.**

G. Each injection site produces a unique pattern of distribution of anesthesia **(2)**.
   1. **Interscalene anesthesia** is most reliable and dense on the upper roots (C5-7) and includes sensory anesthesia of the cervical plexus (C2-4). Occasionally, anesthesia is ineffective in the C8-T1 dermatome (ulnar side of arm) distribution (Figure 12.2). This technique is therefore **best suited for shoulder and upper arm surgery.**
   2. The **supraclavicular block** is performed where the trunks and divisions are most closely approximated in the fascial bundle and before branching

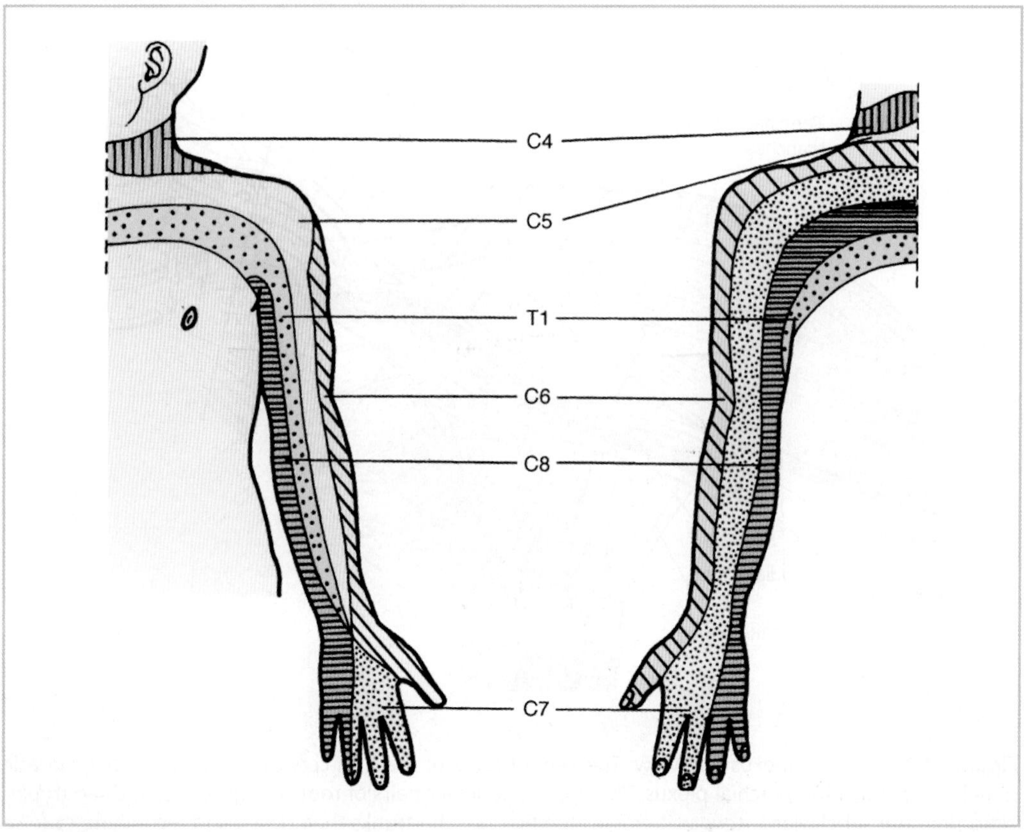

Figure 12.2. Dermatomal distribution of nerve roots in the upper extremity. Interscalene blocks, which are at the level of the roots, will anesthetize the brachial plexus along dermatomal distribution.

occurs, and is therefore the most reliable in **producing sensory anesthesia of the entire forearm and hand.** It does not reliably provide cervical plexus (shoulder) anesthesia.

3. At the target of the **infraclavicular** block, the cords are separated from each other (into lateral, posterior, and middle cords) by the axillary artery below the fascial plane of the perimysium of the pectoralis minor muscle. The **MC** nerve may diverge from the lateral cord above the level of the pectoralis minor. The divergent arrangement of the cords makes complete anesthesia more difficult compared to the supraclavicular block.
4. The **axillary block** is reliable in anesthetizing the three nerves of the hand (radial, median, and ulnar) (Figure 12.3). The MC and medial antebrachial cutaneous nerves and their sensory distribution in the forearm can be spared because these nerves depart from the perivascular bundle high in the axilla.

H. The concept of the "sheath"

1. A proximal **fascial envelope** arises from the lateral extension of the posterior fascia of the AS and anterior fascia of the MS muscles, and extends from the transverse processes for a variable distance in the upper arm.
2. Winnie has popularized the use of this "sheath" to allow **single-injection techniques** for the brachial plexus at all levels in the sheath and has demonstrated extensive spread of solution from single injections (3).

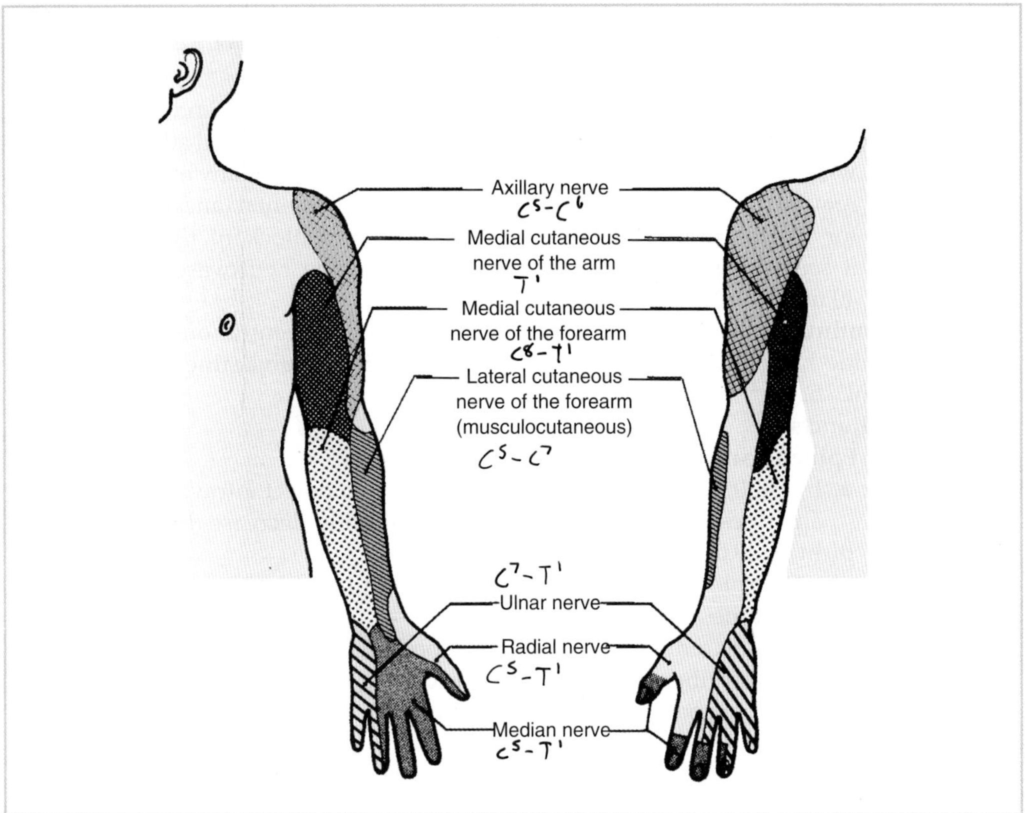

Figure 12.3. Sensory dermatomes of the terminal nerves of the upper extremity. Sensation is provided by the terminal nerves as identified. This pattern is different from the classic dermatomal distribution of the nerve roots (Figure 12.2) and is seen when the brachial plexus is blocked more distally, such as with an axillary block.

3. Distally within this sheath, fascial **septa** may be present (4). Although they do not universally limit the spread of anesthetic solutions (5), they may defeat attempts to produce anesthesia by injection of a single bolus of solution. These septa may account for less than 100% success rate of single-injection axillary anesthesia.

II. Drugs

A. **Local anesthetics (LAs)** are chosen primarily for the **duration** of the anesthetic block.
   1. **Lidocaine** 1% or 1.5% may provide 3 to 4 hours of anesthesia.
   2. **Mepivacaine** 1.5% may provide 4 to 5 hours of anesthesia.
   3. **Bupivacaine, levobupivacaine,** or **ropivacaine** (0.5%) will provide 12 to 14 hours of analgesia.
   4. There is **no need for higher concentrations in brachial plexus anesthesia**, and there is a risk of exceeding maximum recommended doses if they are employed.

B. The **volume** to be injected has been subject to debate. A 25 mL of solution injected directly in the neighborhood of a nerve stimulation or paresthesia will provide anesthesia for most patients.

1. **The upper limit is generally recognized as 50 mL** because this quantity represents the maximum milligram dose of most of the LAs employed.
2. A 30 to 40 mL dose is more commonly used.
3. Although larger volumes may give slightly earlier onset and further spread and are advocated by some (2), studies have demonstrated adequate spread with 40-mL volumes in all areas of injection. Because many of the techniques require an additional 5 or 10 mL of supplemental anesthetic solution for intercostobrachial branches or peripheral block of the ulnar nerve, it seems appropriate to limit injection into the neurovascular bundle to 40 mL.

C. Continuous catheter techniques employ dilute concentrations of long-acting amide LAs such as **0.2% ropivacaine** or **0.125% bupivacaine** at rates of 6 to 8 mL/h.

D. Adjuncts

1. **Epinephrine**
   a. In 1:400,000 dilution, epinephrine helps to detect intravascular injection and does not prolong duration (may slightly decrease duration).
   b. In 1:200,000 dilution, epinephrine:
      (1) Prolongs duration of block, especially with lidocaine and mepivacaine
      (2) May reduce peak systemic blood levels
      (3) May increase risk of nerve damage in patients with underlying neuropathy or with intraneural injection **(6)**
2. **Clonidine**
   a. May prolong analgesia in a dose-dependent manner.
   b. Side effects are minimal if dose is limited to 150 μg.
   c. When added to mepivacaine, an additional 4 hours of analgesia can be provided (7).
3. **Sodium bicarbonate**
   a. Hastens **onset of block** by raising the pH of the solution closer to the pKa of the LA (more molecules in nonionized form to cross the nerve sheath and membrane).
   b. This faster onset is more evident when added to commercially prepared LAs with epinephrine because these solutions are marketed with a lower pH.
   c. In plain LAs (with or without freshly added epinephrine), it may not significantly speed onset and may decrease duration.
   d. **Precipitation of solution can occur if too much bicarbonate is added,** especially with ropivacaine and bupivacaine.
   e. For lidocaine and mepivacaine, 1 mL of 8.4% sodium bicarbonate is added to every **10 mL of LA.**

III. Techniques

A. Interscalene block

This approach is ideal for upper arm and shoulder (acromioplasty, etc.) operations. Although the incidental cervical plexus (C2-4) anesthesia may be advantageous, **"ulnar" (C8-T1) sparing may occur**, such that this block may require supplementation in the axilla or above the elbow if used for hand surgery. US guidance is effective for this block, although traditional peripheral nerve stimulator or paresthesia techniques work well.

1. **US-guided interscalene block.** With US, real-time imaging of the needle may allow a more effective and efficient method to place the needle tip in close proximity to brachial plexus within the interscalene space. Additionally, US allows for real-time observation of LA distribution around the brachial plexus and can potentially guide more purposeful needle tip redirections if necessary (8).
   a. The **patient is positioned** supine, with the head turned slightly to the side opposite the surgical site. A small folded towel is placed under the head, and the ipsilateral hand is held at the side and extended toward the feet.
   b. The **surface anatomy** is identified and marked—the **cricoid cartilage**, the lateral border of the **sternocleidomastoid** (SCM) muscle, and the **interscalene groove**. The latter can be located by asking the patient to raise the head slightly into a "sniffing" position. Two fingers placed along the tense lateral border of the SCM and rolled posterior will drop onto the AS muscle. The scalene muscles lie more posterior than lateral to the SCM and may be harder to appreciate in the heavier patient. The groove between the scalenes can be palpated by gently rolling these fingers further posterior (Figure 12.4).
   c. After sterile **skin preparation** and **draping**, the US probe is prepared. US gel is placed on the transducer and then sterile sleeve is placed

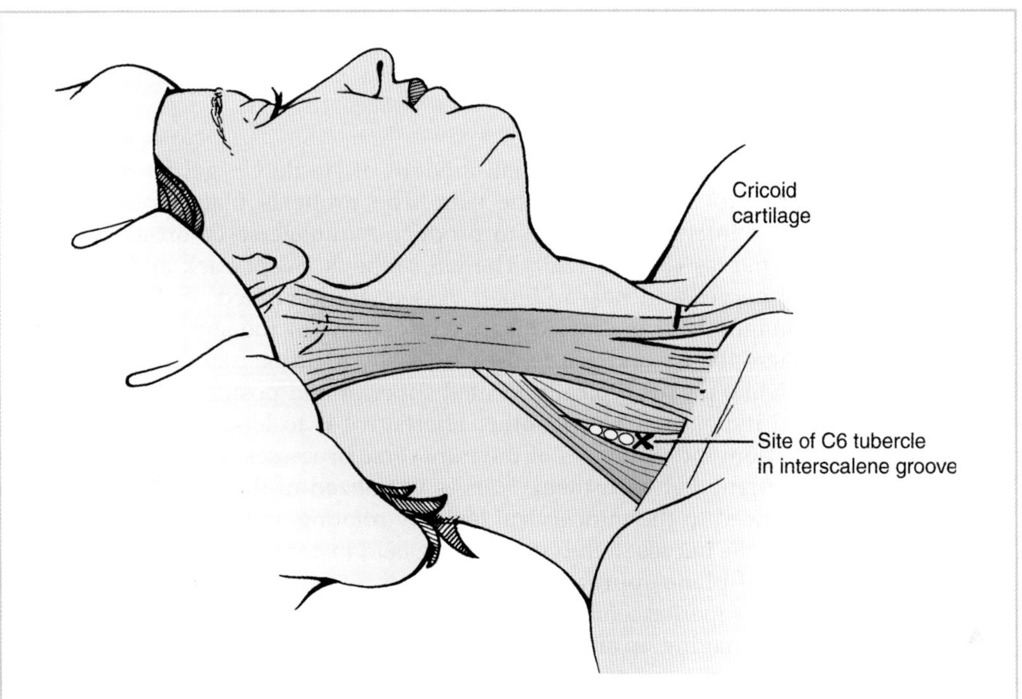

Figure 12.4. Superficial landmarks for interscalene brachial plexus block. The sternocleidomastoid muscle is identified, and the anterior scalene muscle found by moving the fingertips over the lateral border of the larger muscle while it is slightly tensed. The groove between the anterior and middle scalene muscle can usually be felt easily, along with the tubercle of the sixth cervical vertebra, which lies at the level of the cricoid cartilage.

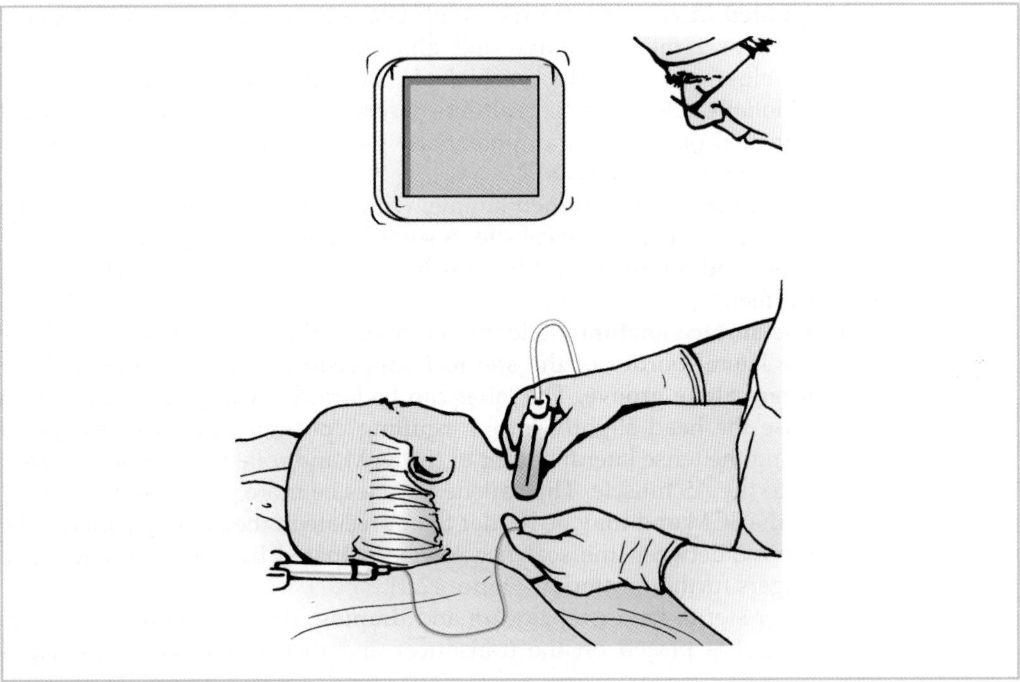

Figure 12.5. Positioning of patient for interscalene ultrasonographic block. The patient is supine, but rolled slightly anterior by placing a blanket or pillow behind the shoulder. When the optimal level of probe placement for nerve visualization is identified, a skin wheal is placed on the posterior edge of the transducer.

over the US probe. A small amount of sterile US gel is then applied either to the probe or the skin. The **probe** is placed perpendicular to the interscalene grove to produce a **transverse (short-axis)** view of the nerves (Figure 12.5). The US probe is swept back and forth until the nerves and nearby blood vessels are identified. If the anatomy is ambiguous, it is easy to start with a view of the supraclavicular area where the rib and artery provide easily identified landmarks, with the brachial plexus typically located superior and posterior to the pulsatile and hypoechoic SA. Another alternative is to look more cephalad for the bony prominences of the transverse processes, with the nerve roots emerging between them. Nerves visualized in these areas can then be followed to the midcervical level by rotating and moving the probe to keep the nerves in the center of the field in a transverse view.

d. Out-of-plane approach. The needle is introduced through a skin wheal at the superior central side of the transducer and advanced, **using real-time imaging**, in an **out-of-plane insertion** into the interscalene groove. The anticipated needle path is now in a caudad direction, but the risk if pneumothorax should be minimized if the needle tip is identified at all times.

e. When the needle appears to lie next to the nerves, a 1- to 2-mL injection should confirm spread of the anesthetic around the nerves. The needle is repositioned and incremental injection is performed until the nerve bundle is surrounded with LA.

f. Nerve-**stimulating needles** may be used, and stimulation may be confirmatory, but not necessary.

g. If an **in-plane** insertion is desired, an approach from the posterior side (through the MS) may be more desirable (to reduce the chance of phrenic nerve injury). If this approach is planned, a towel or blanket should be placed under the ipsilateral shoulder blade to **rotate the patient forward** and allow more room for needle placement (Figure 12.5). Alternatively, the patient can be turned to the lateral position if sufficient pillows are provided to ensure stability.

h. A 50-mm (2-in.) 20- to 22-gauge needle with sterile connection tubing is advanced while injecting 0.5 to 1.0 mL increments of LA to anesthetize the needle tract and optimize needle tip visualization. The needle should be visualized traversing through the levator scapulae and then through the posterior border of the MS muscle (Figure 12.6). As the needle approaches and pushes on the anterior fascia of the MS, the resistance provided by the fascia is seen and felt. Once the needle penetrates the anterior fascia of the MS, the needle tip is within the interscalene space, located on the posterior aspect of the nerve roots. At this point, 1 to 3 mL of LA is injected and the distribution of LA around the brachial plexus elements is observed in real time. After the initial injection, 3 to 5 mL of LA is injected incrementally observing for distension of the interscalene space and more complete LA distribution around the desired components of the brachial plexus.

2. **Continuous interscalene blockade** allows for prolonged postoperative analgesia for procedures such as total shoulder replacement or rotator cuff

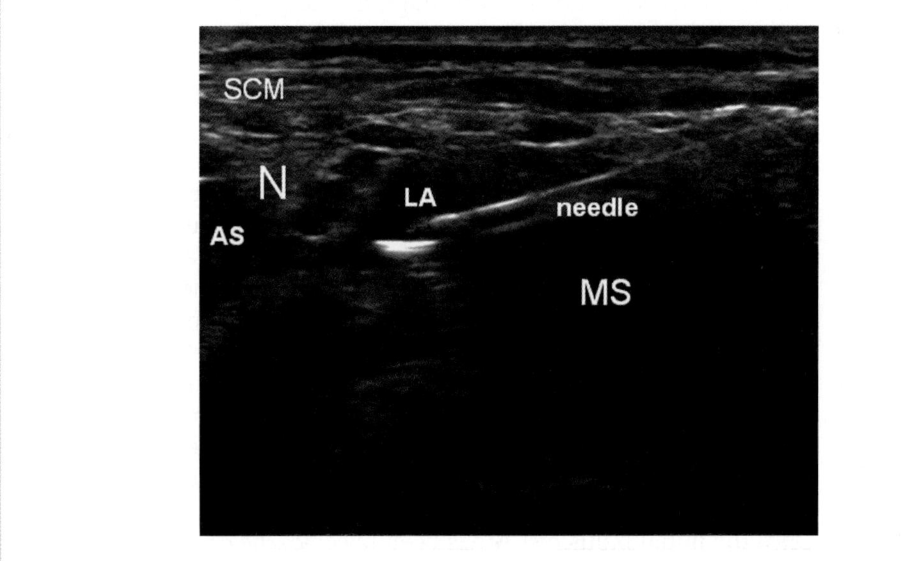

Figure 12.6. Ultrasonographic interscalene block, in-plane. The nerves are identified as hypoechoic circles (*N*) lying between the bodies of the anterior (*AS*) and middle scalene (*MS*) muscles, below the sternocleidomastoid (*SCM*). The needle is introduced from the posterior side through the body of the MS and local anesthetic solution (*LA*) injected to surround the roots/trunks at this level.

repair. There are a number of approaches described (9–11). The authors use an in-plane transverse-MS approach, which allows constant real-time guidance of the needle tip traversing through the posterior aspect of the MS muscle and the anterior fascial plane of the MS muscle located directly posterior to the brachial plexus roots

a. **Position.** The patient is placed supine and a small towel or bump may be placed under the ipsilateral shoulder blade to elevate the shoulder and neck off the bed to facilitate exposure of the posterior aspect of the neck, as in the single-injection in-plane approach.
b. A **preliminary** US view is obtained by placing the US probe just above the clavicle (in the supraclavicular fossa) initially in a coronal plane to the patient. The US probe is then manipulated (rocked back and forth) in a coronal oblique plane to obtain a short-axis view of the SA lying on top of the first rib. Keeping the brachial plexus in the middle of the screen, the US probe is slowly slid superior along the interscalene space until the brachial plexus appears in the form of the hypoechoic roots sandwiched in between the AS and MS muscles. At this point, the probe is typically in an oblique-axial plane to the patient's neck. Finer manipulations of the probe (rotation and tilting/angulation) are performed until an optimal view is obtained. At this point, a footprint of the final probe on the skin surface should be drawn to minimize rescanning after sterile skin preparation and draping have been performed.
c. After **sterile skin preparation** and draping, the transducer is repositioned over the previously drawn footprint and the US view of the brachial plexus is then reacquired. At this point, a small skin wheal of LA is placed 1 cm lateral to the probe (typically over the levator scapulae or the posterior scalene). A 38-mm (1.5-in.) 22-gauge needle with a 3-mL syringe attached is advanced through the skin and into the MS muscle in a posterior to anterior direction toward the brachial plexus with real-time US observation of the entire needle. This allows for anesthesia of the deeper tissues, as well as observation of the correct needle trajectory toward the brachial plexus.
d. A **17-gauge Tuohy needle** (with the bevel pointed laterally) is introduced along the same track **with US guidance (real-time imaging)**. This approach has the needle advanced through the MS muscle and avoids the more superficial cervical fascial layers that often make advancement of a blunt Tuohy needle more challenging. When the needle tip is in the interscalene groove, a 5 to 10 mL of LA solution is injected to "open up" the space and allow easier passage of the catheter (Figure 12.7). This **spread of LA is visualized** with the US probe. Before the block, preparation can include placing the catheter into the needle to the level of the orifice and attaching the syringe of LA to the catheter; this preblock preparation may be helpful to the practitioner placing the block without extra hands available.
e. Once the initial bolus of LA has been injected, the **catheter is threaded approximately 1 to 3 cm (1 in.) and the placement of tip is confirmed by US** with the injection of an additional 5 mL of LA solution to confirm that the injection remains within the interscalene space.
f. When securing the catheter to the skin, tunneling is not necessary with this approach in most patients. A single clear adhesive dressing

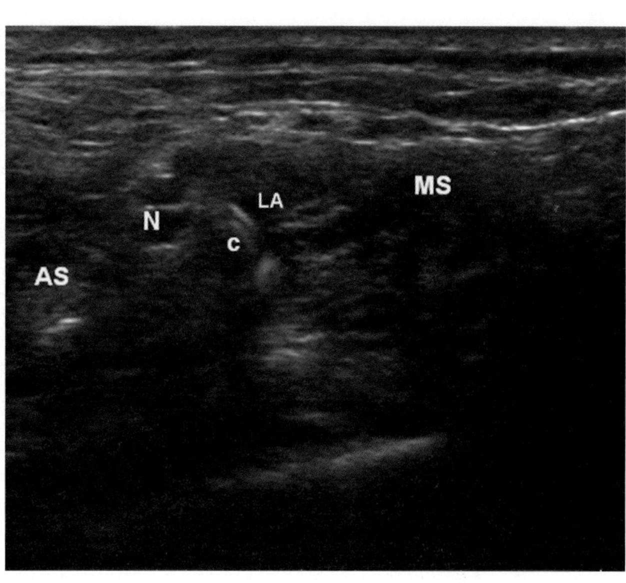

Figure 12.7. Placement of continuous catheter by ultrasonography of interscalene block. The approach is similar to the single injection technique (Figure 12.6), but a larger Tuohy needle is used with a catheter in place as it is advanced. When injection of a small amount of local anesthetic (*LA*) indicates location of the needle tip in the interscalene groove between the anterior scalene (*AS*) and middle scalene (*MS*) near the nerves (*N*), the catheter (*C*) is advanced 1 to 2 cm beyond the needle tip.

(Tagaderm) is usually sufficient. For shoulder surgery, the catheter can be taped posteriorly around the back of the neck to avoid the surgical field.

3. **Paresthesia or peripheral nerve stimulator approach**
   a. The **patient is positioned** supine, as for the single-injection US approach.
   b. The **surface anatomy** is identified and marked as above, but the exact location is more critical for locating the nerves. In addition to the scalene groove, the **tubercle** of the transverse process of the sixth vertebral body (Chassaignac tubercle) should be identified in the base of this groove at the level of the cricoid cartilage, which is commonly also the level at which the external jugular vein crosses the posterior border of the SCM. In virtually all patients, the tubercle can be identified directly, and is a more reliable landmark to identify the location of the nerves. This is not uncomfortable for the patient if done gently. The location of the tubercle should also be marked with an X (Figure 12.4).
   c. After aseptic skin preparation and draping, a skin wheal of LA is raised in the interscalene groove at the level of the "X." A 38-mm (1.5-in.) 22-gauge **needle is inserted in a caudad and posterior direction**, angling toward the tubercle. This requires that the needle be perpendicular to the skin in all planes. A **caudal angulation of at least 50 degrees** will reduce the potential for spinal canal entry (12). The hub of the needle is held between the thumb and forefinger of the dominant hand, the heel of which rests solidly on the clavicle or neck (Figure 12.8). This

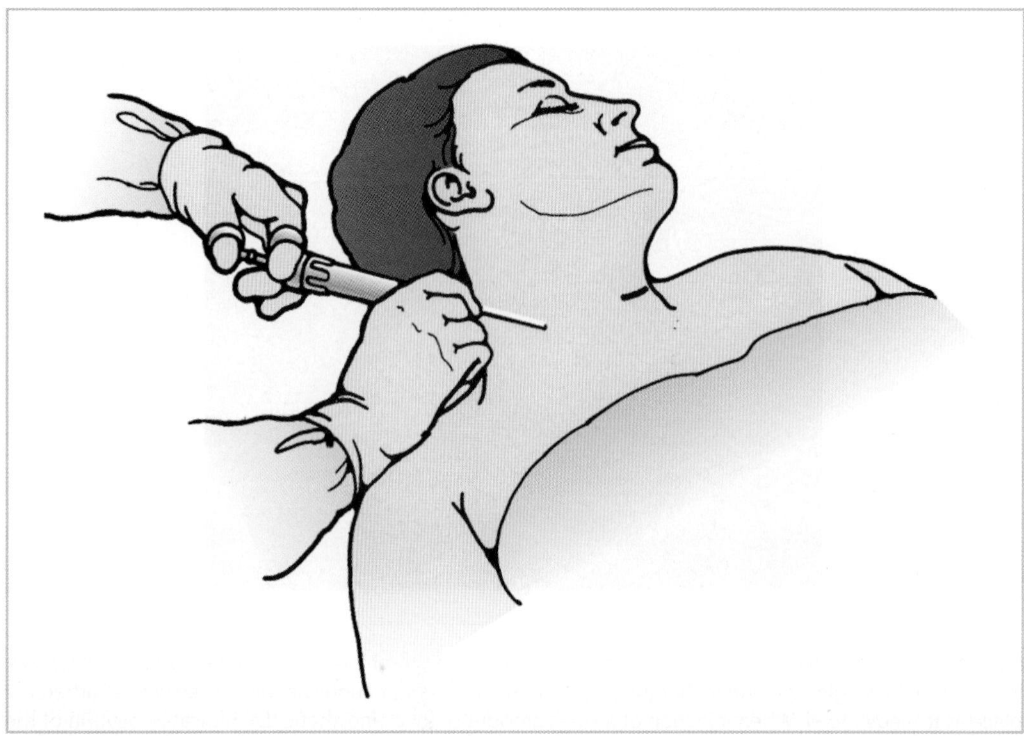

Figure 12.8. Hand position for interscalene block. The needle is introduced into the skin over the interscalene groove at the level of the cricoid cartilage (or the sixth vertebral tubercle, if palpable). It is then directed in a caudad and posterior direction into the interscalene groove with one hand resting on the clavicle exerts constant control of the depth of insertion.

fixation of the needle reduces the chance of accidental movement of the needle when a peripheral nerve stimulator evoked motor response or paresthesia is encountered.

d. The needle is advanced until a stimulator response or paresthesia is obtained or the bone is contacted. If the tubercle is reached before identifying the nerve, the needle is withdrawn almost to the skin and redirected. The path of search for the nerve is in 1-mm steps along a line perpendicular to the presumed course of the nerve (i.e., anterior to posterior); **the needle tip should never be directed cephalad or medially**. This would allow entry into the intervertebral foramen, with the possibility of puncture of the vertebral artery or dura itself. **A more caudad direction will increase the potential for pneumothorax** (Figure 12.9).

e. On obtaining a stimulation or paresthesia in the arm (usually thumb or forearm), gentle aspiration is performed, followed by injection of a 1 mL "test dose." If no cramping or discomfort is produced with this test, a 30 to 40 mL of anesthetic solution is injected incrementally. The needle is held in position with the dominant hand, whereas the 10-mL syringe is detached and refilled. Alternatively, a single 50-mL syringe or a stopcock with an additional 20-mL syringe of LA solution is connected to the needle by a short length of intravenous extension

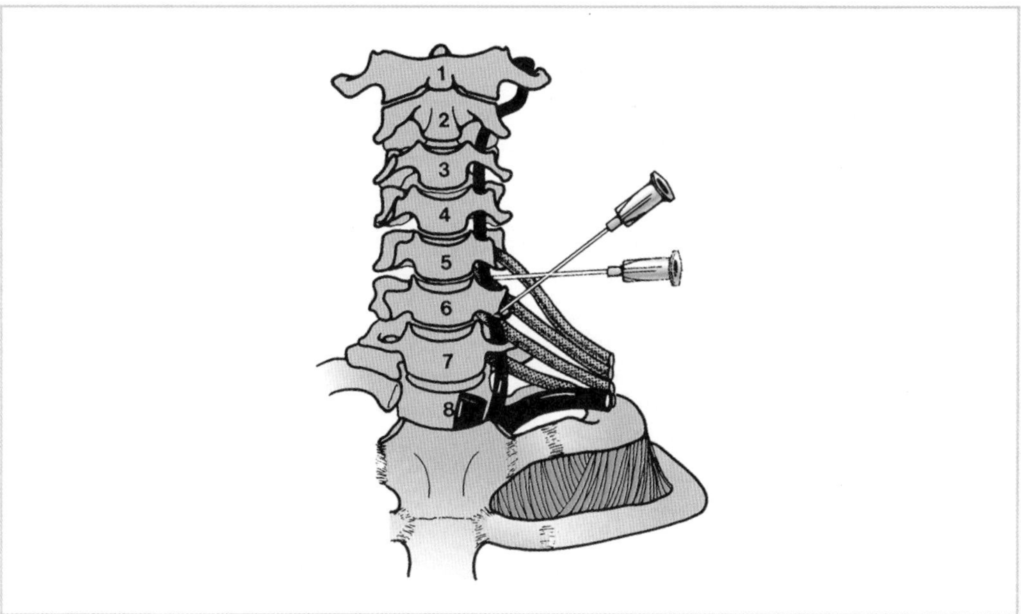

Figure 12.9. Needle direction for interscalene block. The needle is kept in a 45-degree caudad direction; a more caudad direction will contact the pleura, although a medial insertion will allow the point to pass into the intervertebral foramen and produce epidural, spinal, or intra-arterial injection of anesthetic. Note the relation of the vertebral artery and the nerve roots to the transverse processes.

tubing. **Aspiration is performed after each 3- to 5-mL injection, and the patient is observed carefully for signs of intravascular injection.**

f. A **Horner syndrome** occasionally may develop, as well as **ipsilateral phrenic nerve paralysis** (which occurs in 100% of patients with this block) (13) as the solution spreads anterior to the scalene muscles or cephalad in the interscalene groove to the cervical roots (see Section IV).

B. **Supraclavicular block.** This approach relies on the predictable anatomy of the three major trunks of the plexus as they cross over the **first rib** between the insertion of the AS and MS muscles just posterior to the SA. This intersection of nerves with rib occurs behind the midpoint of the clavicle and lies relatively superficially (Figure 12.10). This block provides the best anesthesia of the arm with a single injection, but has been avoided by some because of the risk of pneumothorax. US guidance simplifies the block, and may reduce this risk.

1. **US guidance for the supraclavicular block** has generated a renewed interest in this approach because the **pleura can be directly visualized** and, therefore, avoided (14,15) (Figure 12.11). Theoretically, this should significantly decrease the risk of pneumothorax (assuming the needle's approach is visualized with real-time imaging) because not only can the brachial plexus and SA be visualized but also the first rib and the underlying pleura may be directly visualized in real time.

a. The patient is placed in the **supine position,** with the ipsilateral arm held along the side and extended caudally (as if reaching for the knee) so as to facilitate palpation of the clavicle and scalene muscles.

b. The probe is placed directly **behind the midpoint of the clavicle** in a **coronal oblique plane** and angled to obtain a **short-axis view** of the SA

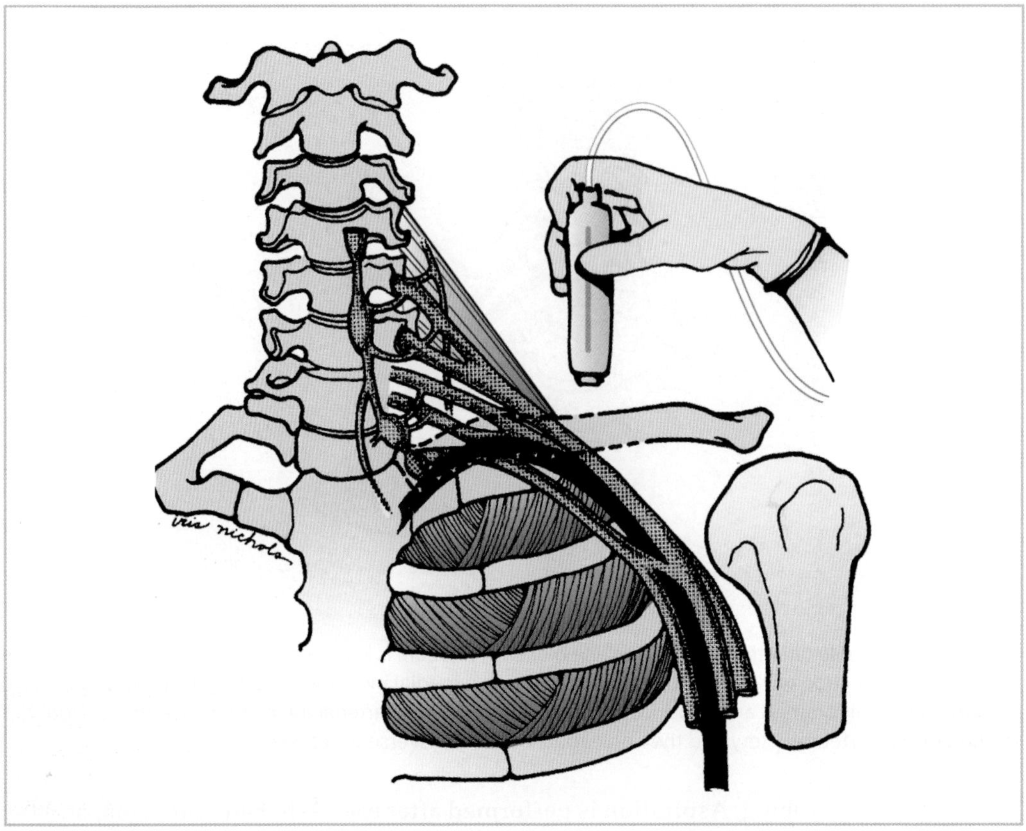

Figure 12.10. Pertinent anatomy of supraclavicular block. The trunks/divisions cross the rib just posterior to the subclavian artery, and can be visualized easily with an ultrasonographic probe placed just behind the clavicle.

lying on the first rib (Figure 12.10). At this point, the brachial plexus is superior and posterior to the pulsatile SA. The brachial plexus may often appear as a cluster of grapes at this level and may either be the trunks or divisions of the brachial plexus.

c. After sterile preparation and draping of the field and the probe, and injection of a skin wheal, the needle is inserted in an **in-plane approach** at 45 degrees, careful once again to **visualize the path of the needle in real-time imaging** (Figure 12.11). A posterior approach usually allows the needle to pass more easily to the posterior and inferior border of the artery where the nerves may lie. Spread of the LA around the nerves confirms appropriate placement. Injection of LA at the inferior aspect of the brachial plexus where it meets the first rib has been shown to provide the most uniform and rapid onset of anesthesia. Alternatively, the needle tip may be repositioned around the brachial plexus after incremental injections of 5 to 10 mL of LA in a deliberate effort to provide a more uniform and complete LA distribution around the brachial plexus.
d. Again, nerve **stimulator** may be used as an adjunct for localization, but is not necessary.

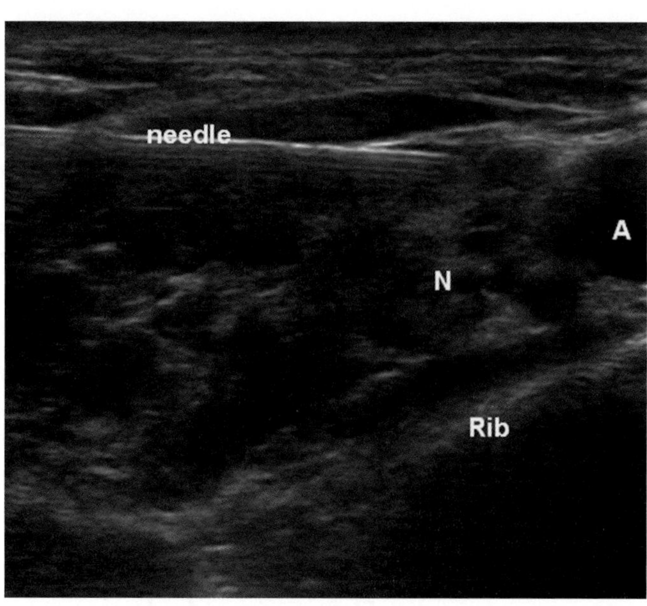

Figure 12.11. Ultrasound (US) guidance for supraclavicular block. With the US probe placed behind the clavicle and parallel to the first rib, the rib is seen as a hyperechoic line (*Rib*) lying under the pulsatile hypoechoic artery (*A*). The nerves appear as three (if still as trunks) to six (if now in divisions) hypoechoic structures (*N*) posterior and superior to the artery. The needle is advanced under US visualization at all times to avoid entry into the artery or lung, and anesthetic injected around the nerves, ideally at the inferior part of the bundle to "lift" the nerves off the rib.

2. **Nerve stimulator or paresthesia approach**
   a. The patient is placed in the same position.
   b. The clavicle and scalene muscles are identified and marked, and an "X" is placed on the skin just posterior to the **midpoint of the clavicle** or in the interscalene groove at this level if it is palpable. The scalene muscles are identified by having the patient lift his or her head to the "sniffing" position. Fingers placed on the taut SCM muscle will then easily roll posterior onto the AS. On a thin patient, the **SA or even the first rib may be identified** at the base of the groove between AS and MS muscles.
   c. After aseptic skin preparation, a skin wheal is placed in the X, and a 38-mm (1.5-in.) 22-gauge needle is introduced in a caudad direction. The syringe is held such that the axis is constantly parallel to the head, ensuring that the **needle direction remains caudad and not directed medially** toward the cupola of the pleura. The hand rests on the clavicle, grasping the hub of the needle between index finger and thumb to prevent unintentional misdirection with patient movement (Figure 12.12).
   d. The needle is advanced to its full depth. If the first rib is not contacted, the needle is redirected in 4-mm steps laterally to locate the rib (a "safe" search pattern). If the rib does not lie lateral to the "X," then careful 2-mm step exploration is performed medial to the mark. In the occasional heavy or "bullnecked" patient, a 50-mm (2-in.) needle may be required to reach the rib. **If a sharp chest pain associated with a cough is produced,**

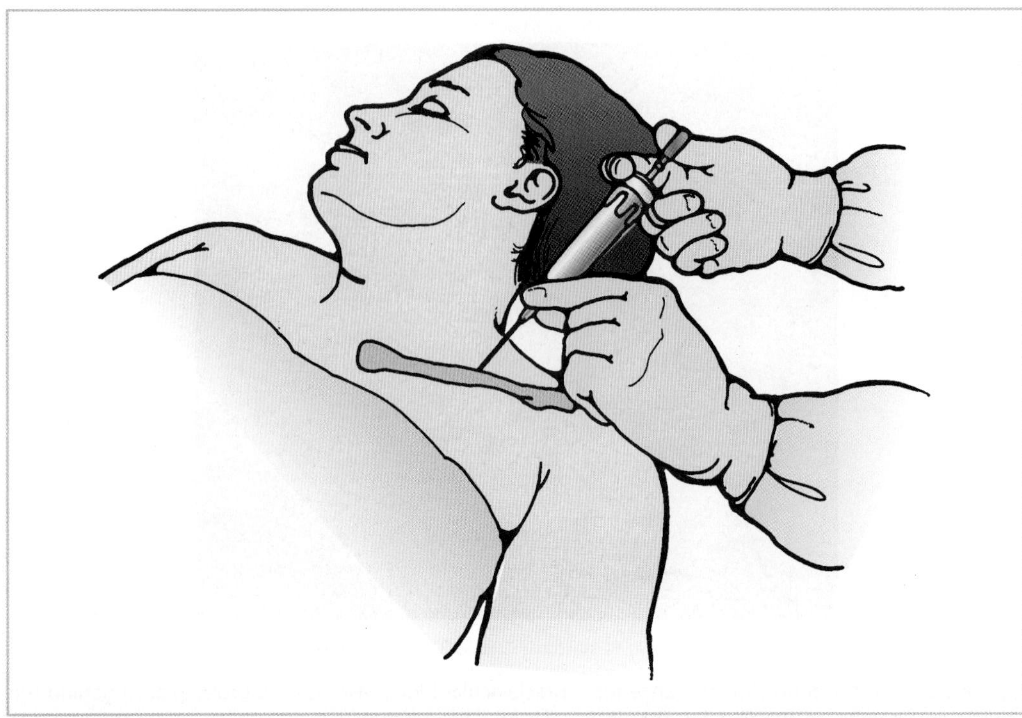

Figure 12.12. Hand position for supraclavicular block. The needle is directed caudad behind the midpoint of the clavicle in the interscalene groove. Again, control of depth is maintained by the hand resting on the clavicle. The syringe is kept in the sagittal plane parallel to the patient's head to prevent medial angulation, which increases the chance of pneumothorax.

the technique is abandoned and a chest x-ray obtained to evaluate for pneumothorax.

e. **Once the rib is contacted,** if nerve localization does not occur the needle is withdrawn almost to the skin and is **redirected 1 to 2 mm posteriorly** and reinserted to gently contact the rib. Vigorous repeated periosteal contact inflicts pain in the patient and dulls and barbs the needle point. The needle direction change needs to be achieved with almost complete withdrawal to skin; partial withdrawal may only succeed in pushing the superficial nerve bundle ahead of the advancing needle (Figure 12.13).
f. The **rib follows an anteroposterior course in this area**. The path of exploration is directly posterior and is therefore in the sagittal plane parallel to the longitudinal axis of the body. This is also perpendicular to the course of the nerve bundle at this point. **Medial direction of the needle can only serve to identify the lung.** The needle is "walked" posteriorly until it falls off the posterior angle of the rib; at this point, direction is reversed and it is "walked" anteriorly until it passes the anterior angle of the rib or the SA.
g. A **stimulation** or **paresthesia** may be elicited at any time. **Sensations in the back or chest wall should not be accepted;** successful anesthesia is greater when eliciting a motor response or paresthesia in the hand or forearm. The patient must be instructed beforehand to report a paresthesia verbally but not to move. The needle is immobilized immediately

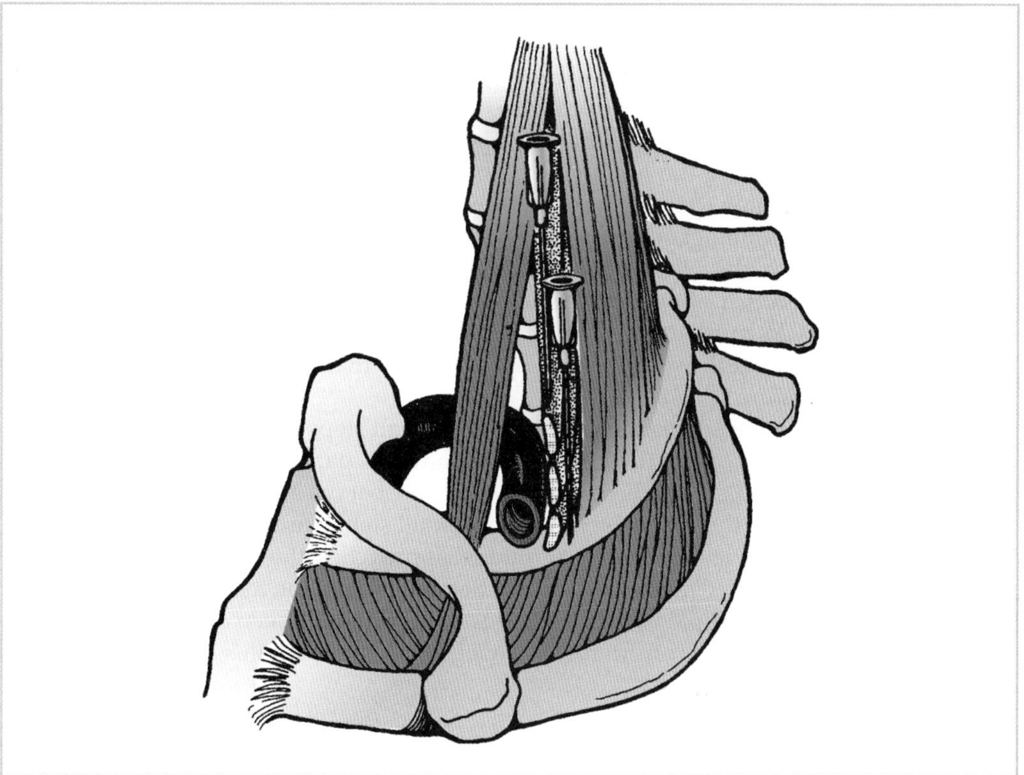

Figure 12.13. Needle direction for supraclavicular block, lateral view. The needle is directed downward onto the first rib, where it can be expected to contact the three trunks of the brachial plexus as they cross over the rib. The rib at this point lies along the anterior-posterior plane of the body. The syringe is kept in the sagittal plane of the body. If the needle contacts the rib without identifying the nerve, it should be withdrawn almost completely to the skin before redirection because short steps along the bone may simply "push" the nerves ahead of the needle.

on the patient's report or a motor response, and LA is injected slowly. If the patient complains of a cramping pain, the needle is withdrawn 1 mm and the injection is repeated. **Aspiration** is performed after each 3 to 5 mL of **incremental injection** to avoid intravascular injection.

h. A **total of 30 to 40 mL is injected** in the neighborhood of the first response. The septa that limit diffusion in the axillary sheath are rarely present at this level, and solution reliably spreads to the major branches of the plexus.

i. If no response is obtained in the first 10 minutes, the landmarks are reexamined and the attempt is repeated. **The nerves usually lie posterior to the initial contact of the rib if difficulty is encountered.** If no paresthesias are obtained, a "wall" of LA may be created by a series of four to five injections of 6 to 7 mL each as the needle is withdrawn from the rib in 3-mm steps "marching" posteriorly from the artery. This is less likely to succeed, and the alternative of an interscalene, axillary, or intravenous block should be considered.

j. If a tourniquet is to be used during surgery, a subcutaneous wheal across the axilla may be necessary to anesthetize the skin of the inner aspect of the upper arm innervated by **the intercostobrachial branches**. This can be achieved with 5 to 10 mL of anesthetic solution injected subcutaneously along the axillary skin crease.

3. **The "plumb-bob" approach** is one of the alternative approaches to the supraclavicular block that have been devised as attempts to reduce the risk of contacting the lung. The plumb-bob approach relies on the anatomical information that the **nerves always lie superior to the lung** (16).
   a. Positioning and preparation are the same as for the traditional approach.
   b. With the patient lying supine, the needle is introduced through the skin just above the clavicle at the point of the lateral insertion of the SCM muscle, but it is **directed downward toward the floor (posteriorly), following the gravitational line that a plumb bob would follow** (Figure 12.14).
   c. If the needle is then redirected in small steps in a 15-degree arc caudad, it will contact the nerves and produce a paresthesia or motor response. Radiologic studies suggest that the nerves will always be contacted before the rib or the lung. Very small steps are critical.

C. The **infraclavicular block** technique approaches the neurovascular bundle from below the clavicle, but still at the point where the major cords are in close proximity. Multiple variations of this approach have been described, reflecting that the nerves lie considerably deeper from the skin in this area, and are not as

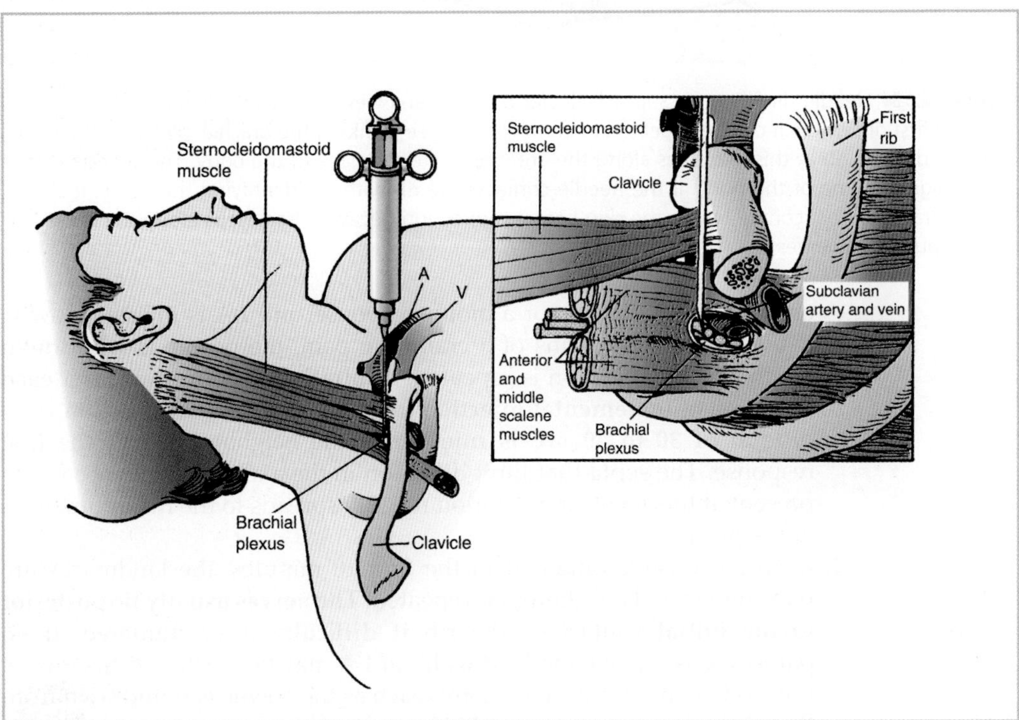

Figure 12.14. The "plumb-bob" approach to the supraclavicular block. The needle is introduced at the midpoint of the clavicle at a position directly posterior. If the nerves are not encountered at the first insertion, the needle is rotated in a caudad direction in very small steps, and will encounter the neurovascular bundle before encountering the lung.

reliably associated with clear landmarks. The **original description by Raj** used the C6 tubercle and the brachial pulse to create a line that would identify the midpoint of the clavicle, where a needle was inserted and directed 45 degrees laterally. This medial landmark maintains the risk of pneumothorax. On the basis of radiologic imaging, **a modified approach** with a more lateral insertion point and a 45- to 60-degree needle angulation may be preferred (17), especially for continuous catheter techniques (see Section III.C.3.). A simpler approach uses the coracoid landmark.

1. For **US guidance** there is no single best approach at this time. The approach is based on visualizing and obtaining a **short-axis view** of the anechoic pulsatile **artery,** as well as recognizing the importance of the fascial planes of the **pectoralis muscles** (especially the pectoralis minor) (18).
   a. The patient is placed supine with the head facing opposite the side of the block. A 5-cm linear array high-frequency probe (7–10 mHz) is placed inferior to the clavicle and just medial to the coracoid process in the parasagittal plane to obtain the short-axis view of the axillary artery.
   b. This is a deeper block than the interscalene or supraclavicular approaches. Therefore, the machine settings should be adjusted to obtain deeper depth of penetration (typically 3–6 cm) and consequently, the frequency may have to be decreased to 7 to 10 mHz to obtain optimal images of the infraclavicular neurovascular bundle (Figure 12.15).
   c. The probe should be adjusted to allow real-time visualization of the pulsatile **axillary artery** located deep to the pectoralis minor muscle fascial plane. In contrast to the interscalene approach where the nerves often appear hypoechoic in cross section, the cords often appear here as **hyperechoic**. The **lateral cord** is most often seen positioned superior (cephalad) to the axillary artery, the **posterior cord** posterior to the artery, and, if visible, the **medial cord** is inferior to the artery often between the artery and axillary vein (Figure 12.15).
   d. After skin preparation and draping, the long axis of the transducer probe positioned just medial to the coracoid process in the parasagittal plane. A skin wheal is made just superior to the superior edge of the transducer, and a 10-cm (4-in.) needle is inserted for the **in-plane approach**. The needle is inserted in an approximately **45-degree angle to the skin** and advanced in a **posterocaudad direction**. The trajectory of the needle is adjusted based on real-time observation of the needle tip. On the basis of magnetic resonance imaging (MRI) studies in volunteers and US-guided neurostimulation blocks, the ideal target for needle tip (and catheter tip placement for continuous techniques) is **posterior to the axillary artery** in close proximity to the posterior cord, which corresponds to the 6 to 8 o'clock position. Placement of the needle tip in this location facilitates LA distribution to all three cords around the axillary artery (Figure 12.15).
   e. Visualization of the LA solution's spread is important. **If spread is superficial (anterior) to the neurovascular bundle, the success of the block is poor** (Figure 12.15) (19,20).
2. The *coracoid approach* technique uses a more lateral point with a vertical needle insertion **(21)** (Figure 12.16).
   a. The patient is positioned supine, with the arm in any comfortable position, including resting at the side. The **coracoid process is identified**

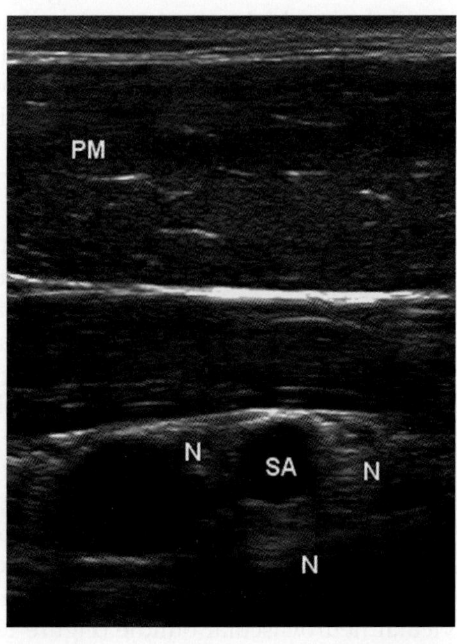

Figure 12.15. Ultrasonographic (US) guidance for the infraclavicular block. The probe is placed below the clavicle and aligned perpendicular to the presumed path of the axillary artery and the accompanying nerves. On the US image, the needle traverses the thick pectoralis major (*PM*) muscle and is inserted posterior to the pulsating hypoechoic artery (*SA*). The nerves (*N*) are present as lateral and medial cords (in those respective locations relative to the artery), whereas the posterior cord is behind the artery and is often confused with the echo shadow of the artery itself. Injection of the local anesthetic should produce a pattern that surrounds the posterior cord and appears to push the artery and the other two cords forward.

and marked on the skin. An "X" is placed 2-cm (0.75-in.) caudad and 2-cm (0.75-in.) medial to the lateral aspect of the coracoid surface mark.

b. A skin wheal is raised at this point, and a 5-cm (2-in.) **needle introduced perpendicular to the skin** (a 90-degree angle). **The average depth of the bundle is 4.2 cm** (1.5 in.; range, 2.25–7.75 cm) **(21)**. In heavier or more muscular patients, an 8- to 10-cm (3.5- or 4-in.) needle may be required.
c. The nerves can be identified by either a **nerve stimulation** or **paresthesia** in the hand. In locating the plexus, the needle should always be directed along a cranial-caudad path. Redirecting the needle medially may increase the risk of pleural puncture and subsequent pneumothorax.
d. When using a peripheral nerve stimulator, direct stimulation of the **pectoralis muscle** that occurs as the needle passes through the muscle can be uncomfortable for patients. Reducing the output on the nerve stimulator during that time may be helpful.
e. **Identifying the RN with a twitch response of wrist or finger extension will result in the highest rate of success** (22).
f. **MC (biceps twitch) and axillary nerve (deltoid twitch) responses are not reliable**as these nerves may branch away from the cords at this point and lie outside the neurovascular bundle. The **MC** nerve may require a **separate injection**.

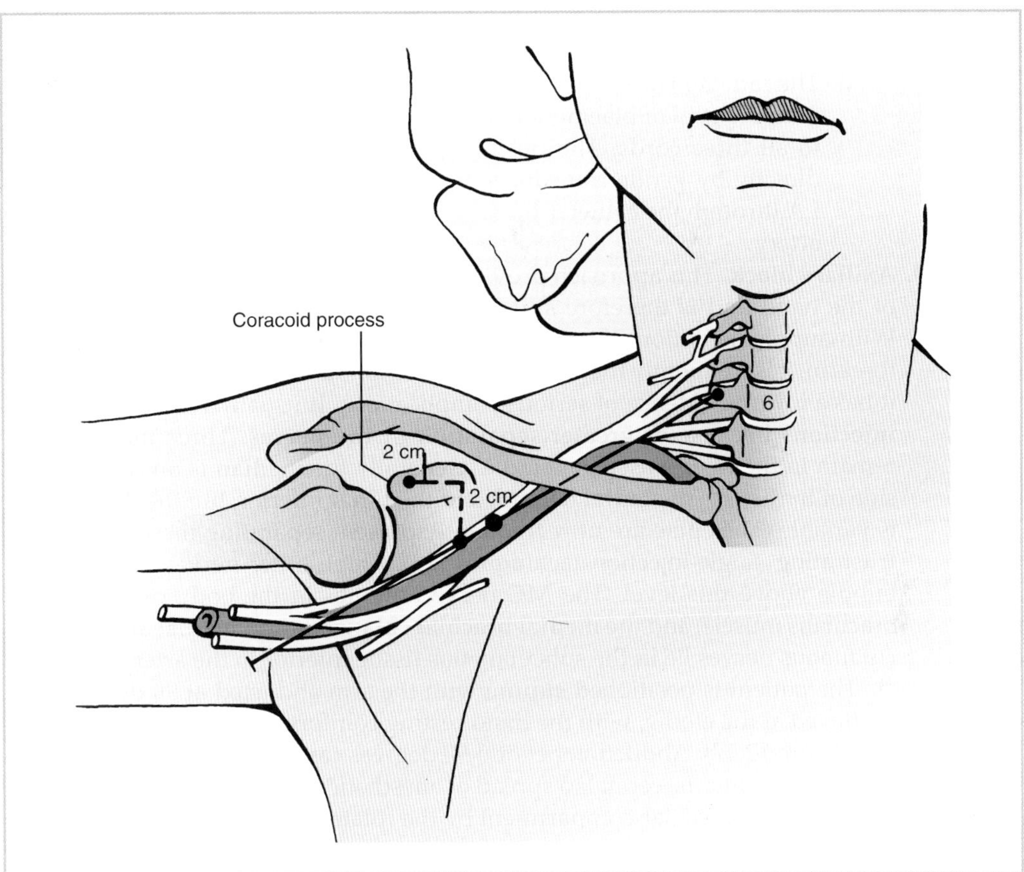

Figure 12.16. Infraclavicular approach. The original description of this technique used the midpoint of the line between the C6 tubercle and the axillary artery (*A*) to mark the insertion point of a needle directed 45 degrees laterally. A lateral approach 2 cm medial and inferior to the coracoid process allows a more perpendicular approach, which may reduce the chance of pneumothorax.

- **g.** Once the twitch is identified, a 30 to 40 mL of LA is incrementally injected. This block has a longer onset time than the other blocks of the brachial plexus.
- **h.** For continuous catheter placement, this approach is more challenging because of the 90-degree turn the catheter needs to make as it passes from the needle orifice.

3. Continuous US infraclavicular block. US guidance greatly facilitates placement of an infraclavicular catheter.

- **a.** The approach is the same as for the single-injection technique previously described.
- **b.** For the US-guided continuous infraclavicular technique, a **17- to 18-gauge Tuohy needle** is used to allow the passage of a 19- to 20-gauge perineural catheter. The use of the larger gauge Tuohy needle is advantageous in that the larger needle improves visualization at deeper depths typically required to reach the cords.
- **c.** After placement of the needle tip **posterior to the axillary artery,** a 15 to 20 mL of LA is incrementally injected through the Tuohy needle,

which distends the space posterior to the artery and facilitates catheter advancement through the needle tip.

d. The catheter is advanced no more than 2 to 3 cm (1 in.) past the needle tip, with the goal of placing the catheter tip to facilitate uniform distribution to all three cords. The position of the catheter tip may be visualized directly by gentle transducer manipulation, or conversely, injection of LA through the catheter tip observing for LA distribution relative to the artery.

D. **Axillary block.** This approach provides anesthesia to the three terminal nerves of the hand and is therefore **suited for most procedures on the hand** itself. With supplementation, it can be used to provide sensory anesthesia for the forearm. It is frequently the block of choice in ambulatory surgery units because it has a lower incidence of serious complications. It usually **requires multiple injections because of greater separation of the nerves**. Three major nerves remain in the neurovascular bundle. Generally the **median** is on the superior side of the artery, the **radial** behind, and the **ulnar** inferior, but the distribution is variable (1). Septae are now frequently present separating these nerves and frustrating single-injection techniques (23). Three other nerves have left the bundle above this level. The **MC** nerve now lies in the body of the coracobrachialis muscle, and the **medial brachial cutaneous** and **medial antebrachial cutaneous** nerves lie in the subcutaneous tissue inferior to the artery.

1. The patient is positioned **supine** with the arm abducted at 90 degrees and flexed at the elbow, with the hand resting comfortably on a towel or pillow (Figure 12.17). Abduction beyond 90 degrees can obscure the axillary pulse and also limit the cephalad spread of anesthetic solution because of pressure on the perivascular compartment by the rotated humeral head.

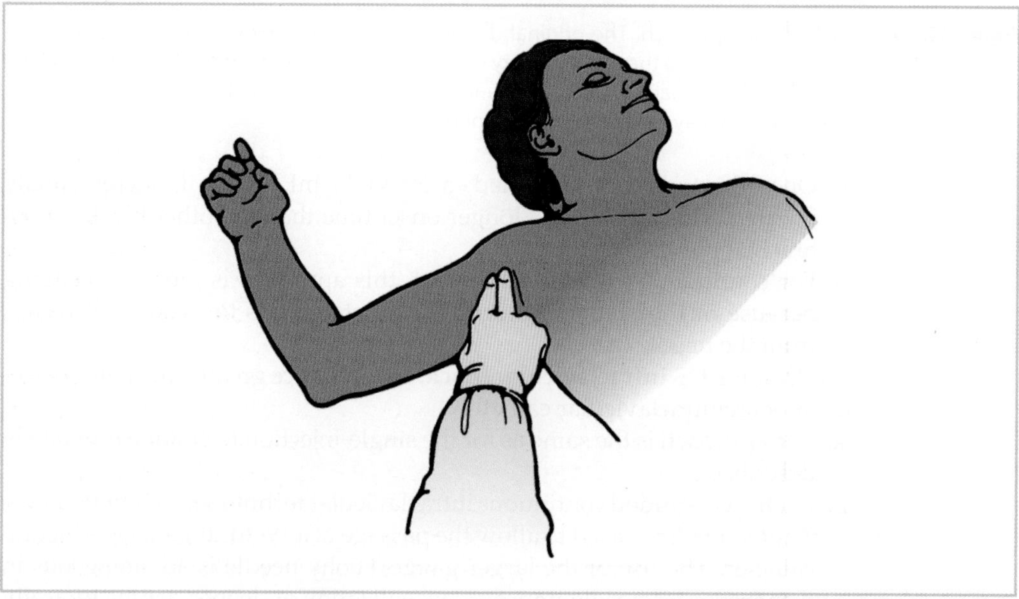

Figure 12.17. Position for axillary block. The arm is elevated (abducted) at 90 degrees at the shoulder, with the elbow flexed at a 90-degree angle and the forearm slightly elevated on a pillow. More extreme abduction may obscure the pulse, which is the critical landmark, usually easily identified by gentle palpation.

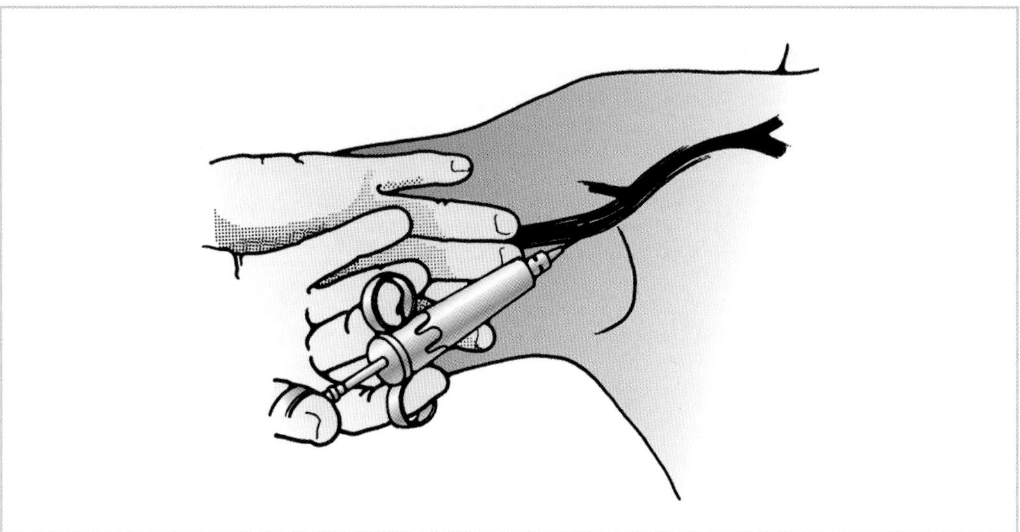

Figure 12.18. Hand position for axillary block. Two fingers of equal length straddle the artery while the needle is introduced along its long axis with a central angulation. The palpating fingers serve not only to identify the vessel but may also compress the perivascular sheath and encourage the spread of anesthetic solution centrally.

2. The **artery** is identified and marked as high as possible in the axilla, usually just lateral to the border of the pectoralis major (PM).
3. After aseptic preparation and drape, the artery is again identified and gently "pinned" between two fingers of equal length on the nondominant hand of the anesthesiologist. The index and middle fingers are commonly used, but the middle and ring fingers are also used (Figure 12.18).
4. A skin wheal is made over the artery, and a 20-mm (5/8-in.) needle attached to a 10-mL three-ring syringe is introduced.
5. At this point, there are several options.
   a. **US** probe guidance is also useful for localization. Use of US may increase success of the block over nerve stimulator techniques (24–26). Nerves are easily visualized around the artery, and the echoes of MC nerve are bright within the coracobrachialis muscle or fascia (Figure 12.19). The needle should be visualized as it approaches each nerve with the **neurovascular bundle** in **short axis,** and the LA solution can be seen spreading around each nerve (Figure 12.19). US has the additional advantage of being able to detect variable anatomy, which is frequent in this area (1), especially the location of the MC nerve, which may be in the coracobrachialis muscle or in a fascial plane outside the muscles.
   b. If US is not used, the simplest technique is **perivascular infiltration** on opposite sides of the artery (23). The needle is advanced as close as practical to one side of the artery while aspirating. If no blood is obtained at a depth felt to be just beyond the vessel, the needle is withdrawn slowly while 3 to 4 mL of anesthetic is injected. The needle is then redirected slightly further away from the vessel, and the process is repeated twice, producing three injections of LA (total of 10 mL) along three parallel lines alongside the vessel, covering a depth from

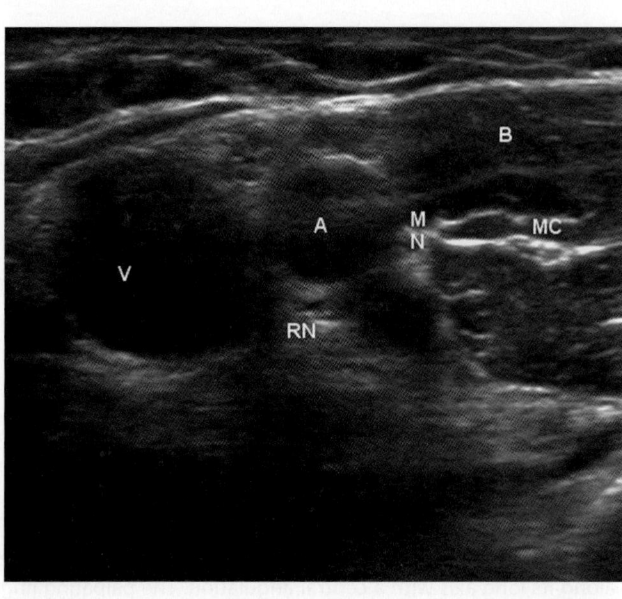

Figure 12.19. Ultrasonographic guidance for axillary block. The axillary artery (*A*) is easily identified as a pulsatile hypoechoic structure lying under the biceps muscle (*B*) and above the hyperechoic shadow of the humerus. It can be distinguished from the veins (*V*), which are easily compressed. The median (*MN*), radial (*RN*) and ulnar nerves surround the artery in a variable pattern. The musculocutaneous (*MC*) nerve lies 1 to 3 cm away from the neurovascular bundle, frequently seen in the fascial plane between the muscles at this level, rather than in the body of the coracobrachialis muscle.

just behind to just in front of the artery (Figure 12.20). The syringe is refilled, and the process repeated on the opposite side of the vessel. After these initial injections, supplemental anesthesia of the other nerves is produced by other injections (see Section III.D.6.). After 5 minutes, evaluation of the distal nerves is performed, and reinjection is made in the areas of nerves that are not yet anesthetized. If at any time the artery itself or a paresthesia is identified, the alternative approaches below are used (Figure 12.20).

c. The **transarterial approach** is also simple and reliable. The needle is advanced intentionally into the vessel with constant aspiration, and the advance halted as soon as blood no longer returns. At this point, the needle is fixed, and 10 mL is injected behind the artery, with intermittent aspiration to ensure that the needle has not migrated back into the vessel. The syringe is then reloaded and withdrawn back through the vessel with **constant aspiration** to indicate when the needle has just exited the anterior side of the artery. At this point, an additional 10 mL of anesthetic is injected, followed by the supplemental nerve injections (see Section III.D.6.).

d. The peripheral **nerve stimulator** can be used in the axilla to identify the three nerves around the artery. Stimulation can be used in the traditional high axillary level, but is also effective distally at the junction of the upper and middle third of the humerus (the "midhumeral" approach),

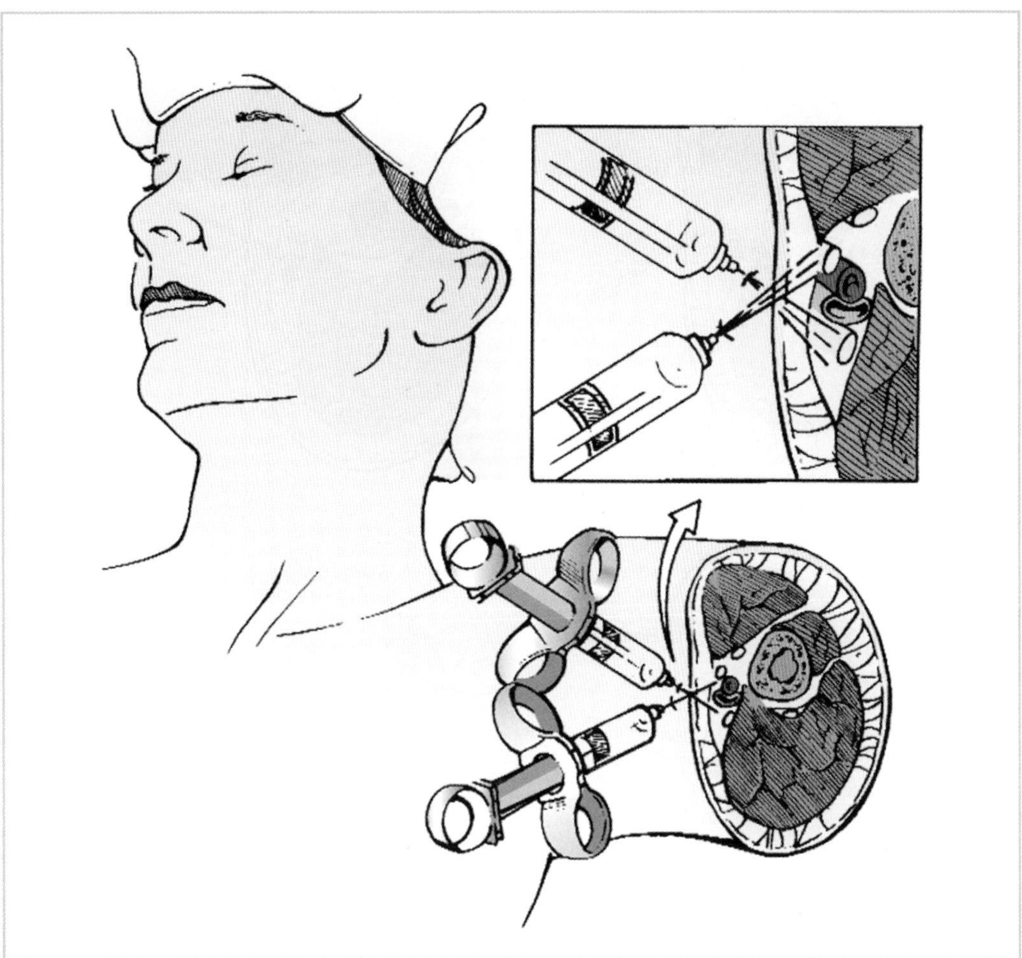

Figure 12.20. Perivascular infiltration approach for axillary block. The needle is introduced next to the artery with constant aspiration, and then injection of multiple small increments is made on withdrawal in a fan-wise pattern moving away from the vessel.

where all four major nerves can be blocked with separate injections (Figure 12.21) (27).

(1) For this approach, the arm is abducted 80 degrees, and the brachial artery is identified, either high in the axilla or at the junction of the upper and middle third of the arm.

(2) First, the **MN** is identified by introducing the stimulator needle next to the brachial artery on the superior side in the direction of the axilla. Stimulation of the MN in this area produces flexion of the wrist or fingers, or pronation of the forearm.

(3) Next, the **ulnar** nerve can be identified by redirecting the needle from the same insertion point in a posterior and inferior direction from the artery. Stimulation of the nerve produces ulnar flexion of the wrist or the last two fingers, or adduction of the thumb.

(4) In the upper axilla, the **RN** is usually stimulated in close proximity to the ulnar. Isolated contraction of the triceps muscle due to direct

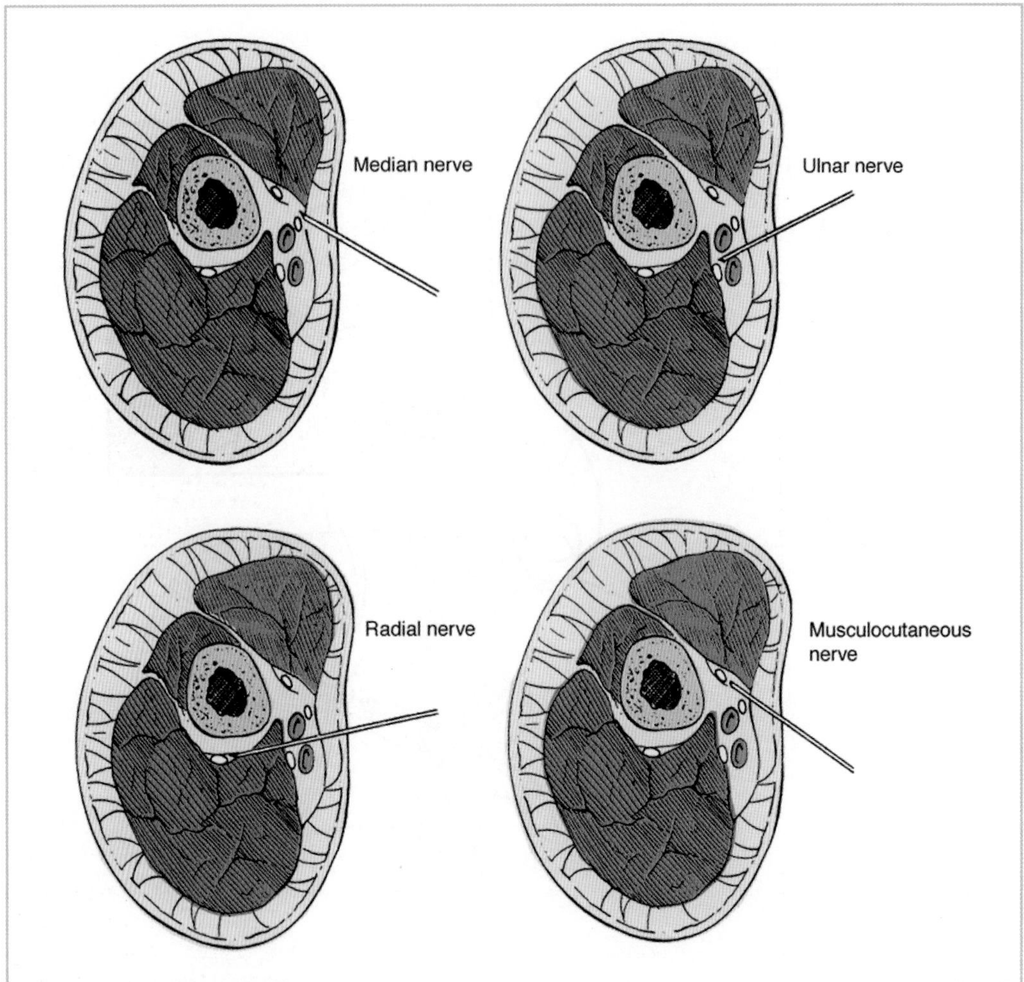

Figure 12.21. The midhumeral approach to axillary block. At this point the nerves are separated more than in the axilla itself, but still allow easy identification with the nerve stimulator.

stimulation can be confusing; therefore, the nerve is better identified by extension of the wrist or fingers.

(5) In the upper axilla, a **separate injection** of the radial or ulnar **may not be necessary** after finding one of these nerves because they generally lie in close proximity and a single injection will usually block both.

(6) If the block is performed at the more distal level, the **RN** is found by redirecting the needle perpendicular to the skin and deep to the artery to the level of the inferior side of the humerus itself to stimulate the RN.

(7) Finally, the needle is redirected superior to the artery to the body of the **coracobrachialis muscle,** where flexion of the elbow identifies the **MC** nerve. Injection of 5 to 10 mL of LA on each of the first three nerves is sufficient, whereas 5 to 6 mL may be adequate for the MC.

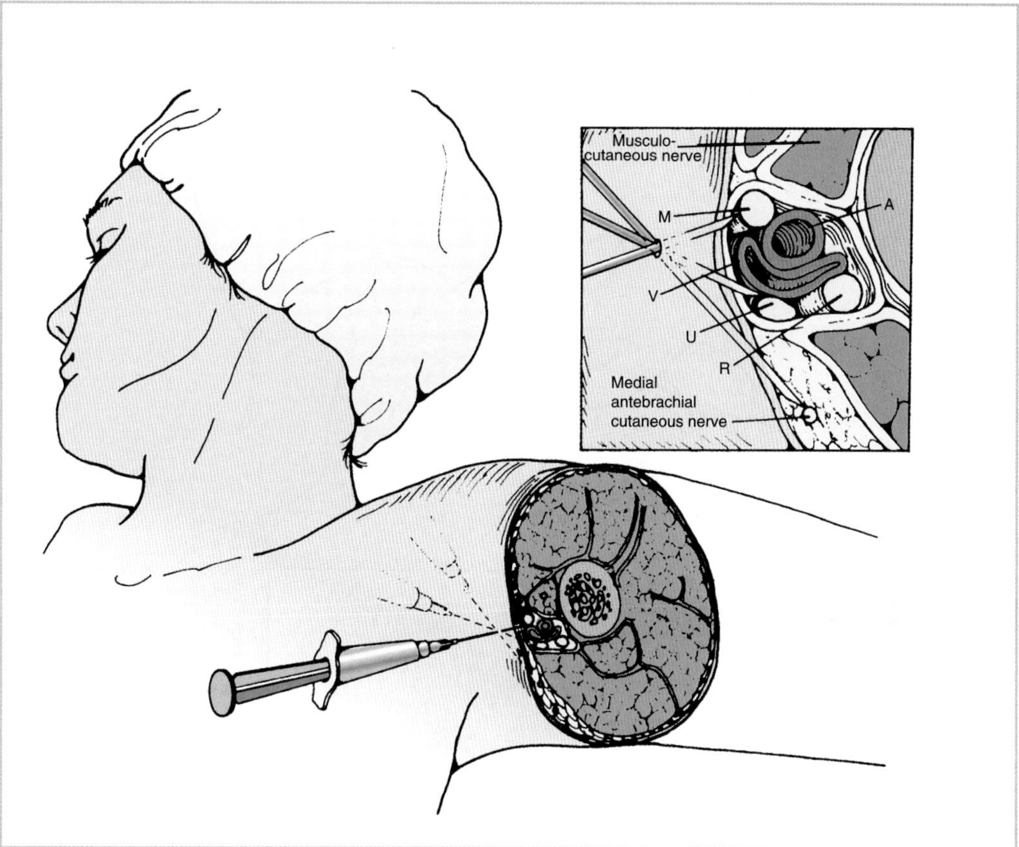

Figure 12.22. Needle position for paresthesia technique of axillary injection. The median (*M*) and musculocutaneous nerves lie on the superior side of the artery (*A*) and vein (v). The latter usually lies within the body of the coracobrachialis muscle at this point. The ulnar (*U*) nerve lies inferior and the radial (*R*) nerve is inferior and posterior to the artery. These positions may vary with individual patients and the medial antebrachial cutaneous nerve usually lies in the subcutaneous tissues just inferior to the neurovascular bundle and is anesthetized by a subcutaneous wheal along that area, along with the intercostobrachial fibers.

e. A fifth approach is the **traditional paresthesia technique**. Paresthesias are sought on either side of the vessel; it should be recalled that the MC nerves and MNs lie superior (consider the arm placed in anatomical position) to the artery in this position and the ulnar nerves and RNs lie inferior (Figure 12.22). Paresthesias should be sought first in the area most likely to affect the surgical field. Success is enhanced by finding **at least one paresthesia on each side of the artery,** although it is difficult to elicit a second paresthesia more than 5 minutes after the first injection, because partial spread of the anesthetic solution may produce hypesthesia of the other nerves. Between 10 and 20 mL of solution should be injected near each paresthesia.

6. With all of these axillary approaches, **supplementation may be required** to anesthetize the MC nerve, medial brachial cutaneous nerve, medial antebrachial cutaneous nerve, and the intercostobrachial branches.

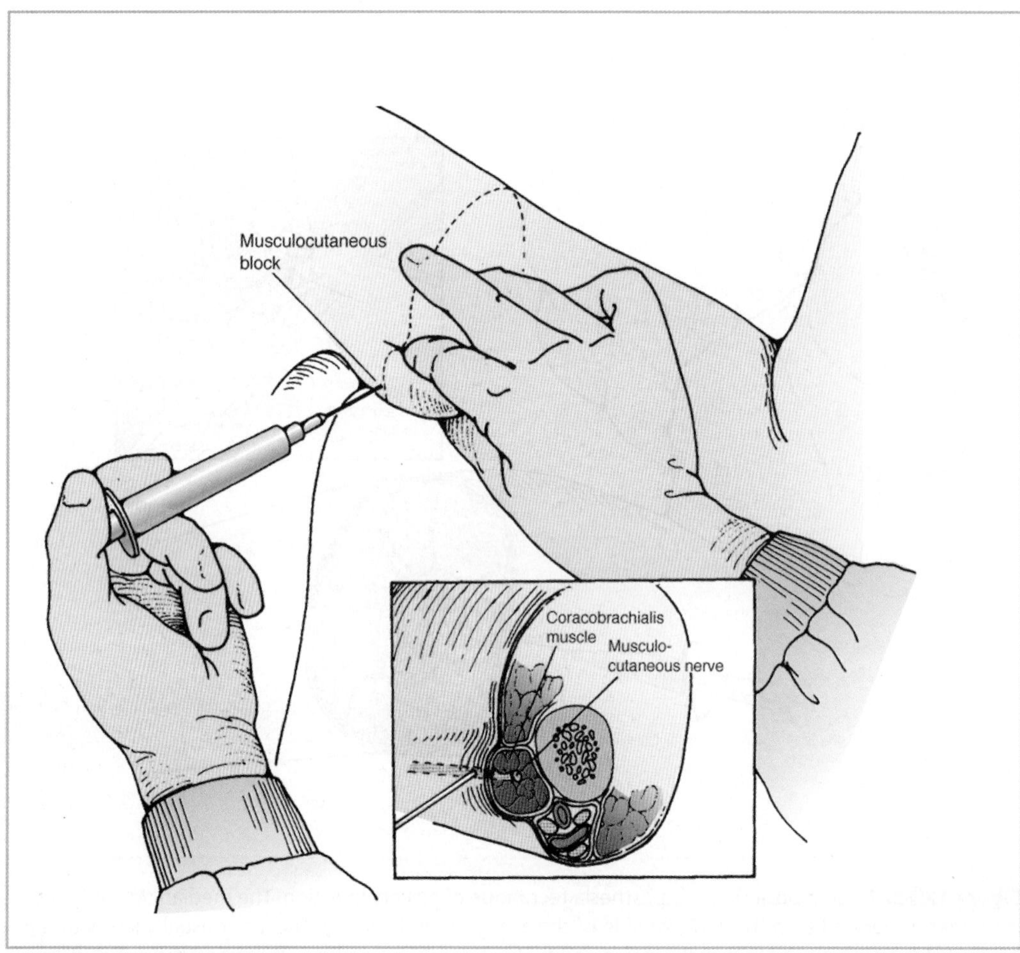

Figure 12.23. Musculocutaneous (MC) nerve. The MC nerve lies in the body of the coracobrachialis muscle. This muscle can be grabbed between the thumb and forefinger of one hand and the nerve blocked by the injection of 5 mL of local anesthetic into the body of the muscle.

a. The **MC nerve** is blocked by a fan-wise injection in the body of the coracobrachialis muscle just superior to the artery. This muscle can be grasped between the thumb and forefinger of one hand at the lateral border of the pectoralis while 5 mL of solution is injected with the other hand (Figure 12.23). Injection frequently produces a dull aching sensation that may resemble a paresthesia, but true nerve localization is rare except with US or nerve stimulation. Larger volume injections in the sheath itself (40 mL) have been recommended to produce MC nerve anesthesia, but this nerve is missed 25% of the time even with high volumes.

b. The **medial antebrachial cutaneous nerve** and its neighbor, the **medial brachial cutaneous nerve**, are blocked by infiltration of the subcutaneous tissues parallel to the axillary skin crease just inferior to the level of the neurovascular bundle with 5 mL of solution. Blockade of these nerves is usually not necessary if surgery is confined to the hand, but they do provide **sensory innervation** of the **ulnar side of the forearm**. The use of an upper arm tourniquet may dictate block of these nerves and **the intercostobrachial nerve** fibers, which is obtained by the same injection.

7. A **continuous axillary technique** has been described for use in patients with anticipated long-duration surgery (such as finger reimplantation with microsurgical techniques), or requirements for prolonged postoperative analgesia or sympathectomy. **Because of its higher failure rate** with MC nerve sparing and with technical difficulties in firmly fixing the catheter in an area that is highly mobile and often sweaty, **this technique has largely been replaced with the infraclavicular continuous technique**.
   - **a.** The original placement of the catheter can be performed by relying on the sensation of "popping" the catheter through the fascial plane of the sheath, although this may be difficult in the heavier patient.
   - **b.** Simple placement of the catheter in the groove between the biceps and triceps muscles alongside the sheath appears to be as effective.
   - **c. Elicitation of a paresthesia or use of a nerve stimulator or US may help confirm the catheter location.** Attempts to localize the sheath exactly, without US guidance, may lead to arterial puncture, potentially producing a hematoma that would interfere with spread of the LA solution.
   - **d.** The use of short 38- to 50-mm (1.5- or 2-in.) catheters may reduce the chance of central spread of anesthetic and increase the frequency of MC nerve sparing. **A 75-mm (3-in.) catheter can be inserted with a flexible guidewire higher in the axilla and threaded proximally, with a greater chance of anesthesia of all four nerves of the forearm**. With appropriate sterile dressing of the catheter entry site, the catheter can be left in place for several days.

IV. Complications

A. Missed nerve blocks occur from 3% to 30% of the time with these techniques (28,29) and usually involve only one or two of the terminal nerves. This can be rectified by repetition of the block (if paresthesias are not relied on and LA toxicity limits are considered), peripheral injection of the nerve (see Chapter 14), or local infiltration by the surgeon. Early identification is essential to allow appropriate correction.

1. **The most common findings are absent C8-T1 anesthesia with the interscalene approach, or residual MC or medial antebrachial cutaneous sensation with the axillary block.** Anesthesia should be assessed as early as 5 minutes after completion of the injection. Onset of anesthesia with all the drugs, including bupivacaine, is within 5 minutes **(2)**, and the absence of some anesthesia in a critical nerve distribution at this time interval should lead to the formulation of alternative plans. Sometimes merely waiting another 5 minutes will allow sufficient diffusion of anesthetic solution to provide analgesia, but alternative plans should be reviewed with the patient and surgeon before an incision.
2. If inadequate anesthesia is discovered at the time of incision (particularly on the forearm), infiltration of the wound with LA by the surgeon or intravenous narcotics by the anesthesiologist may provide the needed supplemental analgesia. General anesthesia should always be considered as a potential necessity in all patients with a regional block.

3. **Testing of the block can be performed quickly and effectively with the "push–pull-pinch–pinch" technique.** The patient is asked to extend (**push**) the forearm against resistance (triceps, RN) and then flex the arm (**pull**), drawing the thumb to the nose (biceps, MC nerve). Sensory anesthesia of the hand to **pinch** on the thenar (MN) and hypothenar (ulnar nerve) areas will confirm block of the other two nerves. This entire sequence can be performed in less than a minute, and the profound loss of radial muscle tone will often give the patient reassurance that the block is working. A full 20 minutes is required for dense anesthesia of the arm, but, fortunately, surgical preparation and draping often provide the needed time interval.
4. **Alkalinization of the LA or performance of the block in a waiting area can further reduce onset time** and improve the depth of anesthesia at the time of incision; the most frequent cause of "failed" anesthesia is premature surgical incision.

B. **Intravascular injection.** Intravascular injection is the most serious potential complication.

1. This is true for the supraclavicular, infraclavicular, and axillary techniques because of their proximity to blood vessels, but it is a **particular concern with the interscalene technique** because of the nearness of the **vertebral artery** to the cervical nerve roots, and the incidence is highest with this technique.
2. **Frequent aspiration, incremental injection, and close observation of the patient are essential.** Resuscitation equipment and intravenous access are mandatory.

C. **Pneumothorax**

1. Pneumothorax occurs rarely in experienced hands, being reported as less than 1% in one series of supraclavicular blocks **(6)**, but it is a risk with this technique. It is also possible to puncture the pleura with the interscalene approach if the needle is directed too far inferiorly. It is also a rare but reported complication for infraclavicular blocks, especially when performed with a more medial approach.
2. Although the complication is not life threatening, it is painful to the patient and a serious inconvenience, particularly if it necessitates unplanned admission of an outpatient to the hospital. The pneumothorax is often small and may resolve spontaneously, and it may not even be symptomatic immediately. Any patient who complains of pain in the chest or shortness of breath should be evaluated with a physical examination and a chest x-ray, and treated with a chest tube if symptomatic.

D. **Neuropathy.** Transient neuropathy is also rare, being reported as 2% or less in several series (see Chapter 3), with **permanent dysfunction extremely rare**.

1. The incidence appears to be higher if paresthesias are sought with sharp (long-beveled) needles or if repeated contact with the nerves is made **(30)**. Particular attention is needed to avoid pinning the nerve roots and trunks against the bony structures during interscalene and supraclavicular blocks.
2. As always, **no injection should be continued if a cramping pain suggests intraneural injection or if there is resistance to injection.**
3. If a postoperative neurologic deficit is detected, **neurologic evaluation should be obtained early.** Precise localization of the injury can help identify if the anesthetic injection itself was related to the deficit. Interscalene injections affect roots and dermatomes, and their effects can be differentiated

from axillary injections, which affect peripheral nerves. Electromyographic testing also can help determine if the injury represents preexisting nerve damage.

4. **Most peripheral injuries resolve spontaneously in 1 to 6 months.** Empathy, close attention to follow-up, and early arrangements for physical therapy will help alleviate patient disability and dissatisfaction, although the long course of recovery is frustrating to physician and patient alike.
5. A unique complication of the interscalene approach is permanent **phrenic** nerve paralysis, which is fortunately rare. The mechanism is unclear, but may involve direct needle injury if the plexus is approached anteriorly through the AS.

E. Vascular injury

1. **Hematoma** formation can occur following supraclavicular or axillary block if the artery is punctured. This is usually of little consequence, but it may discourage performance of these blocks on patients with bleeding disorders.
2. Temporary **vasospasm** of the artery and occlusion of the pulse have been described after puncture, as well as occlusion of the axillary vein. These events are rare, but, again, they suggest that the minimal degree of tissue disruption is the best.

F. Unintentional anesthetic spread is most common with the interscalene approach

1. The most serious problem involves injection of the anesthetic solution **into the epidural or subarachnoid space**, producing a high epidural or total spinal anesthetic. Although bilateral cervical and brachial plexus blocks are the most common events, total spinal anesthesia is a possibility that requires prompt recognition and treatment with ventilatory and cardiovascular support.
2. More frequently, the anesthetic solution spreads to involve the **phrenic nerve**, either at its origin in the cervical roots or along its course on the anterior surface of the AS muscle. Motor blockade of the ipsilateral diaphragm occurs reliably with interscalene block (31). Paralysis of one diaphragm does not represent a problem in the healthy patient, but it may not be well tolerated in the patient with respiratory disease. The sympathetic chain also lies close to the site of injection, and a **unilateral Horner syndrome** is not unusual. **Bronchospasm** caused by sympathetic blockade has also been attributed to spread of interscalene anesthesia.
3. Spread of anesthesia to these structures after supraclavicular anesthesia is less common, and infraclavicular and axillary injections are associated with the least likelihood.

REFERENCES

1 Retzl G, Kapral S, Greher M, et al. Ultrasonographic findings of the axillary part of the brachial plexus. *Anesth Analg* 2001;92:1271–1275.

2 **Lanz E, Theiss D, Jankovic D. The extent of blockade following various techniques of brachial plexus block. *Anesth Analg* 1983;62:55.**

3 Winnie AP, Collins VJ. The subclavian perivascular technique of brachial plexus anesthesia. *Anesthesiology* 1964;25:353.

4 Thompson GE, Rorie DK. Functional anatomy of the brachial plexus sheaths. *Anesthesiology* 1983; 59:117.

5 Partridge BL, Katz J, Benirschke K. Functional anatomy of the brachial plexus sheath: implications for anesthesia. *Anesthesiology* 1987;66:743.

6 Neal JM, Hebl JR, Gerancher JC, et al. Brachial plexus anesthesia: essentials of our current understanding. *Reg Anesth Pain Med* 2002;27(4):402–428.

7 Singelyn F, Gouverneur J, Robert A. A minimum dose of clonidine added to mepivacaine prolongs the duration of anesthesia and analgesia after axillary brachial plexus block. *Anesth Analg* 1996;83:1046.

8 Chan VW. Applying ultrasound imaging to interscalene brachial plexus block. *Reg Anesth Pain Med* 2003; 28:340–343.

9 Pippa P, Cominelli E, Marinelli C, et al. Brachial plexus block using the posterior approach. *Eur J Anaesthesiol* 1990;7:411–420.

10 Boezaart AP, de Beer JF, du Toit C, et al. A new technique of continuous interscalene nerve block. *Can J Anaesth* 1999;46:275–281.

11 Borgeat A, Dullenkopf A, Ekatodramis G, et al. Evaluation of the lateral modified approach for continuous interscalene block after shoulder surgery. *Anesthesiology* 2003;99(2):436–442.

12 Sardesai AM, Patel R, Denny NM, et al. Interscalene brachial plexus block: can the risk of entering the spinal canal be reduced? A study of needle angles in volunteers undergoing magnetic resonance imaging. *Anesthesiology* 2006;105:9–13.

13 Urmey WF, Talts KH, Sharrock NE. One hundred percent incidence of hemidiaphragmatic paresis associated with interscalene brachial plexus anesthesia as diagnosed by ultrasonography. *Anesth Analg* 1991;72(4): 498–503.

14 Kapral S, Krafft P, Eibenberger K, et al. Ultrasound-guided supraclavicular approach for regional anesthesia of the brachial plexus. *Anesth Analg* 1994;78(3):507–513.

15 Williams SR, Chouinard P, Arcand G, et al. Ultrasound guidance speeds execution and improves the quality of supraclavicular block. *Anesth Analg* 2003;97(5):1518–1523.

16 Brown DL, Cahill DR, Bridenbaugh LD. Supraclavicular nerve block: anatomic analysis of a method to prevent pneumothorax. *Anesth Analg* 1993;76:530.

17 Klaastad O, Lilleas FG, Rotnes JS, et al. A magnetic resonance imaging study of modifications to the infraclavicular brachial plexus block. *Anesth Analg* 2000;91:929.

18 Klaastad O, Smith HJ, Smedby O, et al. A novel infraclavicular brachial plexus block: the lateral and sagittal technique, developed by magnetic resonance imaging studies. *Anesth Analg* 2004;98(1):252–256.

19 Porter JM, McCartney CJ, Chan VW. Needle placement and injection posterior to the axillary artery may predict successful infraclavicular brachial plexus block: a report of three cases. *Can J Anaesth* 2005;52(1):69–73.

20 Dingemans E, Williams SR, Arcand G, et al. Neurostimulation in ultrasound-guided infraclavicular block: a prospective randomized trial. *Anesth Analg* 2007;104:1275–1280.

21 Wilson JL, Brown DL, Wong GY, et al. Infraclavicular brachial plexus block: parasagittal anatomy important to the coracoid technique. *Anesth Analg* 1998;87:870.

22 Bloc S, Garnier T, Komly B, et al. Single-stimulation, low-volume infraclavicular plexus block: influence of the evoked distal motor response on success rate. *Reg Anesth Pain Med* 2006;31(5):433–437.

23 Thompson GE. Blocking the brachial plexus. *Anaesth Intensive Care* 1987;15:119.

24 Chan VW, Perlas A, McCartney CJ, et al. Ultrasound guidance improves success rate of axillary brachial plexus block. *Can J Anaesth* 2007;54(3):176–182.

25 Casati A, Danelli G, Baciarello M, et al. A prospective, randomized comparison between ultrasound and nerve stimulation guidance for multiple injection axillary brachial plexus block. *Anesthesiology* 2007;106(5): 992–996.

26 Sites BD, Beach ML, Spence BC, et al. Ultrasound guidance improves the success rate of a perivascular axillary plexus block. *Acta Anaesthesiol Scand* 2006;50(6):678–684.

27 Bouaziz H, Narchi P, Mercier FJ, et al. Comparison between conventional axillary block and a new approach at the midhumeral level. *Anesth Analg* 1997;84:1058.

28 Goldberg ME, Gregg C, Larijani GE, et al. A comparison of three methods of axillary approach to brachial plexus blockade for upper extremity surgery. *Anesthesiology* 1987;66:814.

29 Selander D. Axillary plexus block: paresthetic or perivascular. *Anesthesiology* 1987;66:726.

30 Selander D, Edshage S, Wolff T. Paresthesiae or no paresthesiae? Nerve lesions after axillary blocks. *Acta Anaesthesiol Scand* 1979;23:27.

31 Urmey WF, Gloeggler PJ. Pulmonary function changes during interscalene brachial plexus block: effects of decreasing local anesthetic injection volume. *Reg Anesth* 1993;18:244.

13 Intravenous Regional Anesthesia

Susan B. McDonald

Intravenous regional anesthesia of the extremities is one of the simplest and oldest techniques available, but it still requires understanding of the anatomy, pharmacology, and physiology involved to ensure safe and effective anesthesia.

I. Anatomy

A. Venous plexus of extremities. The peripheral nerves of the arm and leg are nourished by small blood vessels that accompany them. Distension of the venous vessels in these nerves with a local anesthetic solution will cause diffusion of the solution into the nerves and produce anesthesia as long as the concentration in the venous system remains high. This is usually attained by blocking venous flow with a proximal tourniquet, followed by distension of the venous system with a dilute solution of local anesthetic injected through a previously placed venous catheter. **The anesthetic acts on the small nerves and nerve endings** and to a lesser extent on the main nerve trunks.

B. Historically, a form of this technique of venous injection of local anesthetic was first described by August Bier. His original technique required surgical exposure of the veins. The practical application awaited the development of intravenous needles and pneumatic tourniquets, but the technique is still commonly referred to as a *Bier block*.

II. Indications

A. The primary advantages of intravenous regional anesthesia are its simplicity and reliability. It is the **easiest** and **most effective** block of the arm for simple, short procedures, and it is therefore well suited for novices and for ambulatory surgery.

B. Suitable situations for intravenous regional anesthesia

1. Intravenous regional anesthesia is suitable for many operations **on the distal extremities when a proximal occlusive tourniquet can be safely applied.**
   a. **The block is used primarily in the arm.** Although a forearm tourniquet has been employed to reduce the total dose of local anesthetic, the upper arm tourniquet remains the standard.
   b. **In the leg, larger volumes of drug are required and adequate occlusion of vessels is harder to attain** because of thicker muscles and the more irregular shape of the thigh. There are also concerns about intraosseous channels allowing more leakage of local anesthetic solution into the systemic circulation and about the potential of a higher frequency of systemic reactions to anesthetics when the lower limb is blocked with this technique. Although a calf tourniquet has been advocated in reducing the total dose of local anesthetic and has been used successfully, this technique is not as popular as application to the upper extremity.
2. It provides satisfactory anesthesia for foreign body explorations, nerve explorations, surgical repairs of lacerations, and tendon or joint repairs.

3. Although **periosteal anesthesia is not as dense** as with other techniques, it can be used for bunionectomies or reduction of simple fractures.
4. The **rapid recovery of function** in the hand is an advantage.

C. Situations where this technique is less suitable

1. It is not suitable if a condition such as severe ischemic vascular disease contraindicates vascular occlusion with a tourniquet.
2. Some surgeons may also be dissatisfied with the amount of fluid exuded into the surgical field (especially if performing microscopic procedures), but a bloodless field is maintained.
3. The constraints of **anesthetic duration and tourniquet time limit the length of surgery to only short procedures lasting approximately 20 to 60 minutes**.
4. It is not the technique of choice when the benefits of regional block for analgesia postoperatively are recommended.

III. Drugs

A. Local anesthetics

1. **Lidocaine** is the most commonly used drug. A dilute solution is sufficient and is required if the maximum dose is to be avoided with the high volumes necessary for venous distension. **A total of 50 mL of 0.5% lidocaine** is the usual volume for the arm, whereas 100 mL (500 mg) is needed to distend the venous channels of the leg if a thigh cuff is used. In smaller patients, a dose of 3 mg/kg 0.5% lidocaine can be used as a guide for total dose.
2. **Mepivacaine** (5 mg/mL) is also effective (1).
3. **Bupivacaine** (0.25% in similar volumes) has been used for this block, but systemic release of this drug is a **significant concern for cardiotoxicity**.
4. **Ropivacaine** 0.2% is an effective alternative with a greater cardiac safety margin, and may provide some residual analgesia after tourniquet release (2).
5. The amino ester **2-chloroprocaine** is cleared even more rapidly. Its use has been associated with **phlebitis** in one report, but the use of an alkalinized solution produces minimal side effects and analgesia equivalent to lidocaine (3).

B. Additives to the local anesthetic. Numerous studies have evaluated the benefit of adding various agents to the local anesthetic in an effort to improve analgesia both intraoperatively and postoperatively. Except perhaps for the nonsteroidal anti-inflammatory drugs (NSAIDs), studies showing statistically significant benefits are often of questionable *clinical* significance. Risks, such as drug error or unwanted side effects, should be weighed against the slight benefits.

1. **Opioids (meperidine, fentanyl).** Overall as a class of drugs, opioids do not provide much added benefit and may increase postoperative nausea and vomiting **(4)**.
2. **Nonsteroidal anti-inflammatory drugs.** Presumably through a peripheral site mechanism of action, NSAIDs mixed with local anesthetic can provide analgesia for longer duration than when given parentally **(4)**. Twenty milligram ketorolac added to lidocaine for upper extremity surgery is sufficient to reduce the amount of rescue analgesics in the recovery room (5).
3. **Muscle relaxants.** Nondepolarizing agents can provide improved muscle relaxation that may aid in reducing fractures but may also result in prolonged muscle relaxation in that limb (6, 7).

4. α_2-Agonists
   a. **Clonidine** in doses of 1 μg/kg will prolong analgesia after lidocaine block (8), whereas higher doses will also reduce tourniquet pain at the expense of some systemic side effects (9).
   b. **Dexmedetomidine** has also been shown, in limited studies, to improve the analgesic quality perioperatively when added to lidocaine, with minimal side effects (10).
5. **Neostigmine** appears to have no additional benefit (11).
6. **Dexamethasone.** Dexamethasone may provide some analgesic benefit, although there may be concern over potential local irritant effect (12).

IV. Technique

A. Preparation for block

1. The patient is placed in the **supine position, and appropriate monitors are placed**. These include a blood pressure cuff to obtain systolic readings to guide tourniquet settings, and intravenous access in another extremity.
2. An **intravenous catheter is inserted in the hand or foot to be operated on**. This should be a flexible, small, 20- or 22-gauge plastic catheter placed distally from the surgical site and in a position where it will not be dislodged by the Esmarch bandage used for exsanguination. **Distal placement**, rather than in the antecubital fossa, is associated with less probability of leakage under the cuff. The catheter is taped loosely in place and a small syringe or injection cap is fitted over it after a dilute heparin or saline flush is used to clear the lumen.

B. Cuff inflation

1. The tourniquet is placed securely on the proximal part of the extremity to be operated on.
   a. The arm or leg is elevated to promote venous drainage and is then exsanguinated with an **Esmarch bandage** wrapped from the distal end up to the tourniquet itself (Figure 13.1).
   b. The tourniquet is inflated to a pressure 100 mm Hg above the systolic blood pressure, or preferably 300 mm Hg. Tourniquet inflation is checked by balloting the cuff and watching the oscillation of the pressure gauge.
   c. After inflation and removal of the Esmarch wrap, **adequate occlusion is confirmed** by the absence of the radial or posterior tibial pulse.
2. **A constant pressure gas source must be used to maintain inflation of the cuff.** All cuffs have some small-volume leak, and a simple inflation of the standard blood pressure cuff with a bulb will produce a gradual decrease in cuff pressure that will allow leakage of local anesthetic with potentially catastrophic results. The cuffs must be checked before injection and frequently during the procedure.
3. The *"double cuff"* has been popularized for this block to reduce the pressure pain in the unanesthetized skin under the cuff in longer operations (45 minutes or longer).
   a. **Caution regarding the "double cuff."** The presence of two cuffs requires that they both be narrower (5–7 cm) than the standard blood pressure cuff (12–14 cm) used on the arm. Narrower cuffs do not effectively transmit the indicated gauge pressure to deep tissues, and therefore **venous occlusion pressures are less than presumed (13)**. The use of a standard wide cuff may be more desirable and more acceptable if

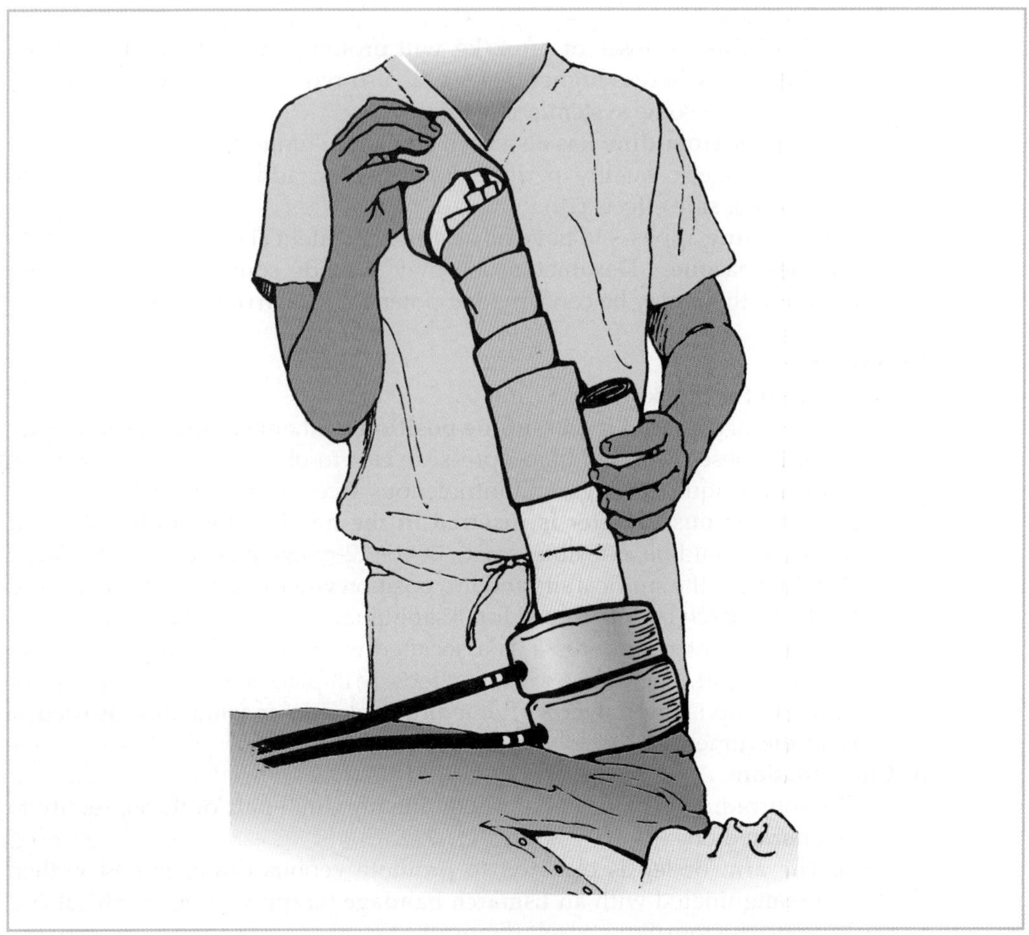

Figure 13.1. Technique for intravenous regional anesthesia. A small intravenous catheter is placed in the hand and the tourniquet is applied to the upper arm. A single tourniquet may be used for shorter operations and may provide more reliable compression of the venous system than the double-tourniquet system shown. Exsanguination of the arm is attained by elevation and wrapping with the Esmarch elastic bandage. The tourniquet is then inflated and the local anesthetic injected.

the procedure is to last less than an hour (about the time for pressure discomfort to develop).

b. If the procedure exceeds 45 minutes, the double cuff may be employed. In this situation, the proximal cuff is inflated for the first 45 minutes of anesthesia. The distal cuff is then inflated over the tissue area that has been numbed by the local anesthetic injection and the proximal cuff (overlying unanesthetized skin) is deflated. The adequacy of the distal cuff must be checked before the proximal cuff is deflated. Although this technique allegedly reduces patient discomfort at the area of the tourniquet, the complex procedure of shifting the inflation **adds the risk of unintentional deflation.**

4. **Injection of local anesthetic solution**

   a. After exsanguination, the limb is returned to the neutral position and the local anesthetic drug is injected through the previously placed catheter.

The **injection is made slowly (90 seconds or more) to produce a peak venous pressure that is not greater than the occluding pressure of the cuff (13).**

b. The patient is warned that this will produce an uncomfortable "pins and needles" sensation for a few seconds. Slow rate of injection may reduce this discomfort.
c. The catheter is removed if surgery will be less than an hour, and pressure is placed over the entry site until it seals. **Adequate sensory anesthesia will ensue in 5 minutes.**
d. If more than 45 minutes have elapsed from the time of injection, anesthesia may begin to diminish. If the surgeon requires more time, the intravenous catheter may be reinjected with local anesthetic solution after 60 to 90 minutes. This is disruptive to the surgery and potentially to the sterile field, and, because of this, for longer procedures, other regional techniques, such as brachial plexus block, are usually a more appropriate plan.

5. **Cuff deflation**
   a. Deflation of the tourniquet can be performed **after 45 minutes with minimal risk** of systemic symptoms of local anesthetic toxicity because the drug binds to the tissues **(14)**.
   b. **If less than 45 minutes have elapsed, a two-stage release is recommended**, where the cuff is deflated for 10 seconds and reinflated for a minute before final release. This allows a gradual washout of anesthetic. Cycling the cuff three times in this manner will delay the onset of peak blood levels, but it does not significantly reduce the level attained with a single deflation (15).
   c. **Under no circumstances is the cuff deflated in the first 20 minutes after injection.** If less than 20 minutes have elapsed, pleasant conversation should be used to fill the time until that interval has passed and a two-stage release can be performed. These steps do not guarantee the absence of systemic toxicity (Figure 13.2).

V. Complications

A. **Systemic toxicity** is the major risk of this procedure.

1. **The greatest danger is from an inadequate tourniquet early** in the procedure when the intravenous volume and concentration are large. Every precaution must be taken to ensure a reliable tourniquet and inflation pressure source.
2. Even with adequate inflation, the narrow cuffs (5–7 cm width) used for the double-tourniquet system will sometimes allow leakage. The use of a standard width adult cuff (12–14 cm) provides more reliable compression of the entire venous system of the extremity, especially in the leg.
3. Leakage is more likely if the injection is made rapidly under high pressure into a vein near the cuff **(13)**.
4. The least leakage occurs when injection is made into a distal vein for more than 90 seconds following exsanguination of the arm and inflation of the cuff to 300 mm Hg pressure. Careful monitoring of mental status is indicated for several minutes, even with an apparently functioning cuff.
5. Tourniquet release inevitably washes drug into the systemic circulation as some local anesthetic remains in the veins at the end of the procedure. **With**

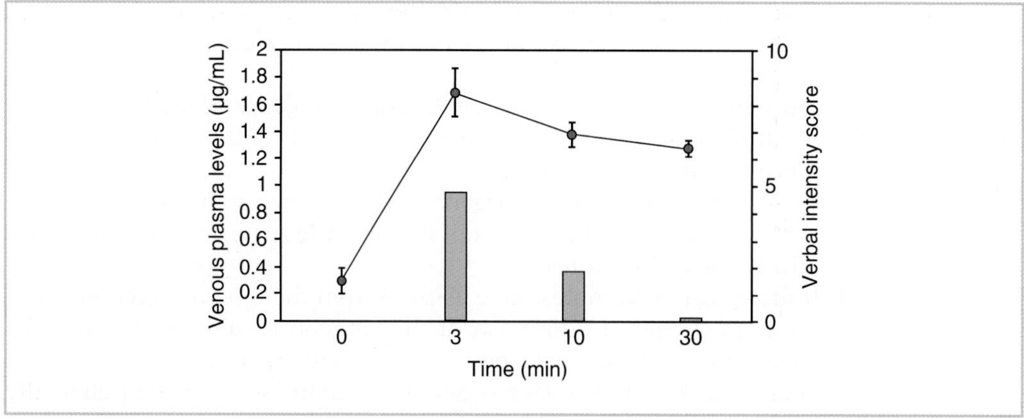

Figure 13.2. Systemic blood levels of 0.5% lidocaine after intravenous regional blockade. After release of the tourniquet, blood levels of local anesthetic increase rapidly, but are also rapidly cleared. After 72 ± 22 minutes of total tourniquet inflation time, the *colored circles* indicate blood levels following injection of 40 mL of 0.5% lidocaine (range to 2 μg/mL). The *solid bars* indicate the verbal numerical intensity score (on scale of 0–10) of central nervous system symptoms of light-headedness, dizziness, and tinnitus at 3, 10, and 30 minutes after deflation. (Adapted from Atanassoff PG, Hartmannsgruber MWB. Central nervous system side effects are less important after iv regional anesthesia with ropivacaine 0.2% compared to lidocaine 0.5% in volunteers. *Can J Anaesth* 2002;49:169–172.)

lidocaine, these levels are subtoxic after 45 minutes, but dangerously high within 20 minutes of injection (14). This is the basis for the guidelines for tourniquet release stated.

6. Because of variability no safety is guaranteed, and all patients having this technique must be monitored closely at all times for possible local anesthetic toxicity. Resuscitation equipment is necessary, and an intravenous access in another extremity is indicated.

REFERENCES

1 Prieto-Alvarez P, Calas-Guerra A, Fuentes-Bellido J, et al. Comparison of mepivacaine and lidocaine for intravenous regional anaesthesia: pharmacokinetic study and clinical correlation. *Br J Anaesth* 2002;88(4):516–519.

2 Hartmannsgruber MW, Silverman DG, Halaszynski TM, et al. Comparison of ropivacaine 0.2% and lidocaine 0.5% for intravenous regional anesthesia in volunteers. *Anesth Analg* 1999;89:727.

3 Lavin PA, Henderson CL, Vaghadia H. Non-alkalinized and alkalinized 2-chloroprocaine *vs.* lidocaine for intravenous regional anesthesia during outpatient hand surgery. *Can J Anaesth* 1999;46:939.

4 Choyce A, Peng P. A systematic review of adjuncts for intravenous regional anesthesia for surgical procedures. *Can J Anaesth* 2002;49(1):32–45.

5 Steinberg RB, Reuben SS, Gardner G. The dose-response relationship of ketorolac as a component of intravenous regional anesthesia with lidocaine. *Anesth Analg* 1998;86:791–793.

6 Elhakim M, Sadek RA. Addition of atracurium to lidocaine for intravenous regional anaesthesia. *Acta Anaesthesiol Scand* 1994;38(6):542–544.

7 Torrance JM, Lewer BM, Galletly DC. Low-dose mivacurium supplementation of prilocaine i.v. regional anaesthesia. *Br J Anaesth* 1997;78(2):222–223.

8 Reuben SS, Steinberg RB, Klatt JL, et al. Intravenous regional anesthesia using lidocaine and clonidine. *Anesthesiology* 1999;91:654.

9 Gentili M, Bernard JM, Bonnet F. Adding clonidine to lidocaine for intravenous regional anesthesia prevents tourniquet pain. *Anesth Analg* 1999;88:1327.

10 Memis D, Turan A, Karamanlioglu B, et al. Adding dexmedetomidine to lidocaine for intravenous regional anesthesia. *Anesth Analg* 2004;98(3):835–840.
11 McCartney CJ, Brill S, Rawson R, et al. No anesthetic or analgesic benefit of neostigmine 1 mg added to intravenous regional anesthesia with lidocaine 0.5% for hand surgery. *Reg Anesth Pain Med* 2003;28(5):414–417.
12 Bigat Z, Boztug N, Hadimioglu N, et al. Does dexamethasone improve the quality of intravenous regional anesthesia and analgesia? A randomized, controlled clinical study. *Anesth Analg* 2006;102(2):605–609.
13 Grice SC, Morell RC, Balestrieri FJ, et al. Intravenous regional anesthesia: evaluation and prevention of leakage under the tourniquet. *Anesthesiology* 1986;65:316.
14 Tucker GT, Boas RA. Pharmacokinetic aspects of intravenous regional anesthesia. *Anesthesiology* 1971;34:538.
15 Sukhani R, Garcia CJ, Munhall RJ, et al. Lidocaine disposition following intravenous regional anesthesia with different tourniquet deflation technics. *Anesth Analg* 1989;68:633.

14 Peripheral Nerve Blocks of the Upper Extremity

Susan B. McDonald

Occasionally, anesthesia of a single nerve of the shoulder, forearm, hand, or digit is required. More commonly, supplementation of a single terminal branch is required after a partially successful brachial plexus block. Central block is more effective, but peripheral approaches are possible and sometimes easier for a single nerve distribution.

I. **Anatomy**

A. **Proximal branches**

1. **Suprascapular nerve**
   - **a.** The suprascapular nerve arises from the superior cord formed by the fifth and sixth cervical roots and passes obliquely laterally under the trapezius to cross through the supraspinous notch to the back of the scapula.
   - **b.** Sensory innervation is to the shoulder joint, but only a small area of surface sensory anesthesia on the shoulder.
   - **c.** Motor innervation is to the supraspinatus muscle, which assists the deltoid in elevating the arm and to the infraspinatus muscle, which externally rotates the humerus (a useful marker for nerve stimulator localization).
2. **Musculocutaneous nerve.** A branch of the lateral cord of the brachial plexus, this nerve branches off before the axilla (see Chapter 12).

B. **Terminal nerves.** The three terminal nerves to the hand travel mostly in muscle compartments, but they have reliable bony landmarks at the elbow and wrist, where the muscles are less prominent as they cross the joints.

1. **At the elbow**
   - **a.** The ulnar nerve is superficial in the groove of the medial condyle of the humerus and the olecranon process. Paresthesias are so easily elicited with pressure that this area is well known as the *funny bone.*
   - **b.** The median nerve is deeper, but it reliably passes just medial to the brachial artery above the skin crease of the antecubital fossa.
   - **c.** The radial and lateral cutaneous nerves of the forearm cross the elbow joint laterally between the biceps tendon and the insertion of the brachioradialis. The former lies close to the humerus itself in this groove, whereas the latter is superficial and has already begun to branch into terminal distribution fibers.
2. **At the wrist, on the palmar surface**
   - **a.** The ulnar nerve crosses the wrist joint by passing above the ulnar styloid in company with the ulnar artery.
   - **b.** The median nerve lies in the middle of the wrist, deep between the tendons of the palmaris longus and flexor carpi radialis (the prominent tendons when the wrist is flexed), and is easily visualized with ultrasonography.
   - **c.** The radial nerve begins branching proximal to the wrist, but it can be found in company with the radial artery and with several of its branches

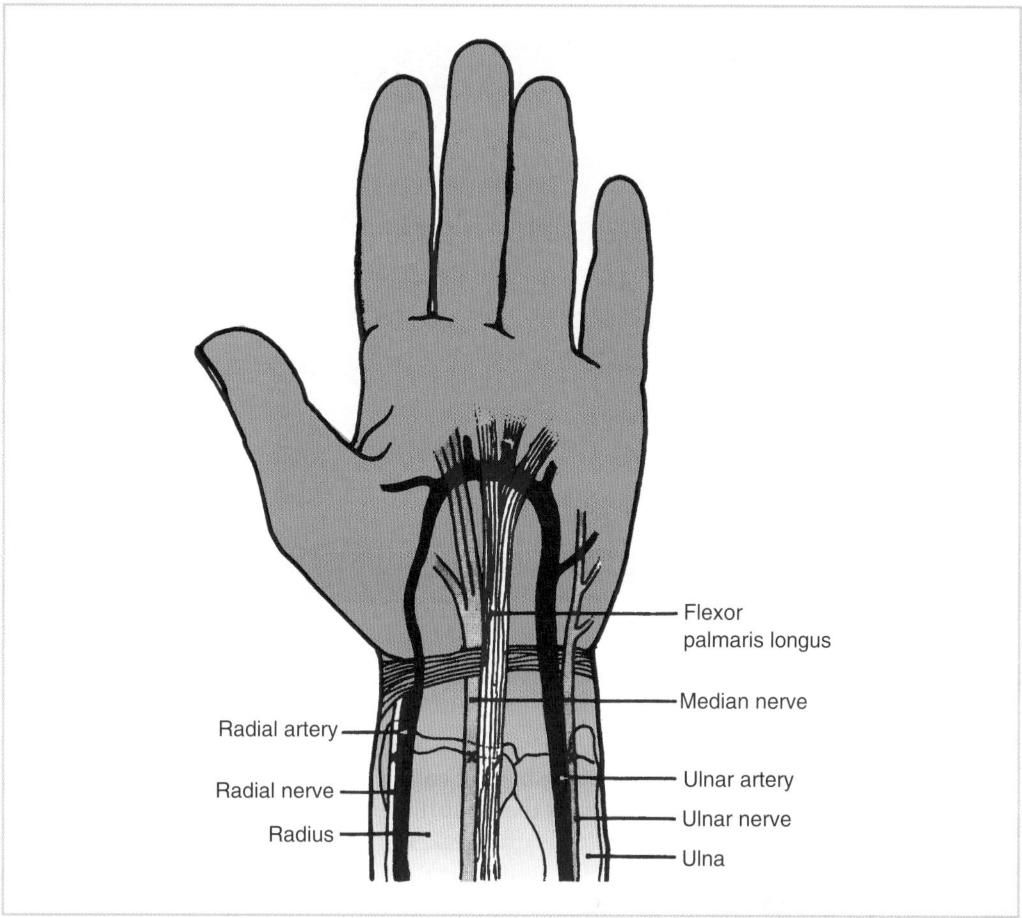

Figure 14.5. Terminal nerves at the wrist. The median nerve lies just to the radial side of the flexor palmaris longus. The ulnar and radial nerves lie just "outside" their respective arteries. The radial nerve has already begun branching at this level and must be blocked by a wide subcutaneous ridge of anesthetic.

C. **Wrist block.** Three separate areas on the palmar surface of the joint must be injected (Figure 14.5).

1. The **ulnar nerve** is blocked with a 25-gauge needle inserted just on the ulnar side of the ulnar artery and advanced between it and the flexor carpi ulnaris to the ulnar styloid. As the needle is withdrawn, 3 to 5 mL of solution is injected.
2. For the **median nerve**, the tendons of the flexor palmaris longus and the flexor carpi radialis are identified by flexing the wrist. A needle is inserted between them to the deep fascia and 3 to 5 mL is injected again as the needle is withdrawn. If ultrasonography is used, an even smaller volume can be used to completely encircle the nerve under direct visualization (Figure 14.6).
3. The **radial nerve** has already branched as it reaches the wrist. In addition to injecting 3 mL of solution along the lateral border of the radial artery two fingerbreadths above the wrist, a superficial ring of solution must be laid from this point extending dorsally over the border of the wrist and into the "snuffbox" area created by the extensor tendons of the thumb.

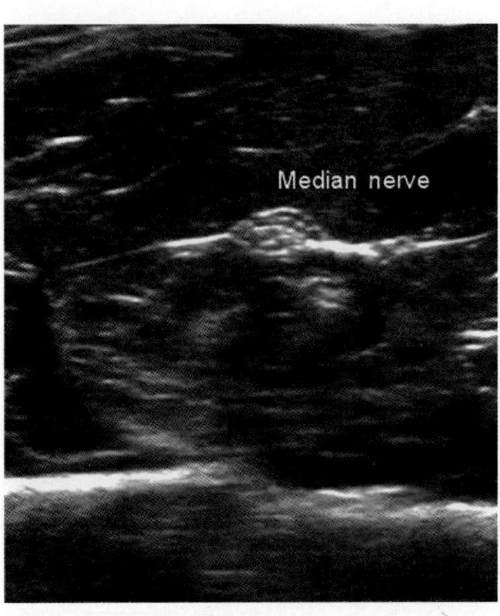

Figure 14.6. Ultrasonographic view of median nerve at wrist.

D. **Digital block.** The terminal nerves of the fingers are similar and can be blocked by injections on each side of the base of each digit. **The most common problem with this form of anesthesia is that insufficient time is allowed for anesthesia to develop** before a procedure is undertaken. Ten to 15 minutes may be required for adequate analgesia.

1. The patient's hand is rested on a flat surface with the palm down and the fingers extended. For each finger, an "X" is placed on the skin of the web space between the metacarpal heads. This is usually at the point where the skin texture changes from the rough character of the dorsal hand to the smooth texture of the palm. A 25-gauge needle is introduced here and directed down toward the metacarpal head of the digit to be blocked. Then 1 to 2 mL of solution is injected along the ventral head and 1 mL is injected along the dorsal head to anesthetize both the dorsal and ventral branches (Figure 14.7). **Both sides of each digit must be blocked**. For the "outside" aspects of the index and little fingers, the injection is made along the appropriate borders of the hand at the level of the metacarpal heads.
2. For the thumb, similar injections are made on each side of the metacarpal head.
3. **No epinephrine is used in the terminal digit blocks.**

V. Complications

A. **Ischemia.** Ischemia of the digits is the most serious complication, and it can be **prevented by avoiding vasoconstrictors and excessive volumes of injection** in digital blocks.

B. **Neuropathy.** Neuropathy with any of these techniques is more likely if paresthesias are sought, **especially in a nerve that may be partially anesthetized** (as in the case of "rescuing" a block) **(6)**. Ultrasonographic localization *may* reduce

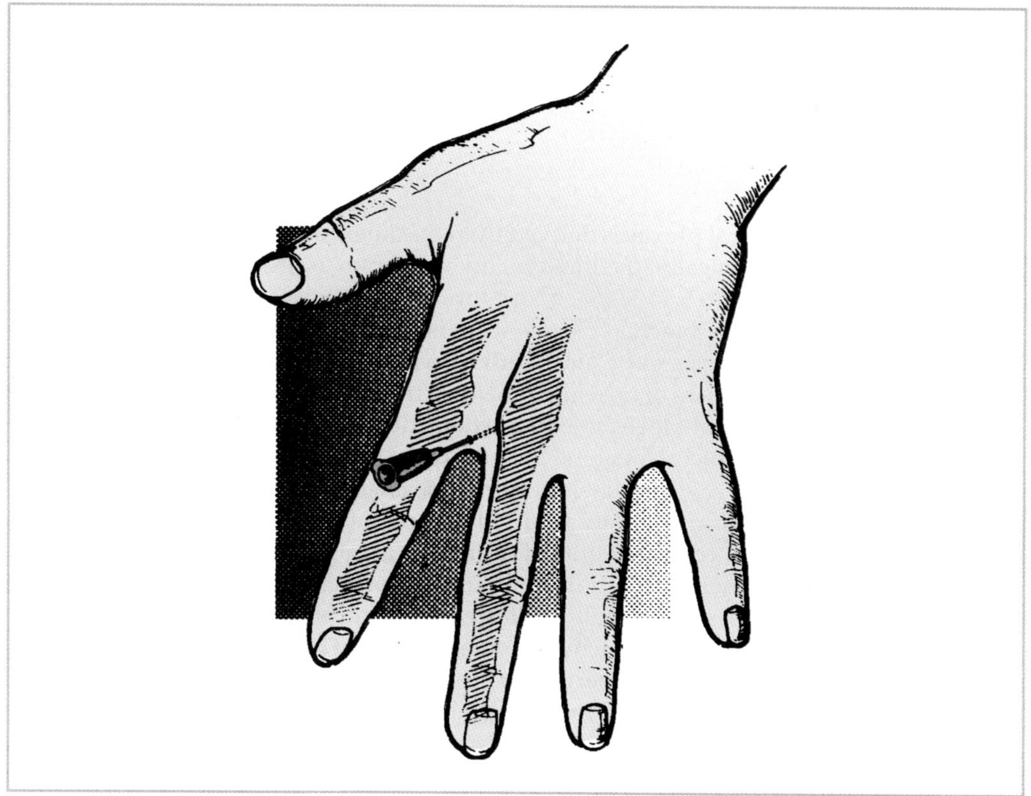

Figure 14.7. Digital nerve block. A 25-gauge needle is inserted into the dorsal aspect of the web space at a 45-degree angle at the level of the change in skin texture and advanced until the bone is gently contacted. The needle is withdrawn 3 to 4 mm, and 2 mL of solution *without epinephrine* is injected in a volar direction and a third milliliter is injected along the dorsal aspect of the phalanx.

this risk. Higher concentrations of anesthetic solutions may be implicated in their occurrence (see Chapter 3). Intraneural injection (which may be heralded by resistance or pain on injection) increases this possibility.

REFERENCES

1 Ritchie ED, Tong D, Chung F, et al. Suprascapular nerve block for postoperative pain relief in arthroscopic shoulder surgery: a new modality? *Anesth Analg* 1997;84:1306–1312.

2 Singelyn FJ, Lhotel L, Fabre B. Pain relief after arthroscopic shoulder surgery: a comparison of intraarticular analgesia, suprascapular nerve block, and interscalene brachial plexus block. *Anesth Analg* 2004;99: 589–592.

3 Neal JM, McDonald SB, Larkin KL, et al. Suprascapular nerve block prolongs analgesia after nonarthroscopic shoulder surgery but does not improve outcome. *Anesth Analg* 2003;96:982–986.

4 **Gray AT, Schafhalter-Zoppoth I. Ultrasound guidance for ulnar nerve block in the forearm. *Reg Anesth Pain Med* 2003;28:335–339.**

5 **Foxall GL, Skinner D, Hardman JG, et al. Ultrasound anatomy of the radial nerve in the distal upper arm. *Reg Anesth Pain Med* 2007:32;217–220.**

6 **Neal JM, Hebl JR, Gerancher JC, et al. Brachial plexus anesthesia: essentials of our current understanding. *Reg Anesth Pain Med* 2002;27:402–428.**

15 Lumbar Plexus Blocks

Francis V. Salinas

I. **General overview**

A. The **lumbosacral plexus** is derived from the anterior rami of the T12 to S3 spinal nerves. Anatomically, the lumbar and sacral plexus are connected through L4 as it bifurcates to join with L5 and form the lumbosacral trunk (Figure 15.1). In contrast to the brachial plexus, there is **no technique that allows the entire lumbosacral plexus to be anesthetized with a single injection.** Therefore, for functional purposes of providing lower extremity anesthesia and analgesia, the lumbar and sacral plexus are **distinct entities** and must be blocked separately to provide complete unilateral lower extremity anesthesia.

B. The ability to provide reliable surgical anesthesia or continuous postoperative analgesia (with a spinal or epidural catheter) of the lower extremity with a single-injection central neuraxial technique is more familiar with anesthesiologists. Nevertheless, the unilateral anesthesia that lumbar and sacral plexus blocks provide is occasionally indicated or a central neuraxial technique is contraindicated, such as the increased potential risk of **central neuraxial hematoma** with the increased use of perioperative venous thromboembolism prophylaxis. Additionally, continuous lower extremity plexus and peripheral nerve **catheter techniques** have been shown to provide superior **postoperative analgesia** to traditional systemic opioid-based therapy and comparable postoperative analgesia to lumbar epidural infusions after major lower extremity surgery.

II. **Anatomy of the lumbar plexus**

A. The clinically relevant motor and sensory innervation of the lower extremities arises from the anterior rami of the **second lumbar through the third sacral spinal nerve roots**. The upper segments (L2-4) form the **lumbar plexus**, which give rise to the **lateral femoral cutaneous, femoral,** and **obturator** nerves (Figure 15.1). As soon as the L2-4 nerve roots emerge from the intervertebral foramina, they become embedded **within the substance of psoas major muscle**. This is because the origin of the psoas major muscle is attached to the lateral surfaces of the vertebral bodies and intervertebral discs and the transverse processes of the lumbar vertebrae (**1**, 2). The intervertebral foramina lie anterior to the transverse processes and posterior to the muscular attachments to the vertebral bodies. Therefore, the nerve roots enter the psoas muscle directly (**1**–3). Within the psoas muscle, the anterior rami **divide into anterior and posterior branches**, which reunite to form the individual nerves of the lumbar plexus.

B. The **lumbar plexus** is situated in the posterior aspect of the psoas muscle between the junction of the posterior third and the anterior two thirds of the muscle. The lumbar plexus descends vertically within the substance of the psoas, and at the L4-5 level, the terminal nerves have been formed. On the basis of anatomic dissections and computed tomography imaging, the terminal nerves are **arranged in medial-to-lateral orientation**, with the obturator nerve most medial, the lateral femoral cutaneous nerve (LFCN) most lateral, and the femoral nerve (FN) in between (**1**, 2). Although all three terminal

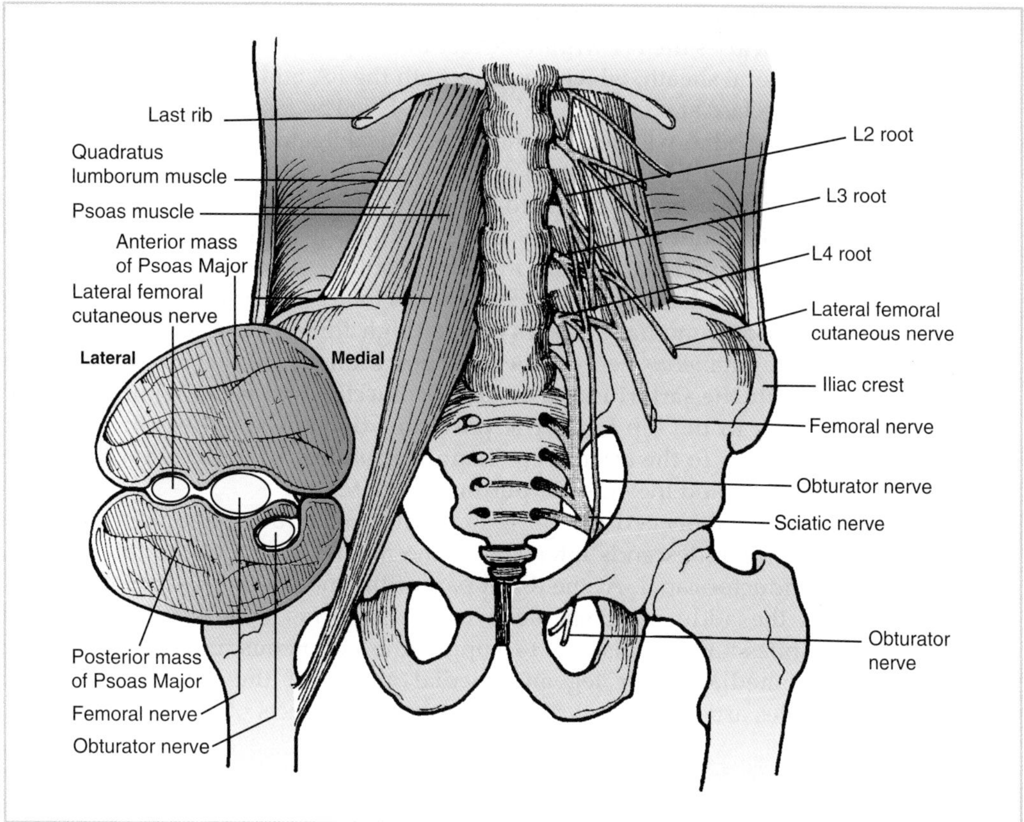

Figure 15.1. Overview of the lumbosacral plexus. The origin of the lumbosacral plexus is broader than the brachial plexus in the cervical region. The roots of the lumbar plexus emerge from their foramina within a fascial plane located between the posterior third and anterior two thirds of the psoas muscle. Within the substance of the psoas muscle, the roots form the terminal nerves in a medial to lateral orientation, with the obturator nerve located most medial, the lateral femoral cutaneous nerve most lateral, and the femoral nerve in between (15.1B). The terminal nerves are more likely to be blocked by an injection within the substance of the psoas muscles. The lower sacral roots form the sciatic nerve and require a separate injection.

nerves are consistently within the psoas major muscle, anatomic studies have demonstrated that the **obturator nerve may be separated** from the femoral nerve and LFCN by a muscular fold more than 50% of the time, which may potentially lead to incomplete blockade of the obturator nerve (1–3).

C. The **FN** is derived from the dorsal divisions of the anterior rami of the L2-4 spinal nerve roots.
   1. The FN emerges from the lateral border of the lower part of the psoas muscle within a **musculoskeletal fascial compartment between the psoas and iliacus muscles** deep to the **fascia iliaca**. It descends inferiorly and enters the thigh deep to the inguinal ligament. At the level of the inguinal ligament, the FN lies 1 to 2 cm lateral and posterior to the femoral artery (FA).
   2. As the FN descends a few centimeters caudad to the inguinal ligament, which is often at the level of the inguinal crease (IC), the FN consistently lays directly **lateral to the pulsatile FA**. At either location, the FN is located **deep to the investing fascia of the iliacus muscle, the fascia iliaca,** which

is the key anatomic component for successful block of the FN. The fascia iliaca encloses the FN within the fascial compartment and separates it from the femoral sheath, which contains both the FA and femoral vein (FV) in a separate fascial compartment from the FN. The fascia iliaca thickens as it courses medially to become the iliopectineal ligament, which anatomically separates the FN from the FA and femoral vein residing in the femoral sheath compartment medial to the nerve (4).

3. As the FN courses inferiorly into the thigh, it divides into **anterior and posterior divisions** that arborize to become terminal branches of the FN. The **anterior division** of the FN supplies the **cutaneous innervation to the anterior and medial surfaces of the thigh** through the medial and intermediate cutaneous nerves. The **muscular branches of the anterior division innervate the sartorius and pectineus muscles**, besides providing articular branches to the hip joint. The **posterior division supplies the muscular innervation to the quadriceps femoris muscles, articular branches to the knee joint**, and the **anterior portion of the femur**.
4. The terminal fibers of the posterior branch constitute the **saphenous nerve (SN),** which descends inferiorly in the medial aspect of the thigh within the adductor canal. At the distal part of the medial thigh, the SN emerges from the adductor canal deep to the sartorius muscle (SM) and then continues further distally to supply the **cutaneous innervation to the anteromedial lower leg and medial aspect of the foot.** The SN also provides articular innervation to the medial aspects of the knee and ankle joints.

D. The **LFCN** is derived from the posterior divisions of the anterior rami of the L2-3 spinal nerve roots. It emerges from the lateral border of the psoas major muscle at the level of the inferior margin of L4. It courses **obliquely around the iliac fossa toward the anterior superior iliac spine (ASIS) on the surface of the iliacus muscle** within the fascia iliaca compartment. The LFCN then descends toward the thigh passing deep to the inguinal ligament approximately **1 to 2 cm medial to ASIS dividing into anterior and posterior branches.** It may also pass under the inguinal ligament as much as 7 cm medial to the ASIS or directly through the SM. The LFCN supplies the **skin over widely variable distribution of the lateral and anterior thigh as far distally as the knee**. It has **no motor** innervation (4).

E. The o**bturator nerve** is derived from the anterior divisions of the anterior rami of L2-4 spinal nerve roots. It is a mixed nerve supplying the **motor innervation to the adductor compartment of the thigh and articular branches to both the hip and knee joints**. Additionally, the obturator nerve supplies a **variable cutaneous distribution** to the posterior-medial portion of the distal thigh, which **may be absent in up to 50% of subjects** (5).

1. The obturator nerve emerges from the medial border of the psoas muscle and descends along the sidewall of the pelvis close to the inferior-lateral portion of the bladder wall until it enters the adductor compartment of the medial thigh by passing through the obturator foramen. Shortly after leaving the obturator foramen, the obturator nerve divides into anterior and posterior division.
2. The **anterior division** descends deep to the adductor longus (AL) and pectineus muscles and superficial to the adductor brevis (AB) and obturator externus (5–7). It provides muscular branches to the superficial adductor

muscles (AL, AB, and gracilis) and articular branches to the anterior-medial aspect of the hip joint. Also, it inconsistently provides a cutaneous branch to the posterior-medial portion of the distal thigh.

3. The **posterior division** descends deep to the AB and superficial to the adductor magnus (AM), just slightly lateral to anterior division in the parasagittal plane (5–7). The posterior division descends with the FA within the adductor canal and terminates by exiting the adductor hiatus to enter the popliteal fossa. The posterior division supplies **muscular branches to the AM and obturator externus,** as well as an articular branch to the posterior aspect of the knee joint (5).

III. Indications

A. **Lumbar plexus block through the psoas compartment** approach in conjunction with sciatic nerve block can provide **surgical anesthesia** for the entire lower extremity, excluding the hip joint. For surgical anesthesia of the hip joint, a psoas compartment block (femoral, lateral femoral cutaneous, and obturator nerves) must be combined with a sacral plexus block that not only blocks the sciatic nerve but also the nerve to the quadratus femoris and superior gluteal nerve, which are branches that come off the sacral plexus proximal to classic gluteal approaches to a sciatic nerve block. A lumbar plexus or FN block alone will provide surgical anesthesia for procedures of the superficial anterior thigh. The most common indication for a psoas compartment block is to provide **postoperative analgesia for major hip surgery.** Typically, a single-injection technique will provide sufficient postoperative analgesia for a primary hip arthroplasty, but a hip arthroplasty revision may benefit from the extended analgesia provided by a continuous psoas compartment catheter.

B. An **FN block** is the most commonly performed block of the lower extremity. A single-injection FN block will provide surgical anesthesia for **superficial procedures of the anterior thigh**, and with the use of a long-acting local anesthetic (LA), it will provide **postoperative analgesia for surgical procedures of the femur and knee joint**. The most common indication for either a single-injection or continuous FN block is for postoperative analgesia after major knee surgeries such as total knee arthroplasty (TKA) or anterior cruciate ligament reconstruction.

C. **LFCN block** alone may be used to provide anesthesia for **cutaneous procedures of the lateral aspect of the thigh**. More commonly, it has been used as a **diagnostic nerve block** to confirm the diagnosis of neuralgia of the LFCN, more commonly known as *meralgia paresthetica.*

D. **Obturator nerve block (ONB)** is commonly used to **treat adductor muscle spasm** associated with neurologic disorders such as strokes, multiple sclerosis, or cerebral palsy. ONB is also occasionally indicated to suppress the **obturator reflex associated with transurethral resection of the lateral bladder wall**. Activation of the obturator reflex may result in sudden violent adduction of the ipsilateral thigh, which not only interferes with the surgical procedure but may also increase the risk of bladder wall perforation or vessel laceration by the resectoscope. Additionally, ONB has been demonstrated to provide a decrease in opioid consumption and pain in patients undergoing TKA when added to sciatic and FN blocks.

E. An **SN block** may be used in conjunction with distal sciatic nerve block to provide complete anesthesia of the lower leg. The advantage of this approach

Table 15.1 Local anesthetic choices for posterior lumbar plexus (psoas compartment) block

Local anesthetic	Onset (min)	Duration of anesthesia (h)	Duration of analgesia (h)
Lidocaine 2% with HCO_3 and 1:400 epinephrine	10–20	5–6	5–8
Mepivacaine 1.5% with HCO_3 and 1:400 epinephrine	10–15	3–5	3–6
Ropivacaine 0.5%	15–20	4–6	6–10

is surgical anesthesia of the lower leg, ankle, and foot without blocking either the hamstrings (with a more proximal sciatic nerve block) or the quadriceps (with FN block).

IV. **Choice of local anesthetic**

The choice of LA for the major lumbar plexus blocks (psoas compartment and femoral-fascia iliaca) is dependent on the requirements for onset of anesthesia and duration of analgesia for single-injection techniques. With the advent of continuous **peripheral perineural catheter techniques**, the anesthesiologist has the advantage of providing a rapid onset of surgical block by injection of the shorter-acting LAs (Table 15.1) through the needle or catheter tip (the primary anesthetic block). Subsequently, an **infusion** of a dilute LA that possesses sensory motor dissociation (the most commonly used being ropivacaine 0.2% or bupivacaine 0.125%) (Table 15.2) may be used to provide the optimal balance of postoperative analgesia with less motor block to facilitate postoperative rehabilitation and recovery. Alternatively, if a central neuraxial technique is chosen as the primary anesthetic, a loading dose (10–15 mL) of the analgesic infusion of ropivacaine 0.2% may be started intraoperatively. The typical postoperative regimen consists of running the analgesic infusion at 4 to 8 mL/h with or without a patient-controlled bolus of 2 to 3 mL every 20 minutes.

V. **Techniques**

The most common techniques for anesthetizing the lumbar plexus and its individual branches are described in the subsequent text. Peripheral nerve stimulator techniques that focus on surface landmarks and evoked motor responses (EMRs), as well as ultrasound (US)-guided techniques (when available) will be discussed. Additionally, both single-injection and continuous peripheral perineural catheter

Table 15.2 Local anesthetic choices for femoral-fascia iliaca block

Local anesthetic	Onset (min)	Duration of anesthesia (h)	Duration of analgesia (h)
Lidocaine 2% with HCO_3 and 1:400 epinephrine	10–20	2–5	3–8
Mepivacaine 1.5% with HCO_3 and 1:400 epinephrine	10–15	3–5	3–8
Ropivacaine 0.5%	15–30	4–8	6–12
Bupivacaine 0.5%	15–30	5–15	8–24

techniques will be described. Paresthesia techniques are not commonly used for lower extremity nerve blocks.

A. **Posterior lumbar plexus (psoas compartment) block.** The lumbar plexus is most commonly located (and blocked) within the **substance of the psoas major muscle** and at the junction of the posterior third and anterior two thirds of the muscle (**1**–3). The lumbar plexus is consistently located **within 2 to 3 cm anterior to the transverse process of the lumbar vertebrae** (8–10). Knowledge of these anatomic considerations allows for increased success and decreased potential risk of serious complications. Because this approach is close to the central neuraxial space, it is recommended that patient preparation include standard monitoring (continuous pulse oximetry, electrocardiogram, and intermittent noninvasive blood pressure). Additionally, medications and airway management equipment for emergency resuscitation should be immediately available. The technique of Capdevila et al. using a **peripheral nerve stimulator** is described **(8–10)**.

   1. **Patient position.** The patient is placed in the **lateral decubitus position** with a slight forward tilt, hips flexed with the operative side to be blocked uppermost.
   2. **External landmarks.** The **iliac crests** and the **spinous process of the fourth lumbar vertebrae** (L4) are identified. A line is drawn connecting the iliac crests **(intercristal line)**. A **second line** is drawn through the center of the L4 spinous process perpendicular to the intercristal line. A **third line is drawn parallel to the second line** (representing the spinal column) through the **posterior superior iliac spine (PSIS)**. The needle insertion point is located along the intercristal line at the **junction of the lateral third and medial thirds of the second line** (representing the center of the spinal column) and third line (representing the center of the PSIS) (Figure 15.2).
   3. After aseptic skin preparation and draping followed by LA infiltration of the proposed needle insertion point, a **stimulating needle** (typically

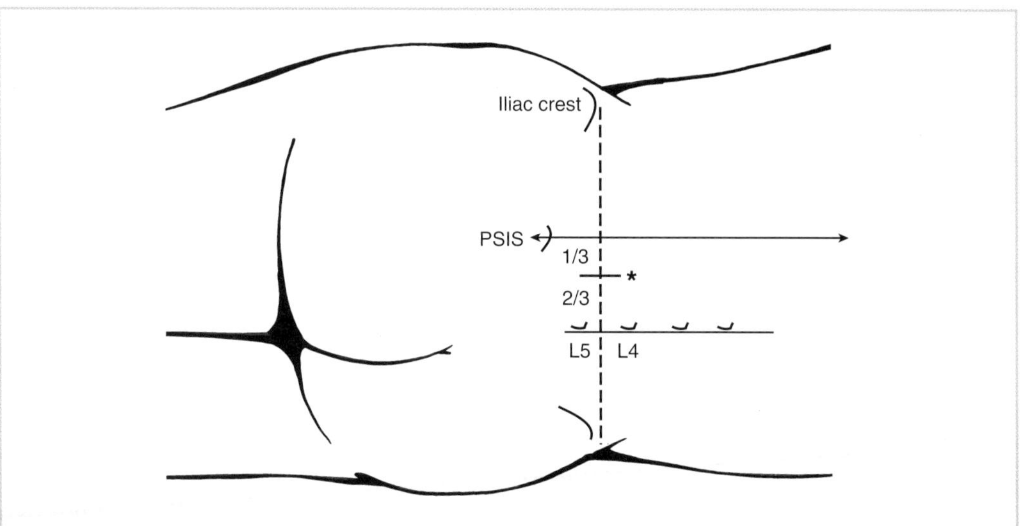

Figure 15.2. Skin landmarks for psoas compartment block. (Reproduced from Capdevila X, Macaire P, Dadure C, et al. Continuous psoas compartment block for postoperative analgesia after total hip arthroplasty: new landmarks, technical guidelines, and clinical evaluation. *Anesth Analg* 2002;94:1606–1613.)

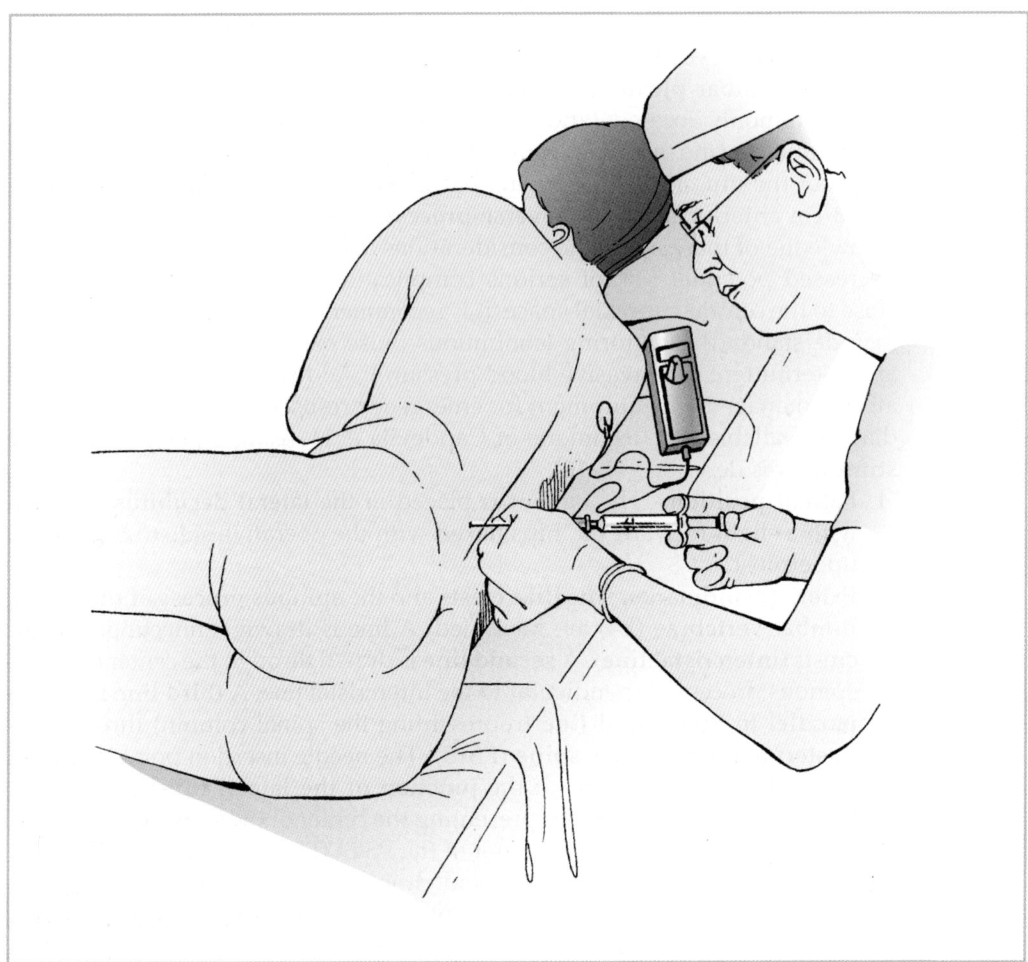

Figure 15.3. Psoas compartment block. A 4-in. needle is advanced perpendicular to the skin until a loss of resistance (similar to an epidural injection) is obtained. At this point, compartment entry can be confirmed by eliciting a response to a nerve stimulator. A catheter can be inserted if continuous analgesia is desired.

100–150 mm [4–6 in.], 20–21 gauge) is slowly advanced at right angles to the coronal plane of the body (Figure 15.3). The stimulating needle is attached to a peripheral nerve stimulator (typical settings of 1.5–2.0 mA, 2 Hz, 100 μs) and to a syringe of LA.

4. The goal is to advance the needle until **contact with lumbar transverse process** (presumably L4) is made. The rationale for attempting to locate the transverse process is as follows. The distance from the skin to the lumbar plexus is typically 60 to 100 mm depending on gender and body mass index (BMI). In contrast, the **distance from the transverse process to the lumbar plexus ranges between 15 and 20 mm** with a median value of 18 mm, **regardless of gender or BMI**.
5. After contact with the transverse process is made, the needle is withdrawn 0.2 cm and redirected under the transverse process and advanced until the desired EMR is elicited. The desired EMR is **quadriceps muscle contractions** (QMCs) and the position of the stimulating needle (or catheter) tip is judged

to be adequate when the current output is 0.5 to 1.0 mA. If the QMC is not elicited after advancing the needle **20 to 30 mm past the transverse process,** the needle is withdrawn and redirected in 15-degree increments in a medial-to-lateral plane (perpendicular to cephalad-caudad course of the FN within the psoas muscle) until QMCs are elicited.

6. After optimizing the stimulating needle tip position, aspiration and a 3-mL test dose are performed to confirm the absence of either an intravascular or central neuraxial location of the LA injection. Typically, **25 to 35 mL of LA** is incrementally injected with frequent aspirations to reduce the potential risk of intravascular injection. A typical onset time for anesthesia is 15 to 30 minutes depending on the type and total mass of LA injected.
7. A **continuous catheter technique** may be utilized to provide extended duration analgesia. The approach is exactly the same as for the single-injection technique except for the following. A larger bore (17- to 18-gauge) insulated stimulating Tuohy needle is typically used to localize the lumbar plexus. After localization of the lumbar plexus with the single-injection technique, a 19- to 20-gauge catheter is inserted through the Tuohy needle and advanced no more than 2 cm past the needle tip. The needle is then withdrawn over the catheter and fixed in place with a sterile clear adhesive dressing. The proximal end of the catheter is then connected to an automated infusion pump.
8. **Clinical pearls**
   a. Contact with the **transverse process** is a key safety step. Advancing the needle tip more than 20 to 30 mm deep to the transverse process significantly increases the potential for retroperitoneal injection.
   b. The correct EMR must be obtained. Stimulation of the obturator nerve will result in an EMR of the adductor muscles and should not be accepted for two reasons: (i) The obturator nerve may be in a separate muscle-fascial plane from the FN and LFCN (1, 2), and (ii) the obturator nerve EMR places the needle tip more medially within the psoas muscle. The distance between the internal border of psoas muscle and the median sagittal plane is only 2.7 ± 0.6 cm (2). Therefore, medial placement of the needle tip may increase the potential risk of unintended central neuraxial anesthesia. Elicitation of sacral EMR (such as hamstring contractions, dorsiflexion, or plantarflexion at the ankle) indicates that the needle tip is too caudal at the level of the lumbosacral trunk, potentially resulting in a failed or incomplete block of the lumbar plexus.

B. Anterior lumbar plexus block. The **FN** may be blocked by a variety of methods. A **paravascular approach** several centimeters caudad to the inguinal ligament using a peripheral nerve stimulator technique is still the most commonly used technique. An **US-guided approach** directly visualizing the paravascular location of the FN (typically just lateral to the FA) deep to the fascia iliaca is gaining increased popularity. Lastly, the **fascia iliaca approach** simply relies on appreciating the "loss of resistance" or "double-pop" sensation when a blunt needle is passed through the fascia lata and then the fascia iliaca. Despite the seemingly different approaches of these three techniques, they all share one common key anatomic component. The FN is always located deep to fascia iliaca in a separate fascial compartment from the FA and vein (which are located within the femoral sheath, but superficial to the fascia iliaca).

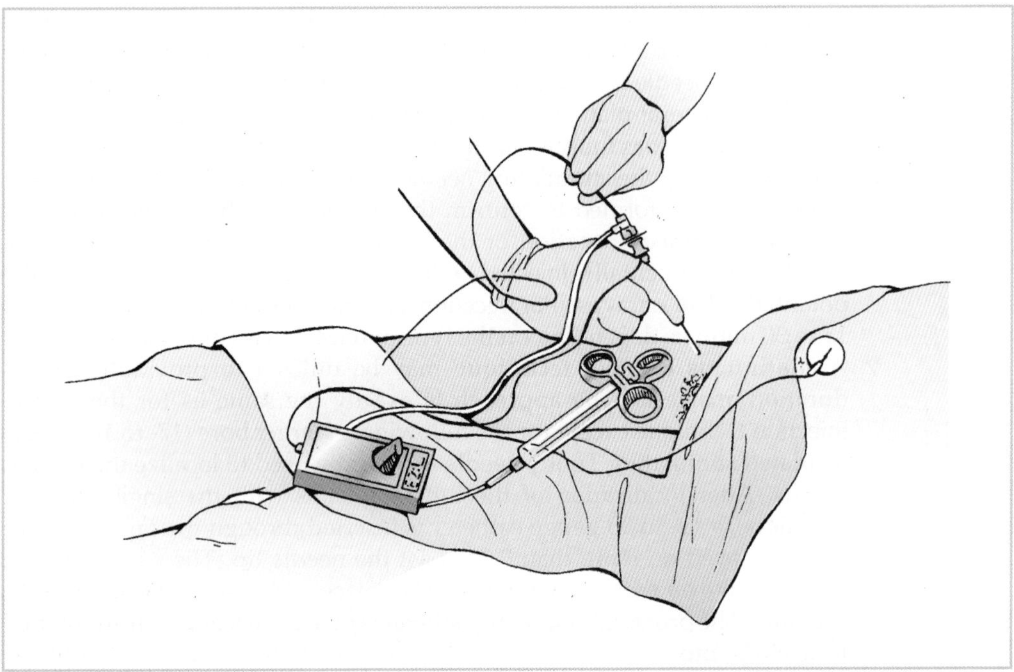

Figure 15.4. Femoral nerve block, nerve stimulator. The needle is introduced lateral to the artery and a motor response or a paresthesia is sought. If a large needle is used, a continuous catheter can be inserted.

1. **FN block (peripheral nerve stimulator approach)** (Figure 15.4)
   a. **Patient position.** The patient is **supine** with the operative leg slightly abducted 10 to 20 degrees.
   b. **External landmarks.** The inguinal crease (**IC**) is identified, typically located 2 to 5 cm caudad to the inguinal ligament, and from medial to lateral has superior-lateral course. The needle insertion site is located along the IC **just lateral (1–2 cm) to the palpable pulse of the FA**. At this level the FN is consistently located lateral to the FA, and is both shallower and wider compared to its location at the level of the inguinal ligament **(11)**.
   c. After aseptic skin preparation and draping followed by LA skin infiltration of the proposed needle insertion site, a 50-mm (2-in.) 22-gauge **stimulating needle** is attached to a peripheral nerve stimulator (typical settings of 1.5–2.0 mA, 2 Hz, 100 μs) and to a syringe of LA.
   d. One hand is used to maintain a finger on the FA pulsation. The other hand introduces the needle **just lateral to the FA pulsation** in a 45- to 60-degree angle to the skin. The needle is slowly advanced deeper in a slight cephalad direction while observing for EMRs. Often the first EMR observed is contraction of the SM, which typically results in contraction of the anterior-medial aspect of the thigh, but without visible quadriceps contractions. **Sartorius EMR should not be accepted** as this indicates that the needle is too shallow as the anterior division of the FN innervates the SM, and the anterior division of the FN is typically located superficial to fascia iliaca.
   e. If a sartorius EMR is elicited, a stepwise and systematic approach is suggested. The first step should be advancing the needle slightly deeper

(typically not more than 1–2 cm) until a QMC is elicited. QMC is confirmed by visible and palpable cephalad movement of the patella ("patellar twitch"). If QMCs are not elicited by simply advancing the needle deeper, the needle is withdrawn until sartorius EMRs return. The needle is then redirected slightly lateral and advanced 1 to 2 cm until QMCs are elicited. If QMCs are not elicited after several lateral redirections, the initial needle is repositioned to the original insertion and angle and then redirected slightly medial until QMCs are elicited.

f. The final needle position is adjusted until QMCs are still elicited at a current output between 0.2 to 0.5 mA. At this point, aspiration and a 3-mL test dose are performed to confirm the absence of an intravascular location of the LA injection. Typically, a **20 to 30 mL of LA is incrementally injected** with frequent aspirations to reduce the risk of intravascular injection. A typical onset time for FN block is 10 to 30 minutes depending on type and total mass of LA used. For example, 20 mL of lidocaine 2% with 50 μg of epinephrine will have an onset of 10 to 20 minutes, 2 to 5 hours of surgical anesthesia, and 4 to 8 hours of postoperative analgesia. In contrast, 20 mL of plain ropivacaine will have an onset 10 to 20 minutes, but 5 to 10 hours of surgical anesthesia, and 8 to 24 hours of postoperative analgesia.

g. If postoperative analgesia beyond 12 to 24 hours is desired, a **continuous femoral perineural catheter technique** is indicated. The landmarks for a continuous femoral catheter technique are the same as for the single-injection technique. A larger bore (17- to 18- gauge) insulated stimulating Tuohy needle is typically used to localize the femoral nerve. After localization of the FN is achieved, a 19- to 20-gauge catheter is inserted through the Tuohy needle and advanced no more than 3 to 5 cm past needle tip. The needle is then withdrawn over the catheter and the latter fixed in place with a sterile clear adhesive dressing. The proximal end of the catheter is then connected to an automated infusion pump.

h. Clinical pearl. The key to successful FN block is placement of the needle (and catheter) tip **deep to the fascia iliaca.** Attempts to thread the catheter 10 to 20 cm past the needle tip to reach the more proximal portions of the lumbar plexus branches (the classic but anatomically incorrect "3-in-1" lumbar plexus block) should not be attempted. Clinical studies have shown that the catheter tip will often travel medial or lateral away from the FN and will not result in blockade of the obturator nerve (12). Additionally, threading the catheter this far past the needle tip may theoretically increase the risk of the catheter curling back on itself and possibly forming a knot.

2. Fascia iliaca block ("loss of resistance or double-pop") technique is the **simplest approach** to provide FN blocks, requiring neither a stimulating needle (with a peripheral nerve stimulator) nor an ultrasonographic machine. In experienced hands, this technique has an 80% to 90% success rate for FN block (13, **14**).

a. Patient position. The patient is **supine** with the inguinal region of the operative side to be blocked exposed.

b. The landmarks include the **ASIS and the pubic tubercle.** A line is drawn connecting the ASIS and pubic tubercle representing the cutaneous projection of the inguinal ligament. The classically described needle

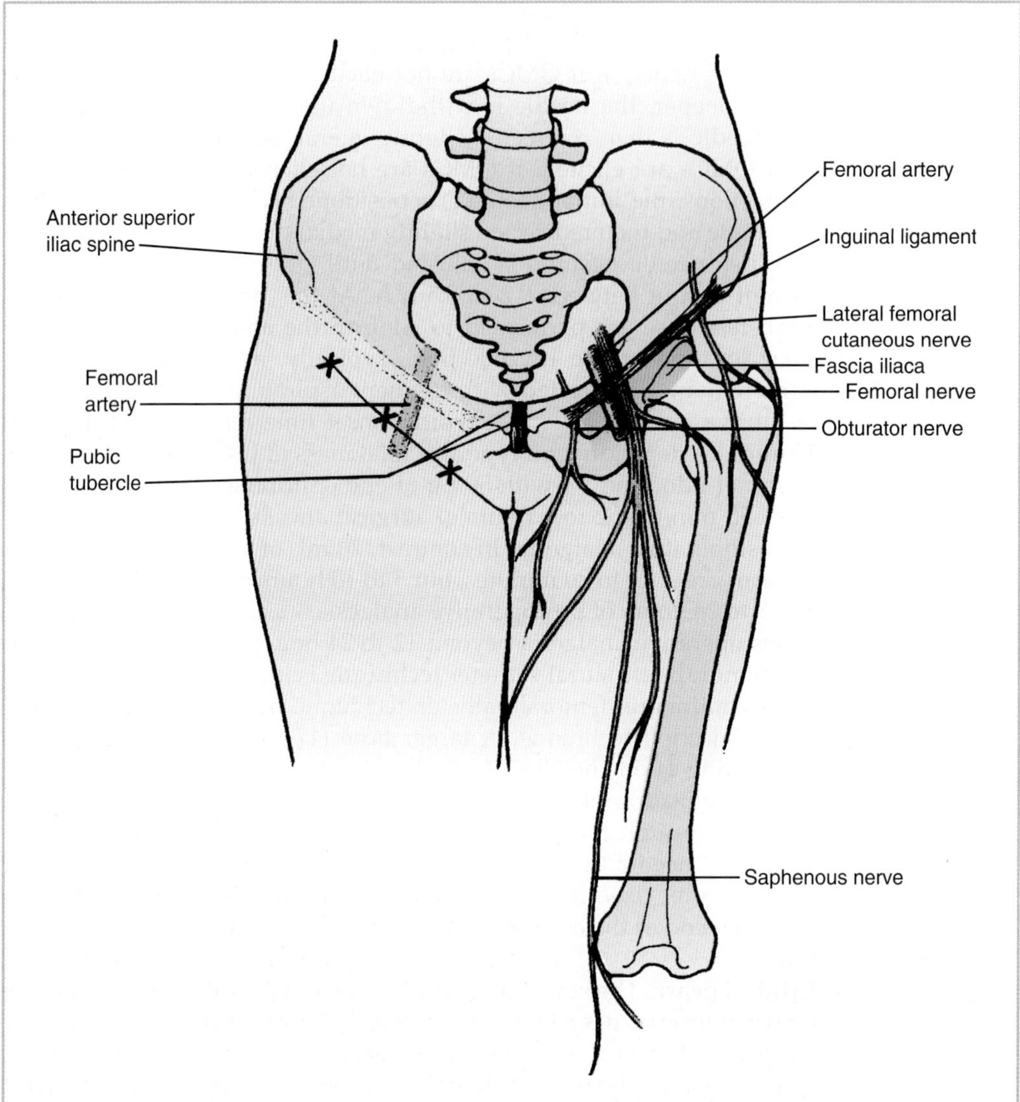

Figure 15.5. Superficial landmarks for anterior lumbar plexus block branches to the groin.

insertion point is located **1 cm below the junction of the lateral third and medial two thirds** of the inguinal ligament (Figure 15.5).

c. After aseptic skin preparation and draping followed by LA skin infiltration of the proposed needle insertion site, a **17- to 18-gauge Tuohy needle** is attached to a syringe of LA.

d. The needle is slowly advanced at a **60- to 80-degree angle** to the skin while feeling for two **distinct losses of resistance** (or a **double-pop**) as the needle first penetrates the fascia lata and then the fascia iliaca. After the **fascia iliaca is penetrated**, the needle angle is decreased to approximately 30 to 45 degrees and advanced a few millimeters further. After aspiration to rule out intravascular placement of the needle tip, 30 ml of LA is incrementally injected. Typically, a larger volume is needed compared to either the peripheral nerve stimulator or US-guided technique to ensure medial spread within the fascia iliaca compartment toward the FN.

e. If a **continuous catheter technique** is desired, a 19- to 20-gauge catheter is inserted through the Tuohy needle and advanced 3 to 5 cm past the needle tip **(14)**. The needle is then withdrawn over the catheter and the latter fixed in place with a sterile clear adhesive dressing. The proximal end of the catheter is then connected to an automated infusion pump.

f. **Clinical pearls.** Appreciation of **two distinct pops** may be difficult. The sensation of "loss of resistance" may be enhanced if the bevel of the Tuohy needle is oriented caudad to allow the blunt portion of the needle tip to penetrate the two fascial layers. For a continuous catheter technique, orient the bevel of the Tuohy needle medial before advancing the catheter past the needle tip, as this may enhance that the catheter tip (and LA) migrates toward the more medially located FN.

3. **US-guided femoral nerve-fascia iliaca block** is one of the **simplest and most successful applications for US-assisted nerve blocks**. Multiple studies have shown that US-guided femoral nerve-fascia iliaca block improves the sensory block and onset time, as well as significantly reducing the minimum effective LA volume compared to peripheral nerve stimulator techniques (15–17). With US guidance the FN may appear **triangular, round, or oval** in shape (Figure 15.6). The FN is consistently located lateral to either the visibly pulsatile FA or profunda femoris artery at the level of the IC. More importantly, the **needle or catheter tip may be observed** in

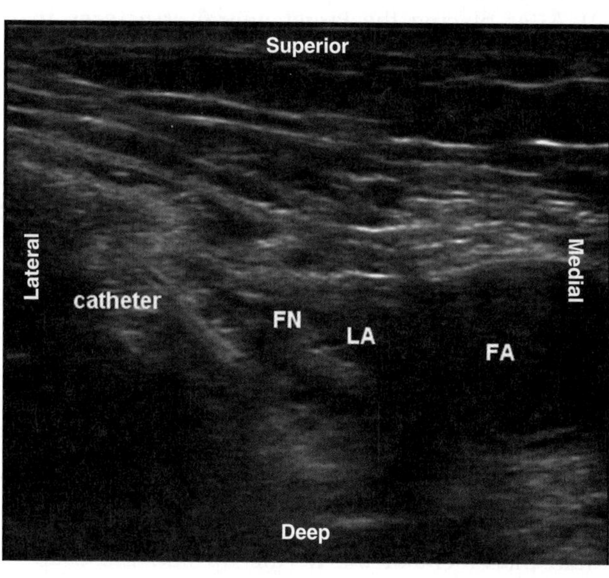

Figure 15.6. Ultrasound anatomy of femoral nerve block. The femoral artery (*FA*) is easily identified in the groin as a hypoechoic pulsatile structure. The femoral nerve (*FN*) lies lateral to it and below the fascia iliaca. A needle correctly inserted from the lateral side will pierce this fascia and the injection of local anesthetic (*LA*) in this plane above the iliacus muscle will "lift" the femoral nerve and surround it with a hypoechoic shadow which will accent the nerve itself.

real time to penetrate the fascia iliaca, and subsequently, LA distribution deep to the fascia iliaca and around the FN.

a. **Patient position.** The patient is **supine** with the inguinal region of the operative side to be blocked exposed.
b. **Probe selection.** A **high frequency linear array transducer (8–12 MHz)** is typically used for this block. A **depth of 3 to 4 cm** is adequate to visualize the FN, fascia iliaca, and FA/femoral vein.
c. **Probe placement and sonoanatomy.** The US probe is placed initially at **a 90-degree angle to the skin and parallel to the IC**.
   (1) The probe position is then adjusted (moved slightly cephalad to caudad, medial to lateral, and cephalad-to-caudad needle angulation) to **optimize the appearance of the target structures**.
   (2) At this point, the most easily recognized structure is the typically **round, pulsatile, noncompressible, and hypoechoic FA**. Medial to the FA is the **larger and easily compressible femoral vein**. The **FN is a hyperechoic structure located just lateral and slightly deeper to the FA**. The **fascia lata** and **fascia iliaca** are seen as hyperechoic linear structures traveling medial-to-lateral, perpendicular to the short axis of the FN and FA (Figure 15.6). The fascia lata is superficial to the fascia iliaca, and the fascia iliaca is superficial to the FN. As the fascia iliaca courses medially, it thickens to become the iliopectineal ligament and is deep to the FA and femoral vein.
d. **Needling technique**
   (1) After aseptic skin preparation and draping followed by LA skin infiltration of the proposed needle insertion site, a 50-mm (2-in.) 22-gauge stimulating needle is attached to a syringe of LA.
   (2) After placing the **target neural structures in the middle of the screen**, the needle is placed just lateral to the lateral aspect of the US probe and advanced **in-plane (to the US beam)** at an appropriate angle toward the target structures. With this technique, the needle will be visualized approaching the FN from superior-lateral aspect of the screen and traveling slightly deeper and medial. Although out-of-plane approaches have been used, the in-plane approach is preferred as this improves visualization of the needle tip passing through the fascia iliaca.
   (3) The **recommended perineural target is needle placement just deep to the fascia iliaca and at the lateral edge of the FN**. At this point, LA is injected and LA distribution deep to the fascia iliaca and around the FN is observed in real time. Typically, a volume of 15 to 25 mL is all that is required to obtain satisfactory LA distribution around the FN.
e. If a **continuous catheter technique** is indicated, a larger bore (17- to 18-gauge) insulated stimulating Tuohy needle is typically used for initial placement of the needle tip and LA deep to the fascia iliaca. After LA distribution around the FN (by injection through the needle tip) is ensured, the US probe is placed aside within the sterile field. A **19- to 20-gauge catheter** is inserted through the Tuohy needle and advanced **no more than 3 to 5 cm past needle tip**. At this point, the US probe is placed over the original site, and an additional 3 to 5 mL of LA is injected through the catheter while observing for LA

distribution around the FN and deep to the fascia iliaca to ensure correct catheter tip position. The needle is then withdrawn over the catheter and the latter fixed in place with a sterile clear adhesive dressing. The proximal end of the catheter is then connected to an automated infusion pump.

C. **Saphenous nerve (SN) block.** The SN can be blocked at multiple levels depending on the anatomic requirements for surgical anesthesia balanced with the desire to minimize significant motor block. Because the SN is the **terminal branch of the posterior division of the FN**, a FN block will provide consistent block of the SN. The major disadvantage of FN approach is the accompanying motor block of the quadriceps muscles. SN block is most often indicated to provide cutaneous anesthesia to the medial aspect of the lower leg, and in conjunction with a distal sciatic nerve block at the popliteal fossa, it provides complete anesthesia for lower leg, ankle, and foot procedures. The traditional approach to block the SN has been as a below-the-knee field block by injecting a **subcutaneous ring of LA** extending from the tibial tuberosity to the dorsomedial aspect of the upper calf. This approach is associated with a high failure rate as the SN has multiple branches at this level, making incomplete block likely **(18)**. Compared with the lower leg, the course of the SN in the distal thigh is more consistent. In the distal thigh, the SN exits the adductor canal in a predictable manner, accompanied by the descending genicular artery. After exiting the adductor canal, the SN and descending genicular artery descend toward the lower leg in a fascial plane deep to the SM adjacent to the vastus medialis. The SN (deep to the sartorius muscle) at this level may be blocked by a peripheral nerve stimulator approach or an US-guided approach (**18**–20). Clinical studies have confirmed that **blockade of the SN at the distal thigh is associated with the highest success rate (18)**. Therefore, the peripheral nerve stimulator and US-guided approach will be described.

1. **Transsartorial peripheral nerve stimulator-guided approach**
   a. **Patient position.** The patient is **supine** with the operative leg to be blocked slightly abducted and externally rotated.
   b. The landmarks are the **sartorius muscles** located just above the medial side of the patella. Identification of the sartorius muscle is facilitated by simply asking the patient to elevate the extended leg 5 to 10 cm. The proposed needle insertion site is **3 to 4 cm superior and 6 to 8 cm posterior to the superior-medial border of the patella**.
   c. After aseptic skin preparation and draping followed by LA skin infiltration of the proposed needle insertion site, a 50-mm (2-in.) 22-gauge stimulating needle is attached to a peripheral nerve stimulator (typical settings of 1.5–2.0 mA, 2 Hz, 100 μs) and to a syringe of LA.
   d. The stimulating needle is inserted slightly caudally at an angle of 45 degrees slightly posterior to the coronal plane through the muscle belly of the SM. The needle is advanced until a slight loss of resistance is felt as the needle passes through the posterior border of the sartorius and enters the subsartorial tissue plane at a depth of 3 to 5 cm. At this point, the patient should report a **paresthesia referred down to the medial malleolus**.
   e. The final needle position is adjusted until paresthesias are elicited at a current output of 0.6 mA or less. After aspiration, followed by injection of a negative test dose of 3 mL of LA, an additional 7 mL of LA is injected.

2. US-guided SN block
   a. **Patient position.** The patient is **supine** with the operative leg to be blocked slightly abducted and externally rotated.
   b. **Probe selection.** A **high frequency linear array transducer** (8–12 MHz) is typically used for this block. A **depth of 3 to 5 cm is adequate** to visualize the muscle planes.
   c. **Probe placement and sonoanatomy.** The US probe is placed initially **perpendicular to the long axis of the operative extremity along the medial thigh 5 to 7 cm proximal the superior border of the patella.**
      (1) The probe position is adjusted until the typical image of the subsartorial tissue plane is visualized (Figure 15.7).
      (2) The sartorius muscle is located posterior to the vastus medialis muscle. Just deep to the sartorius muscle and superficial to the gracilis muscle, the saphenous nerve can be seen as a round or oval hyperechoic structure within the subsartorial compartment sandwiched between these two muscles.
      (3) Directly adjacent to the SN the **descending genicular artery** is identified as a small hypoechoic pulsatile structure, which can be confirmed by using color or pulse-wave Doppler.
   d. **Needling technique**
      (1) After aseptic skin preparation and draping followed by LA skin infiltration of the proposed needle insertion site, a 50-mm (2-in.) 22-gauge stimulating needle is connected to a peripheral nerve stimulator (typical settings of 1.5–2.0 mA, 2 Hz, 100 μs) and to a syringe of LA.
      (2) After placing the target neural structures in the middle of the screen, the needle is placed just next to the anterior-medial aspect of the

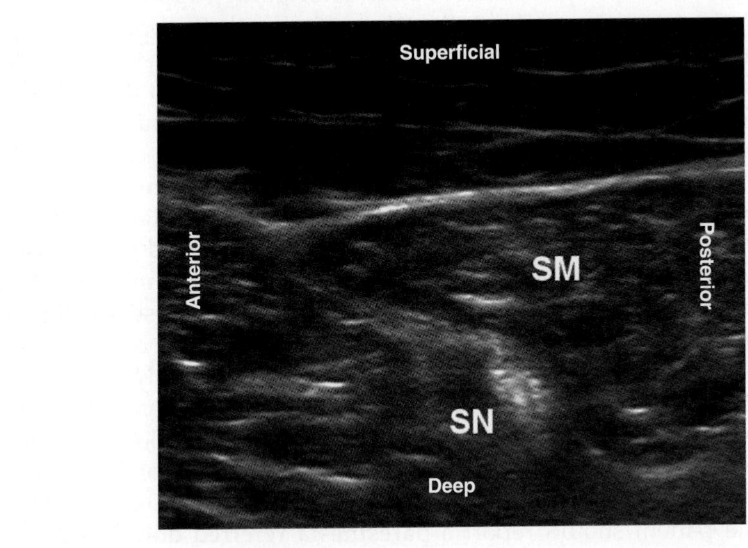

Figure 15.7. Ultrasound anatomy of the saphenous nerve. At the level of the lower thigh the saphenous nerve (*SN*) pierces the adductor fascia and appears as a hyperechoic image under the body of the sartorius muscle (*SM*).

US probe and advanced **in-plane** (to the US beam) in a posterior direction at an appropriate angle toward the target structures.

(3) The **optimal** needle position is **adjacent to the SN when visible or the descending genicular artery (when the SN is not ideally visualized)** within the subsartorial tissue plane. At this point, the peripheral nerve stimulator may also be activated, which should elicit paresthesias referred to the medial lower leg down to the medial malleolus.

(4) After aspiration to rule out intravascular injection, a **5 to 10 mL of LA** is injected. Real-time assessment of LA injection is performed to ensure satisfactory perineural distribution within subsartorial fascial plane.

D. Obturator nerve block

1. The **traditional technique** of performing an ONB utilized the pubic tubercle as the primary landmark. The initial needle insertion point was 2 cm caudal and 2 cm lateral to the pubic tubercle. The stimulating needle was inserted perpendicular to the skin until it made contact with the inferior border of the superior pubic ramus. The needle was redirected further posterior and slightly lateral (in order to walk off the inferior border of the superior pubic ramus) toward the obturator foramen until an adductor EMR is elicited. This approach has been associated with a moderate degree of patient discomfort. Additionally, the obturator vessels and their connection to the external iliac vessels are in close proximity to the obturator foramen and pose a risk of intravascular injection, or if vessel injury occurs, may pose a risk of hematoma or hemorrhage.
2. A new **peripheral nerve stimulator "inguinal approach"** has been described, which is associated with less discomfort and faster block performance compared to the traditional approach (6). Therefore, the inguinal approach to the ONB will be described. Additionally, the newer **US-guided approaches** for ONB place the needle tip in the same location as the peripheral nerve stimulator inguinal approach to the ONB (7). Therefore, both methods complement each other and may be used simultaneously to confirm final needle placement.
   a. **Patient position.** The patient is **supine** with the operative leg to be blocked slightly abducted and externally rotated.
   b. The patient is asked to **flex the hip** and the **IC is identified and marked**. The **AL tendon** is identified as the most superficial palpable tendon in the upper medial part of the thigh. The **femoral pulse** is identified by palpation (or Doppler) over the inguinal crease. The proposed needle insertion point is the **midpoint between the inner border of the adductor longus tendon and femoral arterial pulse** (Figure 15.8). At this level, the obturator nerve has split into its anterior (deep to the AL and pectineus but superficial to the AB) and posterior divisions (deep to the adductor brevis and superficial to the adductor magnus).
   c. After aseptic skin preparation and draping followed by LA skin infiltration of the proposed needle insertion site, a 75 to 100 mm (3–4 in.) 22-gauge stimulating needle is attached to a peripheral nerve stimulator (typical settings of 1.5–2.0 mA, 2 Hz, 100 μs) and to a syringe of LA.
   d. The stimulating needle is advanced in a **30-degree cephalad** direction until an EMR of the **AL or gracilis muscle** is elicited at a current output

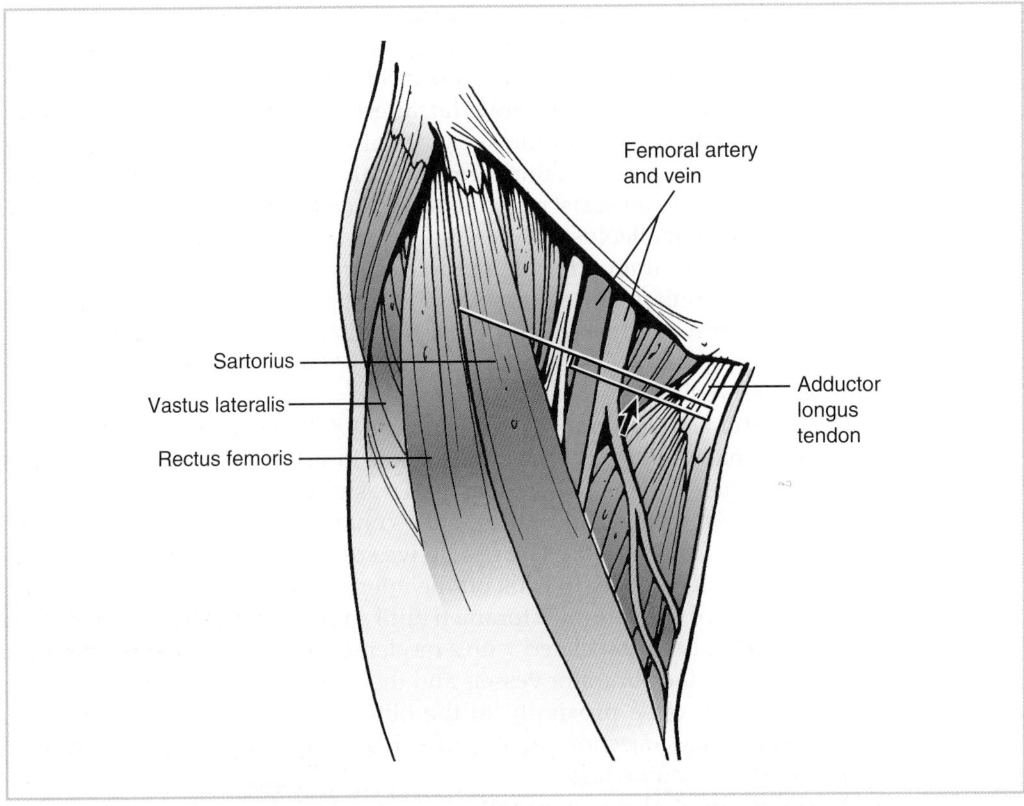

Figure 15.8. Surface anatomy for the obturator block. The inguinal crease (IC) is identified by asking the patient to flex the hip slightly. Along this line, the location of the femoral pulse (FA) and the tendon of the adductor longus (AL) are identified and marked. The midpoint of a line between these two is the starting point for locating the obturator nerve.

at below 0.5 mA (Figure 15.8). This should result in contractions of the anterior part of the inner thigh. The **anterior division is typically located 38 ± 9 mm from the skin**. After aspiration to rule out intravascular injection, 5 mL of LA is injected to block the anterior division.

e. The stimulating needle is slightly withdrawn and redirected **5 degrees lateral** and advanced (with the current output of 1.0 mA) EMR of the adductor magnus are elicited at a current output at or below 0.5 mA. This should result in contractions of the **posterior part of the inner thigh**, along with noticeable adduction of the upper leg. The posterior division is typically located **45 ± 7 mm from the skin**. After aspiration to rule out intravascular injection, 5 mL of LA is injected to block the posterior division.

f. Clinical pearls. Asking the patient to adduct and flex at the hip greatly facilitates **identification of the AL tendon**. Because the cutaneous distribution of the obturator nerve is absent in more than 50% of individuals, the only reliable method to confirm a successful ONB is by testing for decreased hip adduction strength. Do not expect full adductor motor block as the tibial branch of the sciatic nerve supplies the medial aspect of the AM.

3. **US-guided ONB (inguinal)** relies on identification of the muscle layers that surround both the common obturator nerve, as well as the anterior and posterior divisions as they descend further caudad into the thigh (7).
   a. **Patient position.** The patient is **supine** with the leg slightly abducted and externally rotated.
   b. **Probe selection.** A **high frequency linear array transducer** (8–12 MHz) is typically used for this block. A depth of **4 to 5 cm is adequate** to visualize the obturator nerve and surrounding muscular and vascular structures.
   c. **Probe placement and sonoanatomy.** The US probe is placed initially at **a 90-degree angle to the skin and parallel to the inguinal ligament.**
      (1) The probe is then moved **caudally 2 to 4 cm**, while kept parallel to the inguinal ligament cephalad and IC caudad. At this point the **common obturator nerve in short-axis view appears as a hyperechoic, flattened structure** located within a hyperechoic myofascial plane **between the pectineus and AL** superficial to the obturator nerve and the AB located deep to obturator nerve (Figure 15.9). At this level, the pectineus is located lateral to the AL and located just medial to the femoral vein.
      (2) The probe may be moved slightly caudal over the IC to follow the course of the obturator nerve as it splits into the anterior (between

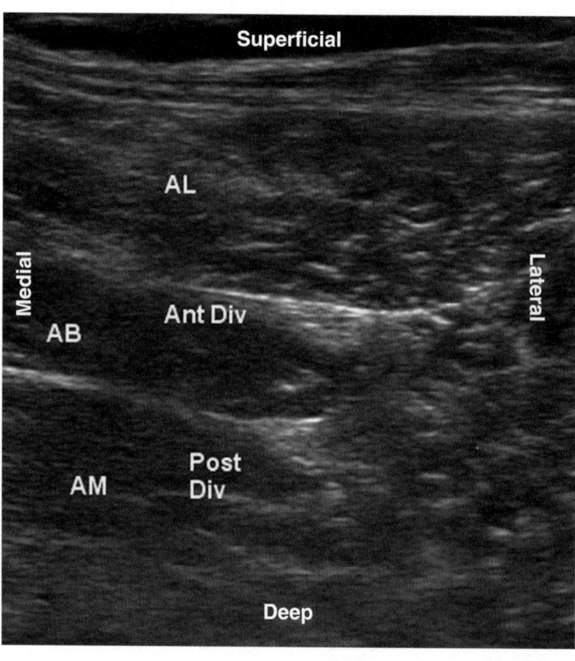

Figure 15.9. Ultrasound anatomy of the inguinal approach to the obturator nerve block. Ultrasound will demonstrate the three adductor muscle layers-the adductor longus (AL), adductor brevis (AB), and adductor magnus (AM). The anterior division of the obturator nerve (Ant Div) lies between AL and AB. The posterior division of the obturator nerve (Post Div) lies between the AB and the AM, which is the desired target for knee joint anesthesia/analgesia.

the AL and the AB) and posterior divisions (between the AB and AM) of the obturator nerve (Figure 15.9).

(3) With this technique, a **combination of compression and tilting cephalad-caudad** of the probe is important to enhance the anisotropy (and sonographic appearance) of the nerve(s) and myofascial structures.

d. **Needling technique**

(1) After aseptic skin preparation and draping followed by LA skin infiltration of the proposed needle insertion site, a 100-mm (4-in.) 22-gauge stimulating needle is attached to a peripheral nerve stimulator (typical settings of 1.5–2.0 mA, 2 Hz, 100 μs) and to a syringe of LA.

(2) After placing the **target neural structures in the middle of the screen**, the needle is placed just medial to the medial aspect of the US probe and advanced **in-plane** (to the US beam) at an appropriate angle toward the target structures. The target is near the anterior and posterior divisions.

(3) At this point, a peripheral nerve stimulator may be attached and turned on simply to confirm that the target structure is a nerve. After aspiration to rule out intravascular injection, 5 mL of LA is injected in proximity to each division. Real-time assessment of LA injection is performed to ensure satisfactory perineural distribution within the appropriate myofascial planes.

E. **Lateral femoral cutaneous nerve block**

1. **Patient position.** The patient is **supine** with the anesthesiologist at the patient's side.
2. The main landmark for the LFCN is the **ASIS**, which is easily palpable in most patients. The proposed needle insertion site is **2 cm medial and 2 cm caudal to the ASIS** (Figure 15.5).
3. After aseptic skin preparation and draping followed by LA skin infiltration of the proposed needle insertion site, a 50-mm (2-in.) 22-gauge stimulating needle is attached to a peripheral nerve stimulator (typical settings of 1.5–2.0 mA, 2 Hz, 100 μs) and to a syringe of LA.
4. The needle is advanced directly posterior **until a loss of resistance** is felt as the needle passes through the fascia lata. Because the perception of the loss of resistance is not consistent, LA should be injected in a fanwise manner from medial to lateral both above and below the fascia lata. Alternatively, the peripheral nerve stimulator may be activated and the needle advanced in the same manner until paresthesia referred to the anterior-lateral aspect of the thigh is elicited.
5. Typically, a volume of 10 mL of LA is injected for this block.

REFERENCES

1 **Sim IW, Webb T. Anatomy and anaesthesia of the lumbar somatic plexus.** ***Anaesth Intensive Care*** **2004;32:178–187.**

2 Farny J, Drolet P, Girard M. Anatomy of the posterior approach to the lumbar plexus block. *Can J Anaesth* 1994;41:480–485.

3 Mannion S, Barret J, Kelly D, et al. A description of the spread of injectate after psoas compartment block using magnetic resonance imaging. *Reg Anesth Pain Med* 2005;30:567–571.

4 Grothaus MC, Holt M, Mekhali AO, et al. Lateral femoral cutaneous nerve: an anatomic study. *Clin Orthop Relat Res* 2005;437:164–168.
5 Bouaziz H, Jochum D, Macalou D, et al. An evaluation of the cutaneous distribution of the obturator nerve. *Anesth Analg* 2002;94:445–449.
6 Choquet O, Capdevila X, Bennourine K, et al. A new inguinal approach for the obturator nerve block: an anatomical and randomized clinical study. *Anesthesiology* 2005;103:1238–1245.
7 Soon J, Schafhalter-Zoppoth I, Gray AT. Sonographic imaging of the obturator nerve for regional block. *Reg Anesth Pain Med* 2007;32:146–151.
8 Capdevila X, Macaire P, Dadure C, et al. Continuous psoas compartment block for postoperative analgesia after total hip arthroplasty: new landmarks, technical guidelines, and clinical evaluation. *Anesth Analg* 2002;94:1606–1613.
9 Awad IT, Duggan EM. Posterior lumbar plexus block: anatomy, approaches, and techniques. *Reg Anesth Pain Med* 2005;30:143–149.
10 Capdevila X, Coimbra C, Choquet O. Approaches to the lumbar plexus: success, risks, and outcomes. *Reg Anesth Pain Med* 2005;30:150–162.
11 Vloka JD, Hadzic A, Drobnik L, et al. Anatomical landmarks for femoral nerve block: a comparison of four needle insertion sites. *Anesth Analg* 1999;89:1467–1470.
12 Capdevila X, Biboulet P, Morau D, et al. Continuous three-in-one block for postoperative analgesia after lower limb orthopedic surgery: where do catheters go? *Anesth Analg* 2002;94:1001–1006.
13 Capdevila X, Biboulet P, Bouregba M, et al. Comparison of the three-in-one and fascia iliaca compartment block in adults: a clinical and radiographic comparison. *Anesth Analg* 1998;86:1039–1044.
14 Morau D, Lopez S, Biboulet P, et al. Comparison of continuous 3-in-1 and fascia iliaca compartment blocks for postoperative analgesia: feasibility, catheter migration, distribution of sensory block, and analgesic efficacy. *Reg Anesth Pain Med* 2003;28:309–314.
15 Marhofer P, Schrogendorfer K, Koinig H, et al. Ultrasonographic guidance improves sensory block and onset time of three-in-one blocks. *Anesth Analg* 1997;85:854–857.
16 Marhofer P, Schrogendorfer K, Wallner T, et al. Ultrasonographic guidance reduces the amount of local anesthetic for 3-in-1 blocks. *Reg Anesth Pain Med* 1998;23:584–588.
17 Casati A, Baciarello M, Di Cianni S, et al. Effects of ultrasound guidance on the minimum effective anesthetic volume required to block the femoral nerve. *Br J Anaesth* 2007;98:823–827.
18 Benzon HT, Sharma S, Calimaran A. Comparison of different approaches to the saphenous nerve block. *Anesthesiology* 2005;102:633–638.
19 Lundblad M, Kapral S, Marhofer P, et al. Ultrasound-guided infrapatellar block in human volunteers: description of a novel technique. *Br J Anaesth* 2006;97:710–714.
20 Krombach J, Gray AT. Sonography for saphenous nerve block near the adductor canal. *Reg Anesth Pain Med* 2007;32:369–370.

16 Sacral Plexus-Sciatic Nerve Blocks

Francis V. Salinas

I. Introduction and general overview

The **sacral plexus** is derived from the ventral rami of the **lumbosacral trunk**, along with the ventral rami of the first, second, and part of the third sacral nerves (Figure 15.1). The **sacral plexus** is formed within the pelvis as the nerve roots converge from their respective exit sites toward the greater sciatic foramen. As the roots coalesce, the plexus forms a **triangular sheet,** the apex of which is oriented toward the infrapiriform foramen, as the sciatic nerve exits (anterior) deep to the inferior margin of the piriformis muscle (Figure 16.1). Within the pelvis, the sacral plexus lies against the posterior pelvic wall anterior to the piriformis muscle and posterior to the internal iliac artery and ureter. The clinically relevant branches of the sacral plexus are the **sciatic nerve and posterior femoral cutaneous nerve (PFCN),** which provide sensory and motor innervation to portions of the entire lower extremity, including the hip, knee, and ankle (Figure 16.2). Additional branches from the sacral plexus proximal to the formation of the sciatic nerve that are important for major hip surgery include the superior and inferior gluteal nerves and the nerve to the quadratus femoris (1).

A. The **lumbosacral trunk** (L4-5) and the **anterior divisions of the S1-3** roots give rise to the **tibial nerve (TN),** whereas the **posterior divisions of S1-3** give rise to the **common peroneal nerve (CPN).** These two distinct nerves unite to form the sciatic nerve. The TN and CPN share a common connective tissue sheath and therefore have the **appearance of a single nerve trunk.**

B. As the sciatic nerve exits the pelvis through the infrapiriform foramen at the inferior border of the piriformis, the **larger TN is medial** and slightly anterior to the CPN. From the point that the sacral plexus first enters the pelvis until the sciatic nerve leaves the gluteal compartment just distal to the ischial tuberosity (IT) and greater trochanter (GT), it is covered by the mass of the gluteus maximus.

C. The sciatic nerve descends to the posterior thigh, **by passing the midpoint between the IT (located medially) and the GT** (located medially). At this level, the sciatic nerve is posterior to the quadratus femoris muscle and anterior to the gluteus maximus (Figure 16.1). As the sciatic nerve descends into the posterior compartment of the thigh, it lies posterior to the lesser trochanter of the femur. Within the proximal posterior compartment of the thigh, just distal to the inferior border of the gluteus maximus, the sciatic nerves lies on the posterior surface of the adductor muscle **immediately lateral to the tendon of the biceps femoris muscle (2)** (Figure 16.3). At this location, the sciatic nerve is relatively superficial and covered only by skin and subcutaneous tissue.

D. As the sciatic nerve descends further down the posterior compartment of the thigh toward the **popliteal fossa**, it lies deep to the biceps femoris muscle. Within the popliteal fossa, the sciatic nerve lies posterolateral to the popliteal vessels. Specifically, the popliteal vein lies medial to the sciatic nerve, whereas the popliteal artery is anteromedial to the sciatic nerve.

E. Although the sciatic nerve may be separated into its two distinct components (but contained within a common connective tissue sheath) as proximal as the

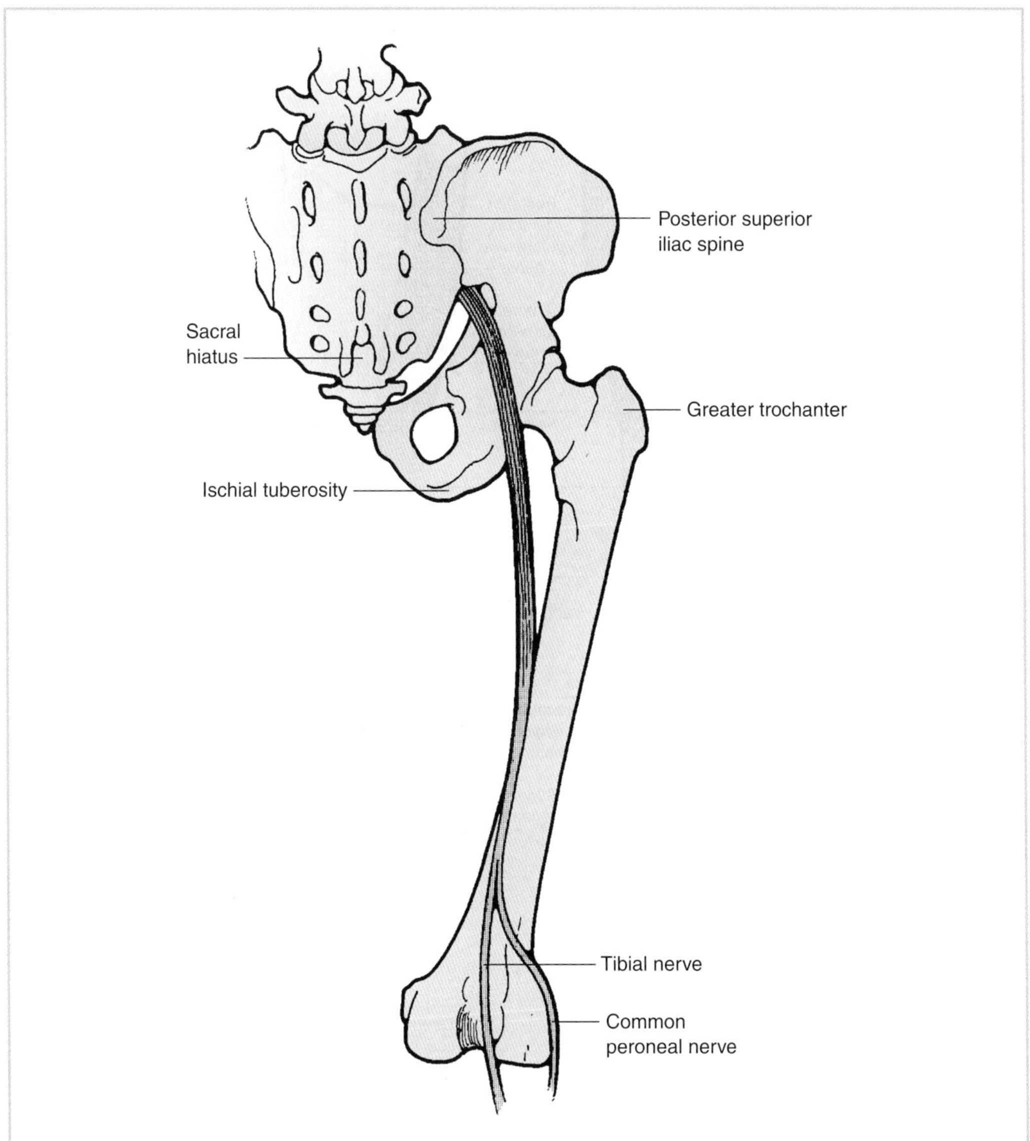

Figure 16.1. Deep anatomy of the sciatic nerve. The nerve exits the pelvis through the sciatic notch and travels behind the femur to bifurcate just above the knee into the tibial and common peroneal nerves.

gluteal region, the **TN and CPN are classically described as separating (from each other)** as individual nerves at the upper aspect of the popliteal fossa. However, evaluation of the division of the sciatic nerve is highly variable and on average occurs at **6 to 9 cm above the popliteal crease,** but with a range of 0 to 14 cm (**3**, 4).

F. The **PFCN** is a purely sensory nerve derived from the ventral rami of the S1 to S3 spinal nerves. Although deep to the gluteus maximus, the PFCN is located medial and superficial to the sciatic nerve. At this level, the PFCN gives off inferior cluneal branches to supply the skin of the lower buttock and perineal branches to supply the skin on the posterior aspect of the external genitalia. The

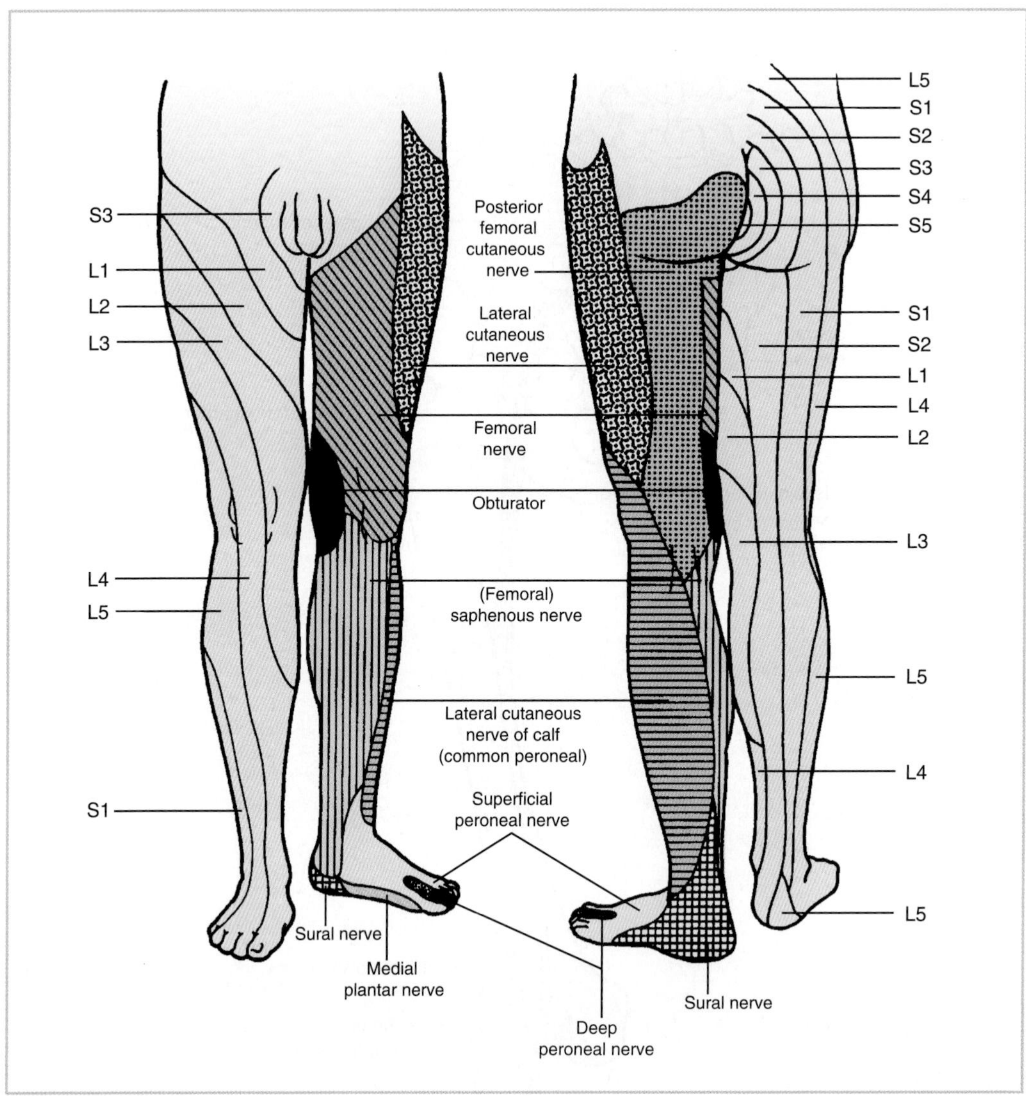

Figure 16.2. Dermatomal and peripheral nerve branches of the leg.

PFCN emerges from the inferior edge of the gluteus maximus to lie within the subcutaneous tissue and descends further along the posterior aspect of the thigh and lower leg to supply the skin of the posterior aspect of the thigh and calf.

II. Indications

The primary indication for sciatic nerve block is to provide **operative anesthesia to the lower leg, ankle, or foot**. In order to provide complete anesthesia to the lower leg, the **saphenous nerve** must also be blocked to anesthetize the skin of the medial lower leg, which is not supplied by the sciatic nerve. In contrast, a continuous sciatic perineural catheter from the level of the sacral plexus down to the popliteal fossa will provide excellent **postoperative analgesia** for painful procedures of the lower leg such as hallux valgus repair, below the knee amputations, and open reduction-internal fixation of ankle and lower leg fractures. For operative

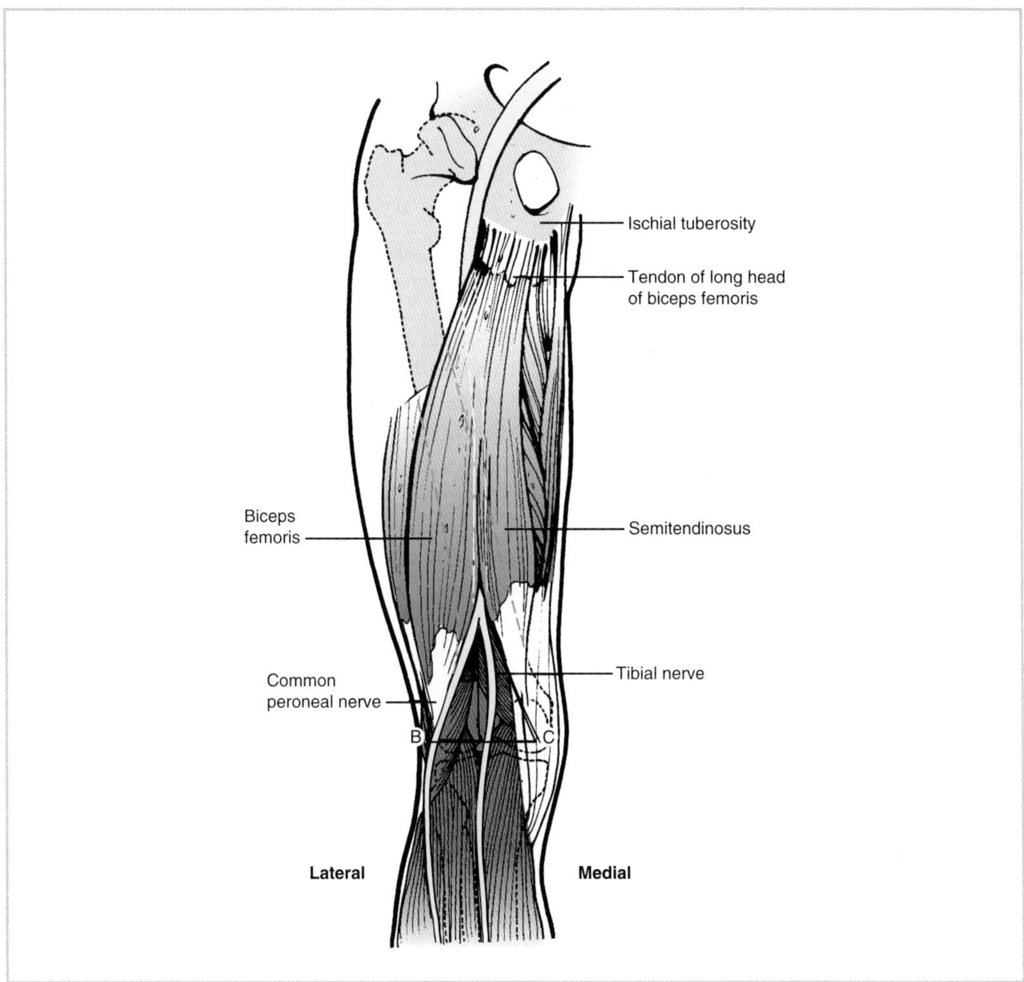

Figure 16.3. Relationship of the sciatic nerve to the muscles of the posterior thigh.

procedures of the femur and knee joint, a sciatic nerve block in combination with a psoas compartment block will provide complete surgical anesthesia for procedures such as total knee replacement, anterior cruciate ligament reconstruction, above-the-knee amputations, and open reduction-internal fixation of femur fractures. A more proximal sciatic nerve block at the gluteal or subgluteal region is commonly indicated for severe **knee pain** after total knee replacement despite a successful femoral nerve block. For operative procedures of the **hip joint** such as total hip replacement, only a parasacral approach in combination with a psoas compartment block will provide complete surgical anesthesia.

III. Choice of local anesthetic

The choice of local anesthetic for the sacral plexus-sciatic nerve block is dependent on the requirements for **onset of anesthesia** and **duration** of analgesia for single-injection techniques, as well the anatomic location where the block is performed. The sciatic nerve block is different from the individual nerve blocks of the lumbar

Table 16.1 Local anesthetic choices for sacral plexus-proximal sciatic nerve block

Local anesthetic	Onset (min)	Duration of anesthesia (h)	Duration of analgesia (h)
Lidocaine 2% with HCO_3	10–20	5–6	5–8
Mepivacaine 1.5% with HCO_3	10–15	4–5	5–6
Ropivacaine 0.5%	15–20	6–12	6–24
Bupivacaine 0.5%	15–30	8–16	10–36

plexus, as the anatomic location of the sciatic nerve block has a significant impact on the total local anesthetic mass requirements.

A. Specifically, the **proximal approaches to sciatic nerve block consistently have a shorter latency** to complete anesthesia (5) and lower total anesthetic requirement compared with the distal popliteal approaches (6,7). Additionally, epinephrine is not routinely recommended for proximal sciatic nerve block because of the possibility of epinephrine exacerbating ischemic injury due to stretching or sitting on the anesthetized sciatic nerve with a prolonged block.

B. With the advent of **continuous peripheral perineural catheter techniques**, the anesthesiologist has the advantage of providing a rapid onset of surgical block by injection of the shorter-acting local anesthetics (Table 16.1 and 16.2) through the needle or catheter tip (the primary anesthetic block). Subsequently, an infusion of a dilute local anesthetic that possesses sensory-motor dissociation (the most commonly used being ropivacaine 0.2% or bupivacaine 0.125%) may be used to provide the optimal balance of postoperative analgesia with less motor block to facilitate postoperative rehabilitation and recovery. Alternatively, if a central neuraxial technique is chosen as the primary anesthetic, a loading dose (10–15 mL) of the analgesic infusion of ropivacaine 0.2% may be started intraoperatively. The typical postoperative regimen consists of running the analgesic infusion at 4 to 8 mL/h with or without a patient-controlled bolus of 2 to 3 mL every 20 minutes.

IV. Techniques

The sacral plexus-sciatic nerve is the **longest nerve in the body** and may be blocked at the sacral plexus, gluteal, subgluteal, and popliteal levels. Although, **posterior approaches to the sciatic nerve are the most commonly performed** techniques, the sciatic nerve may also be blocked from an anterior approach in the proximal thigh, as well as lateral approaches extending from the mid-thigh to just above the popliteal fossa. The choice of technique will be dictated by the requirements for surgical anesthesia and postoperative analgesia, as well as the ability of the patient to assume the appropriate position. Although posterior approaches are the most commonly performed techniques, patient factors (morbid obesity, painful fractures, and the presence of casts-fixation devices) may preclude patients from assuming either the lateral decubitus or prone position. Therefore, either anterior or lateral approaches provide alternative techniques when the patient cannot assume the lateral or prone position. As with lumbar plexus blocks, both **single-injection** and **continuous catheter** techniques are available for all approaches. Additionally, both **traditional peripheral nerve stimulator** (**PNS**) and **ultrasound-guided** (**USG**) approaches will be described. Paresthesia techniques are not recommended for sacral-sciatic nerve blocks.

Table 16.2 Local anesthetic choices for distal popliteal sciatic nerve block

Local anesthetic	Onset (min)	Duration of anesthesia (h)	Duration of analgesia (h)
Lidocaine 2% with HCO_3 and 1:400 epinephrine	10–20	2–5	3–8
Mepivacaine 1.5% with HCO_3 and 1:400 epinephrine	10–15	3–5	3–8
Ropivacaine 0.5%	15–30	4–8	6–12
Ropivacaine 0.75%	10–15	5–10	6–24
Bupivacaine 0.5%	15–30	5–15	6–30

A. **Parasacral nerve block approach (PSNB).** The parasacral technique blocks the sacral plexus proximal enough to reliably provide anesthesia to the **sciatic and PFCN,** as well the superior and inferior gluteal nerves, nerve to the quadratus femoris, and the pudendal nerve (**8**, 9) contained between the piriformis muscle posterior and the pelvic fascia anterior. Therefore, it can be described as true sacral plexus block. In contrast to slightly more distal gluteal approaches, the **PSNB** approach (in conjunction with a psoas compartment block) can provide true unilateral anesthesia for hip surgery (10,11). The only two landmarks that are important are the **posterior superior iliac spine** (**PSIS**) and **IT** (Figure 16.4).

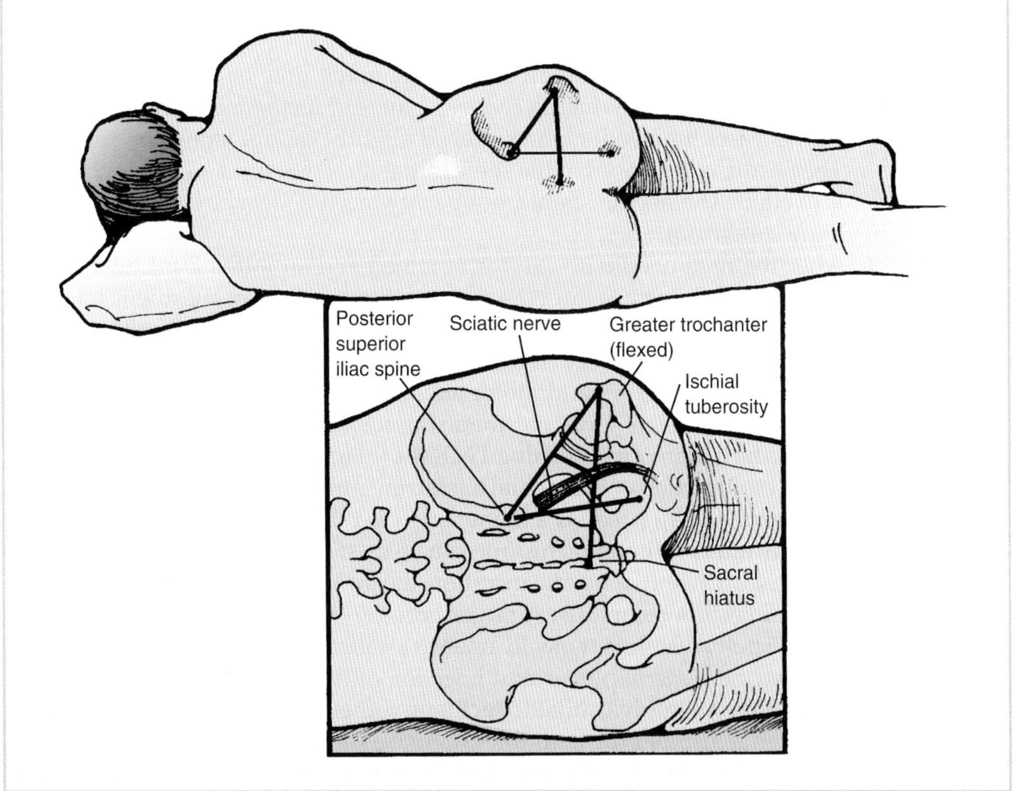

Figure 16.4. Landmarks for posterior sciatic block at the hip.

Therefore, it is a relatively easy block to learn with a high success rate (12). The relative disadvantages of this block include the proximity of structures anterior to the sacral plexus (iliac vessels, ureter, and bladder) and the associated weakness of the hamstrings and adductor muscles. Therefore, for procedures of the lower leg, a more distal approach at the popliteal fossa maybe more appropriate.

1. **Patient position.** The patient is placed in **the lateral position with a slight forward tilt** with the operative side to be blocked uppermost. The dependent limb should be straight and the operative limb should be flexed slightly at both the hip and knee.
2. The **external landmarks are the PSIS and the IT**. A line is drawn connecting the PSIS and IT corresponding to the sacrotuberous ligament. The proposed **needle insertion site is along this line 6 cm caudal to the PSIS**, which allows access to the sacral plexus as it passes through the greater sciatic foramen.
3. After aseptic skin preparation and draping followed by local anesthetic skin infiltration of the proposed needle insertion site, a 100-mm (4-in.) 21-gauge stimulating needle is attached to a PNS (typical settings of 1.5–2.0 mA, 2 Hz, 100 μs) and a syringe of local anesthetic.
4. The stimulating needle is advanced **perpendicular to the skin** in a **parasagittal plane** until a sacral plexus evoked motor response (EMR) is elicited at a current output between 0.2 and 0.5 mA. Acceptable EMR includes not only **plantar flexion** (TN) or **dorsiflexion** (CPN) of the foot or toes but also **hamstring contractions** (biceps femoris, semimembranosus, and semitendinosus) as acceptable endpoints.
5. The upper margin of the greater **sciatic notch** may be encountered as the needle is advanced, which serves as a gauge of further needle advancement. In this case, the needle is introduced slightly caudal along the same line. The needle is advanced in the same initial direction until an acceptable EMR is elicited. The needle should not be advanced 2.5 cm beyond the depth of bony contact **(8)**.
6. After the final needle position is obtained and an initial 3-mL test dose to confirm the absence of intravascular location of the local anesthetic injection, a total of 20 mL of local anesthetic is incrementally injected with frequent intermittent aspirations to reduce the risk of intravascular injection. Typical onset time for sensory and motor anesthesia is 10 to 20 minutes depending on the total mass of local anesthetic injected and the EMR elicited. Clinical studies have demonstrated that TN EMR (plantar flexion at the foot or ankle, as well contraction of the medial hamstring muscles [semimembranosus and semitendinosus]) predicts a higher success rate of anesthesia (13).
7. A **continuous catheter technique** can be used to provide extended duration analgesia. The initial needle insertion site and approach are the same as the single-injection technique. A larger bore (17- to 18-gauge) insulated stimulating Tuohy needle is typically used to localize the sacral plexus. After localization of the sacral plexus and injection of the local anesthetic, the needle is angulated slightly caudal to facilitate catheter passage. A 19- to 20-gauge catheter is inserted through the Tuohy needle and advanced no more than 2 cm past needle tip. The needle is then withdrawn over the catheter and the latter fixed in place with a sterile clear adhesive dressing. The proximal end of the catheter is then connected to an automated infusion pump.

8. **Clinical pearls.** If there is no EMR at a needle depth of 10 cm, the needle direction should be redirected caudally 5 to 10 degrees along the same line. Bony contact is preferred as this serves as an added safety step in judging the adequate depth of needle insertion.

B. **Sciatic nerve block, posterior transgluteal approach.** This is the **classic technique** of sciatic nerve block as initially described by Labat and later modified slightly by Winnie. This approach shares similar indications for both single-injection and continuous perineural catheter techniques, with the exception of not consistently blocking the sacral plexus branches (nerve to the quadratus femoris, superior and inferior gluteal nerves) required for complete anesthesia for hip surgery.

1. **Patient position.** The patient is placed in the **lateral decubitus position with a slight forward tilt,** hips flexed with the operative side to be blocked uppermost. The dependent limb should be straight and the operative limb should be flexed slightly at both the hip and knee.
2. **External landmarks.** The three palpable landmarks include the PSIS, the superior-most aspect of the GT, and the sacral hiatus. A line is drawn between the PSIS and GT. A second line is drawn from the SH and the GT. At the midpoint of the line between the PSIS and GT, a perpendicular line is drawn until it intersects with the line between the SH and GT (Figure 16.4). This third line is known as the *Labat line* and typically intersects the line between the SH and GT at a distance of 4 to 5 cm, and corresponds to the proposed needle insertion point. The proposed needle insertion point corresponds to the lateral border of the sciatic notch.
3. After aseptic skin preparation and draping followed by local anesthetic infiltration of the proposed needle insertion point, a stimulating needle (typically 100–150 mm [4–6 in.], 20–21 gauge) is slowly advanced at right angles to the spherical skin plane of the buttocks. The stimulating needle is attached to a PNS (typical settings of 1.5–2.0 mA, 2 Hz, 100 μs) and a syringe of local anesthetic.
4. The skin and underlying muscular/adipose tissue of the buttock is highly mobile and the skin-to-nerve distance may be substantial, especially in obese patients. Therefore, the fingers of the palpating hand should be firmly pressed on the needle insertion site to decrease the skin-to-nerve distance and skin should be stretched between the index and middle finger to allow greater precision in needle movement.
5. As the stimulating needle is advanced, the initial EMR observed may be **gluteus muscle** contractions, indicating that the needle tip is still too shallow. The needle is advanced further until EMR of the **hamstring muscles, or plantar flexion or dorsiflexion at the ankle or foot** are observed. The final position of the needle tip is judged to be adequate when EMR are elicited at 0.2 to 0.5 mA.
6. If the initial needle pass does not result in nerve localization, then a systematic approach is recommended for needle redirection. If bone is encountered, the depth should be noted as this likely represents the lateral border of the sciatic notch and the sciatic nerve will be located slightly deeper and more medial. Therefore, the needle is withdrawn to just below the skin and redirected with a slight medial angulation and advanced until the desired EMR is elicited. If this step does not elicit a desired EMR, mentally visualize the course of the sciatic nerve as it emerges from the

medial side to the center of the sciatic notch and then curves downward to course midway between the GT and IT. At this point, the needle is redirected in a systematic manner in 5- to 10-degree increments cephalad or caudad along the Labat line.

7. After the final needle position is obtained and an initial 3-mL test dose to confirm the absence of intravascular location of the local anesthetic injection, a total of 25 to 35 mL of local anesthetic is incrementally injected with frequent intermittent aspirations to reduce the risk of intravascular injection. Typical onset time for sensory anesthesia is 25 to 35 minutes depending on the total mass of local anesthetic injected and the EMR elicited. Seeking an EMR of both branches (TN and CPN) of the sciatic nerve and dividing the total local anesthetic injection equally between the two nerves improves both onset time and success of complete sciatic nerve block (14).
8. A **continuous catheter technique** may be utilized to provide extended duration analgesia. The initial needle insertion site and approach are the same as the single-injection technique. A larger bore (17- to 18-gauge) insulated stimulating Tuohy needle is typically used to localize the sciatic nerve. After localization of the sciatic nerve and injection of the local anesthetic, the needle tip is angulated slightly caudal toward the midpoint of the GT and IT to facilitate catheter passage along the course of the sciatic nerve. A 19- to 20-gauge catheter is inserted through the Tuohy needle and advanced no more than 2 cm past the needle tip. The needle is then withdrawn over the catheter and the latter fixed in place with a sterile clear adhesive dressing. The proximal end of the catheter is then connected to an automated infusion pump.

C. **Sciatic nerve block, USG posterior subgluteal approach.** Although **USG sciatic nerve block** at the gluteal level may be attempted, it is **technically challenging** due to the required depth of the sciatic nerve at the ischial spine level, especially in obese patients. A slightly more caudal approach at the level where the sciatic nerve courses **between the GT and IT offers several advantages (15)**. First, the sciatic nerve is likely to be more superficial and inferior to bulkiest portion of the gluteus maximus. Second, the location of the sciatic nerve is consistently observed to be at the midpoint between highly echogenic (and therefore, visible) IT medially and GT laterally. The sciatic nerve is visualized as a hyperechoic, oval to lip-shaped structure found in between the GT and IT. The sciatic nerve is located within the subgluteal space sandwiched directly deep to the fascial plane of the gluteus maximus and superficial to the underlying quadratus femoris muscle (Figure 16.5).

1. **Patient position.** The patient is placed in the **lateral decubitus position with a slight forward tilt**, hips flexed with the operative side to be blocked uppermost. The dependent limb should be straight and the operative limb should be flexed slightly at both the hip and knee.
2. **Probe selection.** A **mid to low frequency curved array transducer (2–5 MHz)** is typically used for this block. The lower frequency allows for a greater depth of penetration and the curved probe provides a **wider field of view required to visualize the GT and IT**.
3. **Probe placement and sonoanatomy.** The ultrasound probe is initially placed at a 90-degree angle to the skin, with the long axis of the probe directly over and parallel to a line drawn between the inner borders of the IT and GT (Figure 16.5).

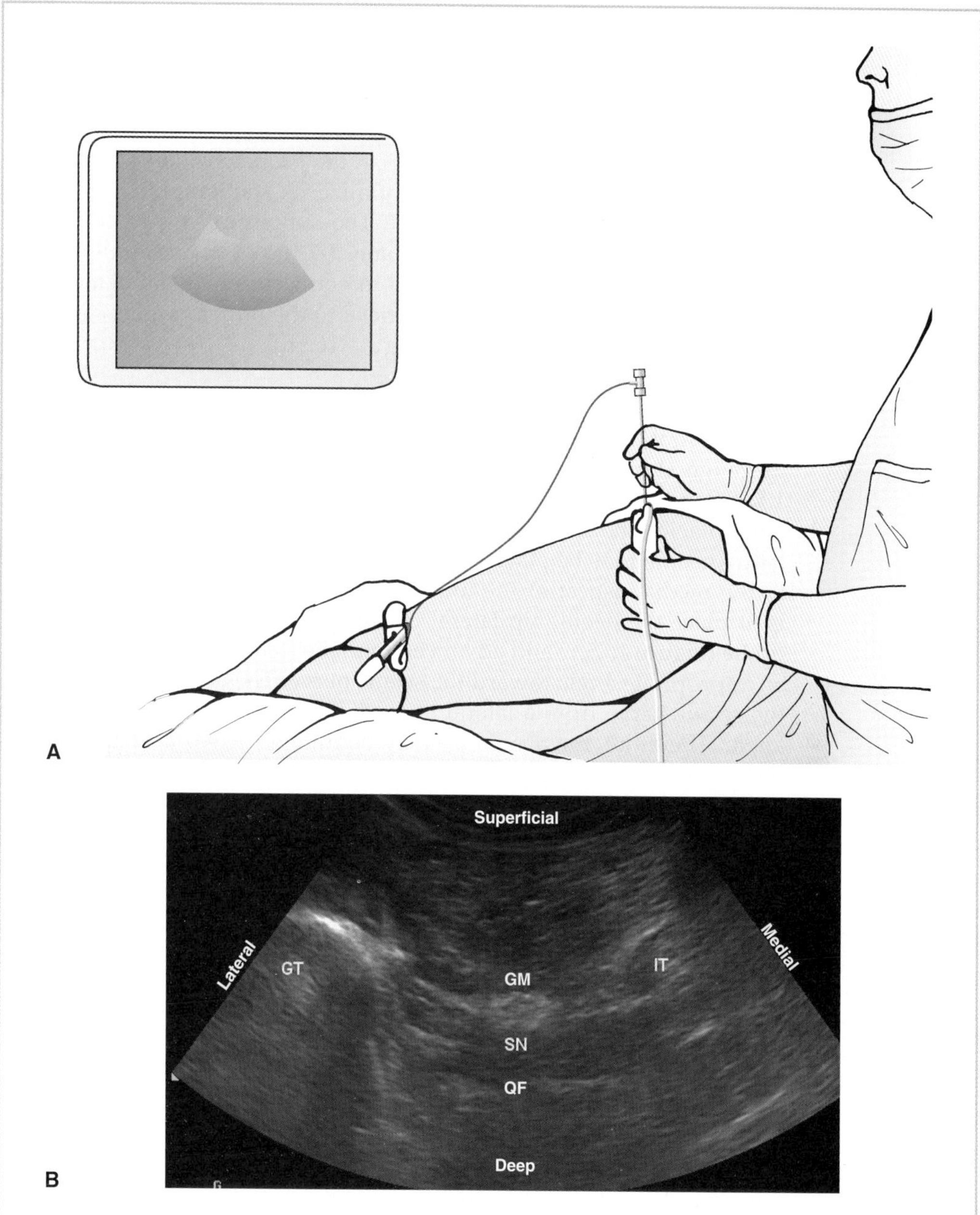

Figure 16.5. Ultrasound visualization of the sciatic nerve *(S)* in the subgluteal region. The patient lies in the lateral position with the hips and knees flexed. The curved array ultrasound probe is placed at the level of the inferior border of the gluteus maximus *(GM)* in the middle of the proximal thigh *(A)*. The image is image is adjusted to show the greater trochanter *(GT)* laterally, the ischial tuberosity *(IT)* medially, and sciatic nerve *(S)* will be visualized between these two landmarks, deep to the *GM* and superficial to the quadratus femoris *(QF)*.

a. Typically, the depth of the sciatic nerve is **5 to 8 cm depending on the body habitus** of the patient.
b. The gain and focal point are adjusted to optimize the appearance of the GT, IT, and subsequently the sciatic nerve.
c. At this point, the sciatic nerve often appears as **hyperechoic, oval to lip-shaped** structure. Slight adjustments in the probe position will enhance the anisotropy of the nerve and optimize its sonographic appearance within the subgluteal compartment. The subgluteal compartment is a fascial compartment bounded medially by the IT and laterally by the GT. The sciatic nerve is sandwiched in between the fascial plane of the gluteus maximus muscle and superficial to the underlying fascial plane of the quadratus femoris muscle (Figure 16.5B).

4. **Needling technique**
   a. After aseptic skin preparation and draping followed by local anesthetic skin infiltration of the proposed needle insertion site, a 100-mm (4-in.) 21-gauge stimulating needle is attached to a PNS (typical settings of 1.5–2.0 mA, 2 Hz, 100 μs) and a syringe of local anesthetic.
   b. After placing the target structures in the middle of the screen, the stimulating needle may be placed either lateral to the lateral aspect or medial to the medial aspect of the ultrasound probe. The preferred approach is to place the needle tip lateral to the lateral aspect of the ultrasound probe (Figure 16.5A) and advanced in plane (to the ultrasound beam) at an appropriate angle toward the sciatic nerve. The needle will approach the sciatic nerve from a lateral to medial direction at a relatively steep angle. Therefore, the needle tip may be difficult to see at it approaches the sciatic nerve. Simply injecting a small amount (0.5–1.0 mL) of local anesthetic will result in the formation of a small hypoechoic collection that is easily visible, thereby providing an indirect but useful assessment of needle tip location. The initial typical target site for the perineural needle placement is the space located between the greater trochanter and the lateral aspect of the sciatic nerve. The needle tip may then be adjusted in real time to achieve a circumferential collection of local anesthetic around the sciatic nerve.
   c. As the needle tip approaches the sciatic nerve, a **visible pop or loss of resistance** is seen and felt as the needle tip penetrates the fascial plane of the gluteus maximus. At this point, the PNS may be activated and the location of the needle tip confirmed by the appropriate sciatic nerve EMR. Local anesthetic is injected and local anesthetic distribution deep to the gluteus maximus within the subgluteal space and around the sciatic nerve is observed in real time. Typically, a volume of 15 to 25 mL is all that is required to obtain satisfactory local anesthetic distribution around the sciatic nerve.
5. If a **continuous catheter technique** is indicated, a larger bore (17- to 18-gauge) insulated stimulating Tuohy needle is typically used for initial placement of the needle tip and local anesthetic within the subgluteal compartment. After local anesthetic distribution (by injection through the needle tip) is ensured the ultrasound probe is placed aside within the sterile field. A 19- to 20-gauge catheter is inserted through the Tuohy needle and advanced no more than 2 to 3 cm past needle tip. At this point, the ultrasound probe is placed over the original site, and an additional 3 to 5 mL of local anesthetic

is injected through the catheter while observing for local anesthetic distribution within the subgluteal compartment around the sciatic nerve to ensure correct catheter tip position. The needle is then withdrawn over the catheter and the latter fixed in place with a sterile clear adhesive dressing. The proximal end of the catheter is then connected to an automated infusion pump.

D. **Sciatic nerve block, posterior infragluteal-parabiceps approach.** Traditional proximal posterior approaches to sciatic nerve block described in preceding text require needle placement deep to the gluteus maximus. This approach may be difficult and painful, especially in obese patients if multiple needle redirections are required. Additionally, the sciatic nerve at the level of the gluteal approaches is in close proximity to the inferior gluteal artery, thereby increasing the potential risk of vascular puncture and/or intravascular injection. A newer proximal posterior approach to sciatic nerve block relies on **two easily identifiable landmarks** (2): the **lateral border of the biceps femoris muscle tendon** and the **inferior border of the gluteus maximus (gluteal crease).** At this location, the sciatic nerve is just lateral to the lateral border of the tendon (Figure 16.3). The infragluteal-parabiceps technique has several advantages, which include a relatively shallow depth (as compared to the traditional approach of Labat), the absence of any muscles or major vascular structures (which should decrease the potential for patient discomfort and intravascular injection of local anesthetic). The technique described in the subsequent text relies on **peripheral nerve stimulation**, although USG techniques may also be used.

1. **Patient position.** The patient is placed in the **lateral decubitus position with a slight forward tilt,** hips flexed with the operative side to be blocked uppermost. The dependent limb should be straight and the operative limb should be flexed slightly at both the hip and knee. Alternatively, the patient **may also be placed prone** to enhance the visibility of the gluteal crease.
2. **External landmarks.** The **gluteal crease** is identified and marked with a line. **The lateral border of the biceps femoris muscle tendon is identified**. A helpful approach to identify the biceps femoris muscle tendon is to first locate its tendinous insertion at the IT. The course of the tendon is palpated as it descends in the posterior thigh. The proposed needle insertion point is **1 cm below the gluteal crease along the lateral border of the biceps femoris muscle tendon**.
3. After aseptic skin preparation and draping followed by local anesthetic infiltration of the proposed needle insertion point, a stimulating needle (typically a 50–100 mm [2–4 in.], 21–22 gauge) is **inserted just lateral to the biceps femoris muscle tendon** with an angle of 70 to 90 degrees to the skin and advanced in a **cephalad manner**. The stimulating needle is attached to a PNS (typical settings of 1.5–2.0 mA, 2 Hz, 100 μs) and a syringe of local anesthetic.
4. As the stimulating needle is advanced, the needle tip passes through skin and subcutaneous tissue until the desired EMR is elicited. Contraction of the biceps femoris muscle is not accepted as this indicates either direct muscle stimulation or stimulation of the motor branch. If this occurs, the needle is advanced slightly deeper. The desired EMR is **inversion or plantar flexion of the foot** (see subsequent text). If plantar flexion is elicited, the needle tip is redirected just lateral to obtain inversion. Alternatively, if the dorsiflexion is obtained, the needle tip should be slightly adjusted medial to elicit inversion. The final position of the needle tip is considered optimal when the desired EMR is still elicited at 0.2 to 0.5 mA.

5. After the final needle position is obtained and an initial 3-mL test dose to confirm the absence of intravascular location of the local anesthetic injection, a total of **25 to 35 mL of local anesthetic** is incrementally injected with frequent intermittent aspirations to reduce the risk of intravascular injection. Typical onset time for sensory anesthesia is 15 to 25 minutes depending on the total mass of local anesthetic injected and the EMR elicited.
6. A **continuous catheter technique** may be utilized to provide extended duration analgesia. The initial needle insertion site and approach are the same as the single-injection technique. A larger bore (17- to 18-gauge) insulated stimulating Tuohy needle is typically used to localize the sciatic nerve. After localization of the sciatic nerve and injection of the local anesthetic, the needle angle is decreased and the **needle tip is oriented toward the midpoint of the GT and IT** to facilitate catheter passage along the course of the sciatic nerve. A 19- to 20-gauge catheter is inserted through the Tuohy needle and advanced no more than 3 to 5 cm past needle tip. The needle is then withdrawn over the catheter and the latter fixed in place with a sterile clear adhesive dressing. The proximal end of the catheter is then connected to an automated infusion pump.
7. **Clinical pearls.** Asking the patient to *"bend the leg"* (flexion at the knee) results in contraction of the hamstring muscles, which helps to accentuate the location of the lateral border of the biceps femoris muscle tendon. Understanding the anatomy of the sciatic nerve is key to interpreting EMR when using a PNS technique (Figure 16.6).
   a. **Plantar flexion** corresponds to stimulation of the TN.
   b. **Dorsiflexion** corresponds to stimulation of the CPN.
   c. **Eversion** corresponds to stimulation of superficial branch of the CPN, located on the lateral aspect of the CPN.
   d. **Inversion** corresponds to stimulation of the TN (contraction of the tibialis posterior muscle) and the deep branch of the CPN (contraction of the tibialis posterior muscle). Therefore, **inversion indicates that the needle tip is central in location** to the sciatic nerve with simultaneous stimulation of both the TN and the deep branch of the CPN. Additionally,

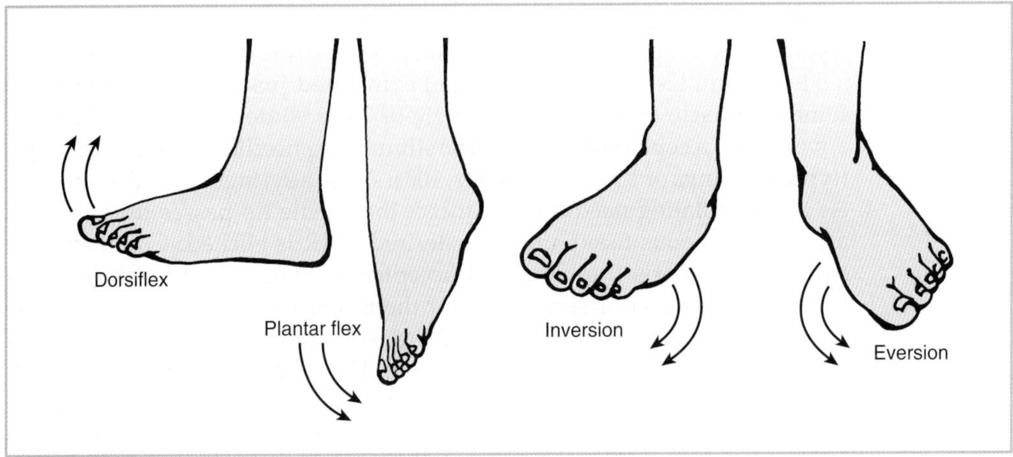

Figure 16.6. Foot movements with sciatic stimulation.

intraneuronal topography of the TN demonstrates that the nerve bundles innervating the tibialis posterior muscle are located within the lateral aspect of the TN **(16)**. Therefore inversion indicates that the needle is near the lateral portion of the portion of the TN, which lies in close proximity to the CPN.

The infragluteal-parabiceps approach will not block the PFCN. Therefore, operative procedures of the posterior thigh will require either a transgluteal or parasacral approach or separate block of the PFCN with a subcutaneous injection just below the gluteal crease.

E. **Sciatic nerve block, USG anterior approach.** The anterior approach to the sciatic nerve is an **advanced peripheral nerve block technique** when using a PNS. This is because the location of the sciatic nerve is **deep** (from the anterior approach), and the sciatic nerve is **often located directly posterior to the lesser trochanter** from the location of the initial needle insertion site with traditional PNS approaches. Multiple descriptions of the anterior approach have been described based on soft tissue (inguinal ligament or crease), vascular (femoral artery), and bony prominences (anterior superior iliac spine [ASIS], pubic tubercle, or pubic symphisis) landmarks. Because of the complexity of the landmarks and the location of the sciatic nerve posterior to the lesser trochanter, the optimal anterior approach is a **USG technique (17)**.

1. **Patient position.** The patient is **supine** with the hip and knee slightly flexed and the hip externally rotated at approximately 45 degrees.
2. **Probe selection.** A **mid to low frequency curved array transducer (2–5 MHz)** is typically used for this block. The lower frequency allows for a greater depth of penetration and the curved probe provides a wider field of view required to visualize the femur and the sciatic nerve.
3. **Probe placement and sonoanatomy.** The ultrasound probe is placed **8 cm distal to the inguinal crease on the anterior aspect of the thigh**. The probe is initially oriented at a 90-degree angle to the skin, with the long axis of the probe perpendicular to the long axis of the thigh (Figure 16.7).
   a. Typically, the depth of the sciatic nerve is **5 to 7 from the anterior surface** of the thigh depending on the body habitus of the patient.
   b. The penetration of the transducer should be adjusted to allow a **depth of field of 6 to 9 cm**. The gain and focal point are adjusted to optimize the appearance of the sciatic nerve and femur.
   c. The sciatic nerve often appears as a **hyperechoic, oval to elliptical structure** posterior and medial to the hyperechoic lesser trochanter. A systematic survey can optimize the appearance of the sciatic nerve. As the ultrasound probe is moved proximally and distally along the thigh, the lesser trochanter is identified as a segment that is wider than the femoral shaft. The sciatic nerve is located deep to the adductor magnus muscle and anterior to the gluteus maximus muscle (Figure 16.7B). The femoral vessels are located within the compartment of the quadriceps muscles anterior and well lateral to the femur. If the lesser trochanter obstructs the visualization of the sciatic nerve, the probe is slid further medially so that path of the ultrasound beam toward the sciatic nerve is no longer obstructed by the hyperechoic shadow cast by the lesser trochanter. Alternatively, the probe can be slid slightly caudal until the path of the ultrasound beam is caudal to the lesser trochanter.

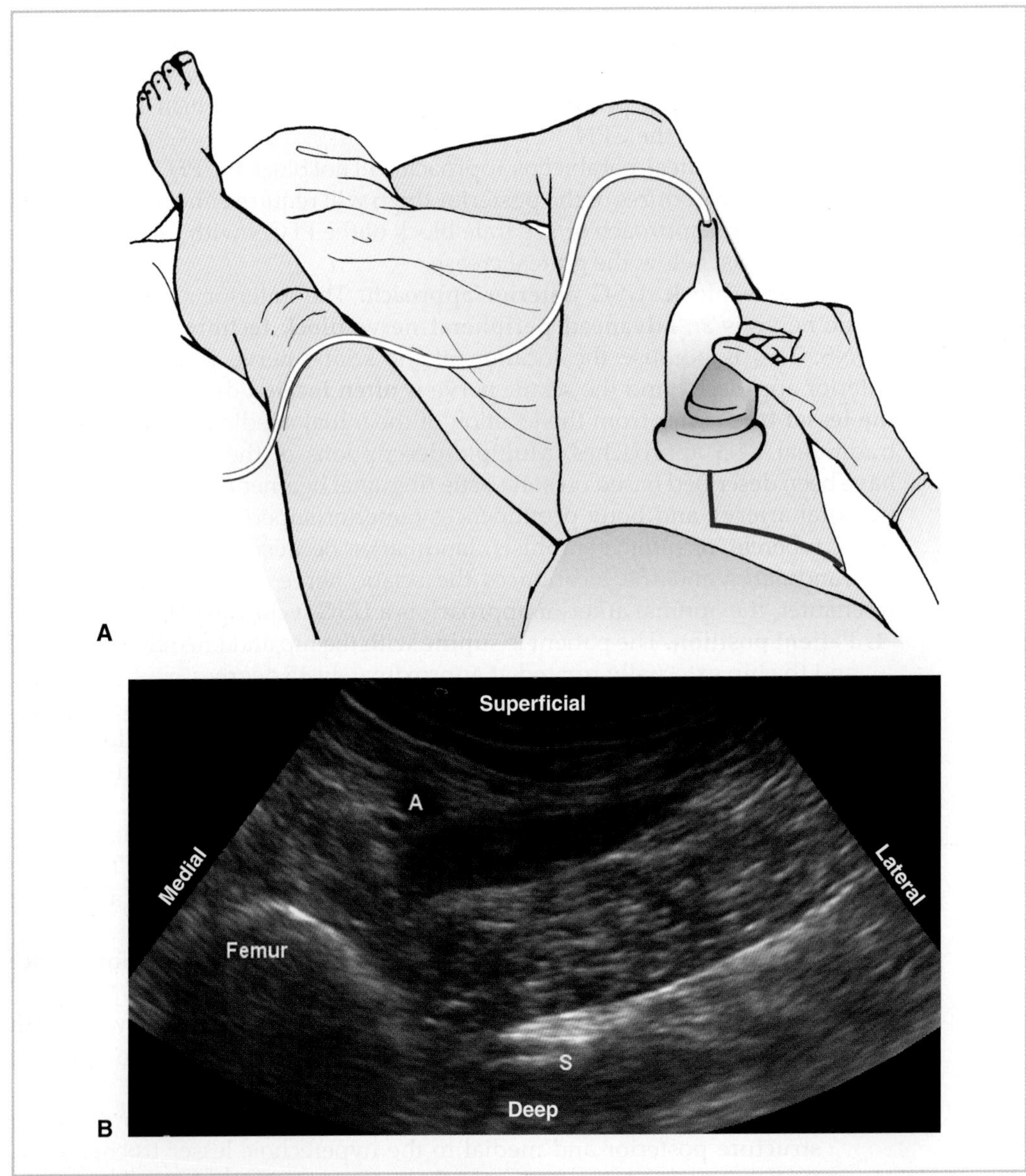

Figure 16.7. Anterior approach to the sciatic nerve. **A:** The patient is placed supine with the knee and hip flexed slightly to allow the leg to rotate 45 degrees externally. The curved array probe is placed on the skin perpendicular to the shaft of the femur at 8 cm distal to the inguinal crease. **B:** The femur appears as a semicircular hyperechoic shadow on the lateral side (*femur*), lying below and slightly lateral to the femoral artery (*A*). The sciatic nerve (*S*) appears as a hyperechoic bundle of fascicles deep and medial to the femur. Needle insertion should be from the more medial side of the thigh to avoid the artery and allow better visualization of the shaft as it is inserted in plane to the transducer.

4. **Needling technique**
   a. After aseptic skin preparation and draping followed by local anesthetic infiltration of the proposed needle insertion point, a stimulating needle (typically 100–150 mm [4–6 in.], 20–21 gauge) is attached to a PNS (typical settings of 1.5–2.0 mA, 2 Hz, 100 μs) and a syringe of local anesthetic.
   b. After placing the target neural structures in the **middle of the screen**, the stimulating needle is inserted just medial to the medial aspect of the ultrasound probe and advanced **in plane** (to the ultrasound beam) at an appropriate angle toward the sciatic nerve. The needle should be **advanced from an anterior-medial to posterior-lateral direction** toward the sciatic nerve. The needle will approach the sciatic nerve at a relatively steep angle. Therefore, the needle tip may at times be difficult to see as it approaches the sciatic nerve. Simply injecting a small amount (0.5–1.0 mL) of local anesthetic will result in the formation of a small hypoechoic collection that is easily visible thereby providing an indirect but useful assessment of needle tip location. Additionally, activating the PNS and eliciting the desired sciatic nerve EMR may also confirm the proximity of the needle tip to the sciatic nerve.
   c. The goal is to incrementally inject local anesthetic around the sciatic nerve represented as hypoechoic fluid collection encircling the nerve. Typically, a **volume of 15 to 25 mL** is required to obtain satisfactory local anesthetic distribution around the sciatic nerve. This may require withdrawing the needle after an initial local anesthetic injection followed by redirecting the needle tip and injection of the remaining local anesthetic volume to ensure uniform spread around the sciatic nerve.

F. **Popliteal fossa sciatic nerve block, posterior PNS approach.** The popliteal fossa is the **most widely chosen site** to block the sciatic nerve. At this location, the sciatic nerve is easily accessible at relatively shallower depths compared to the more proximal approaches. An additional advantage of sciatic nerve block at the popliteal fossa is the ability to provide near complete anesthesia (with the exception of the cutaneous contribution of the saphenous nerve) or **postoperative analgesia to the lower leg** without concomitant block of the hamstring or posterior adductor muscles in the thigh.

1. **Patient position.** The patient is placed **prone** with the feet hanging over the gurney to facilitate evaluation of EMR at the ankle or foot.
2. **External landmarks.** The landmarks include the popliteal crease and the **palpable tendons of the biceps femoris muscle (laterally) and tendons of the semimembranosus and semitendinosus (medially).** Palpation of the tendons can be accentuated simply by asking the patient to **flex the leg** at the knee to contract the hamstring muscles (18). The proposed needle **insertion site is 7 to 8 cm above the popliteal crease** at the midpoint between the tendons. At this point above the popliteal crease, the TN and CPN have not yet separated in most patients (3,4).
3. After aseptic skin preparation and draping followed by local anesthetic infiltration of the proposed needle insertion point, a stimulating needle (typically 50 mm [2 in.], 22 gauge) is inserted at the proposed needle insertion site. The stimulating needle is attached to a PNS (typical settings of 1.5–2.0 mA, 2 Hz, 100 μs) and a syringe of local anesthetic.

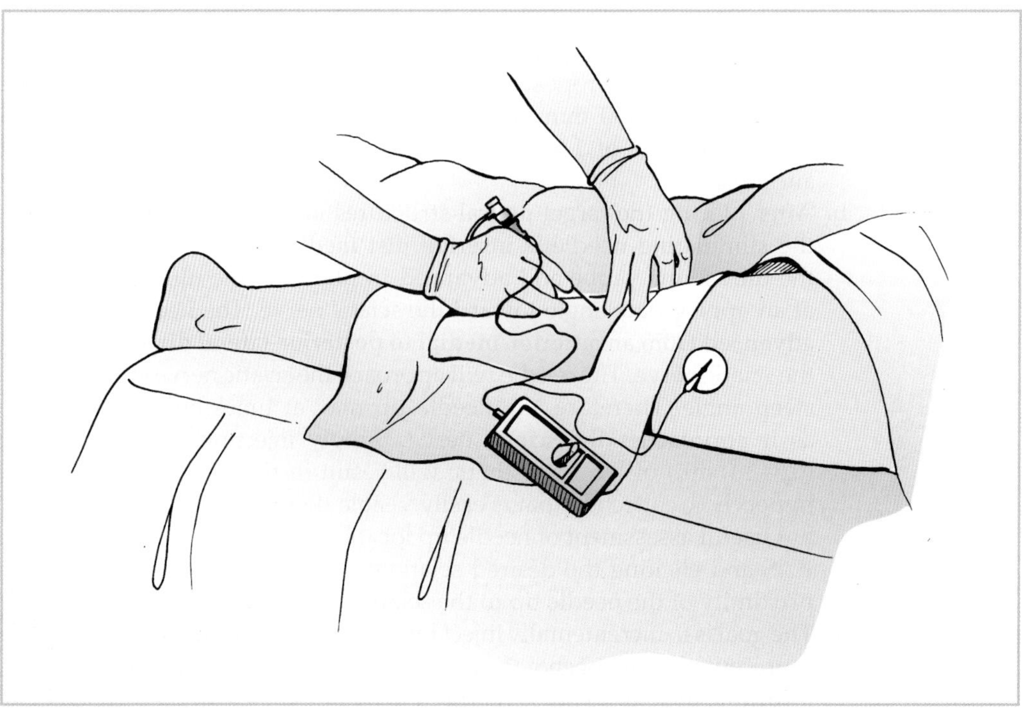

Figure 16.8. Popliteal fossa block, posterior nerve stimulator approach. The needle is inserted and angled 45 degrees cephalad. The nerves will usually be contacted halfway between the skin and the femur.

4. The stimulating needle is advanced with a **slight cephalad angulation** until the desired EMR is elicited (Figure 16.8). The desired EMR is **inversion or plantar flexion** of the foot (see section IV, D, 7). If plantarflexion is elicited, the needle tip is redirected slightly lateral to obtain inversion. Alternatively, if dorsiflexion is obtained, the needle tip should be redirected slightly medial to elicit inversion. The final position of the needle tip is considered optimal when the desired EMR is still elicited at 0.2 to 0.5 mA. If the needle tip is below the bifurcation of the sciatic nerve, inversion may be difficult to elicit. An acceptable approach is to perform a "*double-stimulation*" technique by injection of the half of the total local anesthetic volume after eliciting either a TN or CPN response (19). This is followed by the appropriate redirection (slightly lateral after a TN response or slightly medial after a CPN response) of the needle tip to stimulate the other branch of the sciatic nerve and injection of the remaining volume.
5. After the final needle position(s) is (are) obtained and an initial 3-mL test dose to confirm the absence of intravascular location of the local anesthetic injection, a total of 40 mL (20 mL at each branch of the sciatic nerve if a double-stimulation technique is utilized) of local anesthetic is incrementally injected with frequent intermittent aspirations to reduce the risk of intravascular injection. Typical onset time for sensory and motor anesthesia is 10 to 25 minutes depending on the total mass of local anesthetic injected and the EMR elicited.
6. A **continuous catheter technique** may be utilized to provide extended duration analgesia. The initial needle insertion site and approach are the

same as the single-injection technique. A larger bore (17- to 18-gauge) insulated stimulating Tuohy needle is typically used to localize the sciatic. After localization of the sciatic nerve and injection of the local anesthetic, the needle is **angulated further cephalad** to facilitate catheter passage. A 19- to 20-gauge catheter is inserted through the Tuohy needle and advanced no more than 3 to 5 cm past needle tip. The needle is then withdrawn over the catheter and the latter fixed in place with a sterile clear adhesive dressing. The proximal end of the catheter is then connected to an automated infusion pump.

G. Popliteal fossa, USG prone lateral approach

1. **Patient position.** The patient is placed **prone.**
2. **Probe selection.** A **high frequency (8–12 MHz) linear array transducer** is typically used for this block. The higher frequency allows for a greater resolution penetration as the sciatic nerve is typically located at depth of **2 to 4 cm from the skin surface**.
3. **Probe placement and sonoanatomy.** The **long axis of the ultrasound probe is parallel to the popliteal crease** and slowly moved cephalad (20) (Figure 16.9A).
   a. At this level, the **popliteal artery** is seen as a round, pulsatile hypoechoic structure in the middle of the screen located superficial to the distal femur. The popliteal vein is typically slightly superficial and lateral to the popliteal artery and may not be seen as the pressure of the ultrasound probe easily compresses it (20).
   b. The probe is slowly advanced cephalad observing for the appearance of the TN branch of the sciatic nerve. The **TN should be seen as a hyperechoic structure that is always superficial and lateral to the popliteal artery**. The ultrasound probe is slowly advanced further cephalad until the **CPN becomes visible just medial to the biceps femoris muscle and lateral to the TN**. At this point, the ultrasound probe is advanced further cephalad until the **TN and CPN come together to form the sciatic nerve**, and the location of the probe on the posterior thigh is marked. Note the location of the sciatic nerve in between the convergence of the lateral (biceps femoris) and medial (semimembranosus and semitendinosus) hamstring muscles corresponding to the apex of the popliteal fossa.
4. **Needling technique**
   a. After aseptic skin preparation and draping followed by local anesthetic skin infiltration of the proposed needle insertion site, a 50-mm (2-in.) 21-gauge stimulating needle is attached to a PNS (typical settings of 1.5–2.0 mA, 2 Hz, 100 μs) and a syringe of local anesthetic.
   b. After placing the target neural structures in the middle of the screen, the stimulating needle is placed lateral to the lateral aspect of the ultrasound probe. Insertion of the needle between the tendons of the vastus lateralis and the biceps femoris muscles allows a flatter angle of approach to the sciatic nerve allowing improved visualization of the needle. The needle is advanced in plane (to the ultrasound beam) and the needle tip will approach the sciatic nerve from a lateral to a medial direction. As the needle approaches the sciatic nerve, a visible and palpable "pop" is observed as the needle tip penetrates a fascial plane located just superficial to the sciatic nerve.

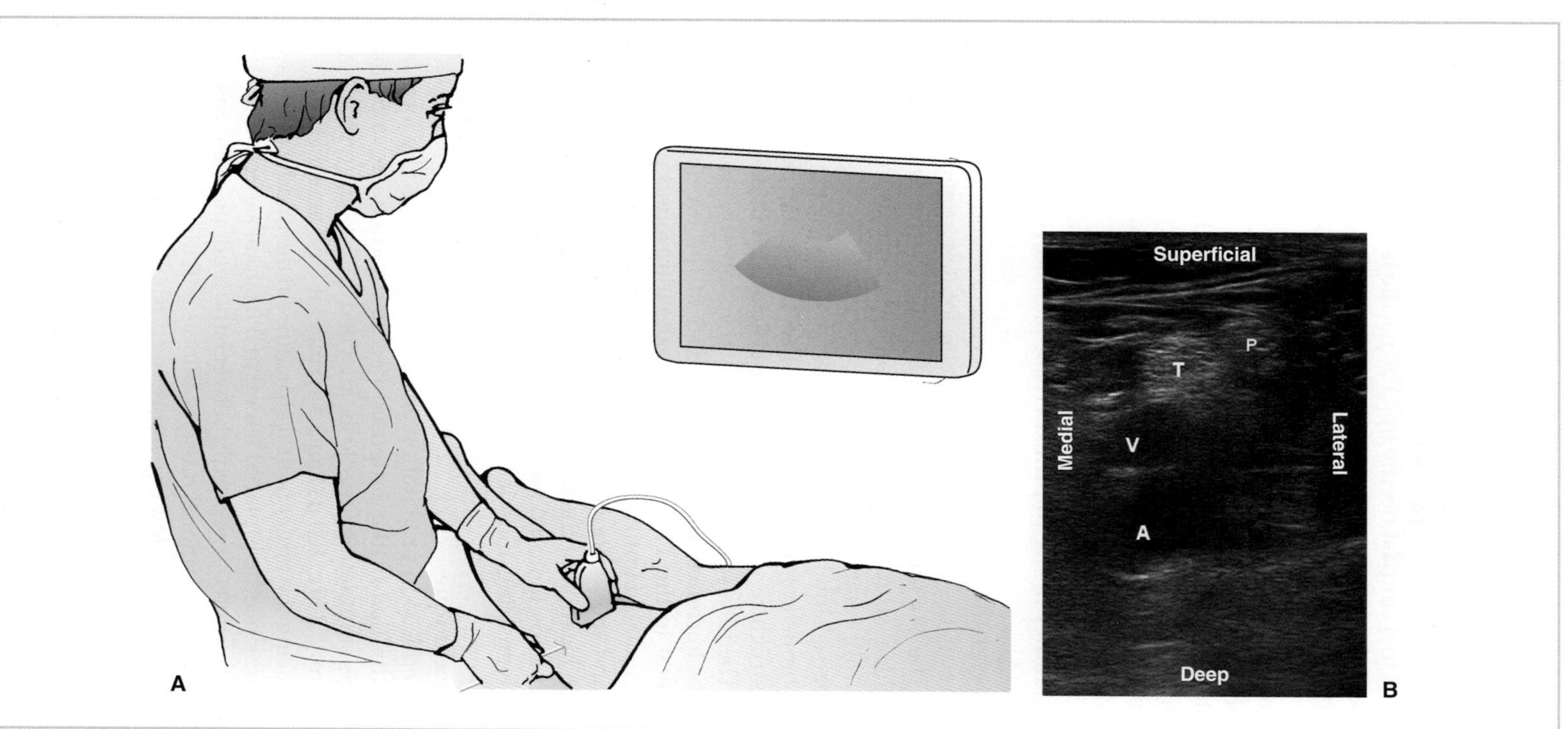

Figure 16.9. Ultrasound block at popliteal fossa, posterior approach. **A:** The patient is positioned prone with a pillow under the ankles to provide some flexion of the knee. The linear array probe is placed at the popliteal crease to locate the popliteal artery. **B:** Tracing the artery cephalad will allow visualization of the tibial (*T*) and peroneal (*P*) nerves, usually lying superficial and lateral to the artery (*A*) and vein (*V*). The nerves will merge into a single sciatic trunk at a variable distance above the crease.

c. The initial target site for the needle tip is lateral to the sciatic nerve. At this point, local anesthetic is injected while observing for the desired local anesthetic distribution as evidenced by a hypoechoic fluid collection around the hyperechoic sciatic nerve. Typically, a volume of 25–40 mL is required to achieve the desired local anesthetic distribution if the needle is not moved. Alternatively, the needle tip may be repositioned superficial, deep, and medial to the sciatic nerve with fractional injection of the total local anesthetic volume in real time to achieve a uniform distribution of local anesthetic around the short axis of the sciatic nerve (*"donut sign"*).

5. If a **continuous catheter technique** is indicated, a larger bore (17- to 18-gauge) insulated stimulating Tuohy needle is typically used for initial placement of the needle tip and local anesthetic around the sciatic nerve. After local anesthetic distribution (by injection through the needle tip) is ensured the ultrasound probe is placed aside within the sterile field. A 19- to 20-gauge catheter is inserted through the Tuohy needle and advanced **no more than 3 to 5 cm** past needle tip. At this point, the ultrasound probe is placed over the original site, and an additional 3 to 5 mL of local anesthetic is injected through the catheter while observing for local anesthetic distribution around the sciatic nerve to ensure correct catheter tip position. The needle is then withdrawn over the catheter and the latter fixed in place with a sterile clear adhesive dressing. The proximal end of the catheter is then connected to an automated infusion pump.

H. **Popliteal fossa sciatic nerve block, nerve stimulator lateral approach** The main disadvantage of the posterior approach to the sciatic nerve block in the popliteal fossa is the need to position the patient prone in order to perform the block. This may preclude certain patients (morbid obesity, painful fractures with cast or fixation devices, or unstable spines) who may otherwise benefit from a sciatic nerve block.

1. **Patient position.** The patient is **supine** and the foot on the side to be blocked should be positioned so that EMR of the sciatic nerve can be easily observed. This is best achieved by **placing the lower leg on a soft bump so that the foot (including the Achilles tendon) extends beyond the bump** (Figure 16.10).
2. **External landmarks.** The landmarks are the **popliteal crease,** the **vastus lateralis muscle, and the biceps femoris muscle.** Palpation of the popliteal crease and the groove between the muscles can be accentuated simply by asking the patient to **flex the leg at the knee** to contract the hamstring muscles. The proposed needle **insertion site is 7 to 8 cm cephalad to the popliteal crease** in the groove between the vastus lateralis and biceps femoris muscles. At this point above the popliteal crease, the TN and CPN have not yet separated in most patients (3,4).
3. After aseptic skin preparation and draping followed by local anesthetic infiltration of the proposed needle insertion point, a stimulating needle (typically 100 mm [4 in.], 21 gauge) is inserted at the proposed needle insertion site. The stimulating needle is attached to a PNS (typical settings of 1.5–2.0 mA, 2 Hz, 100 μs) and a syringe of local anesthetic.
4. The stimulating needle is inserted in a **horizontal plane** between the vastus lateralis muscle and biceps femoris muscles and advanced to gently contact the lateral aspect of the femur. **Contact with the femur** is a key element as it

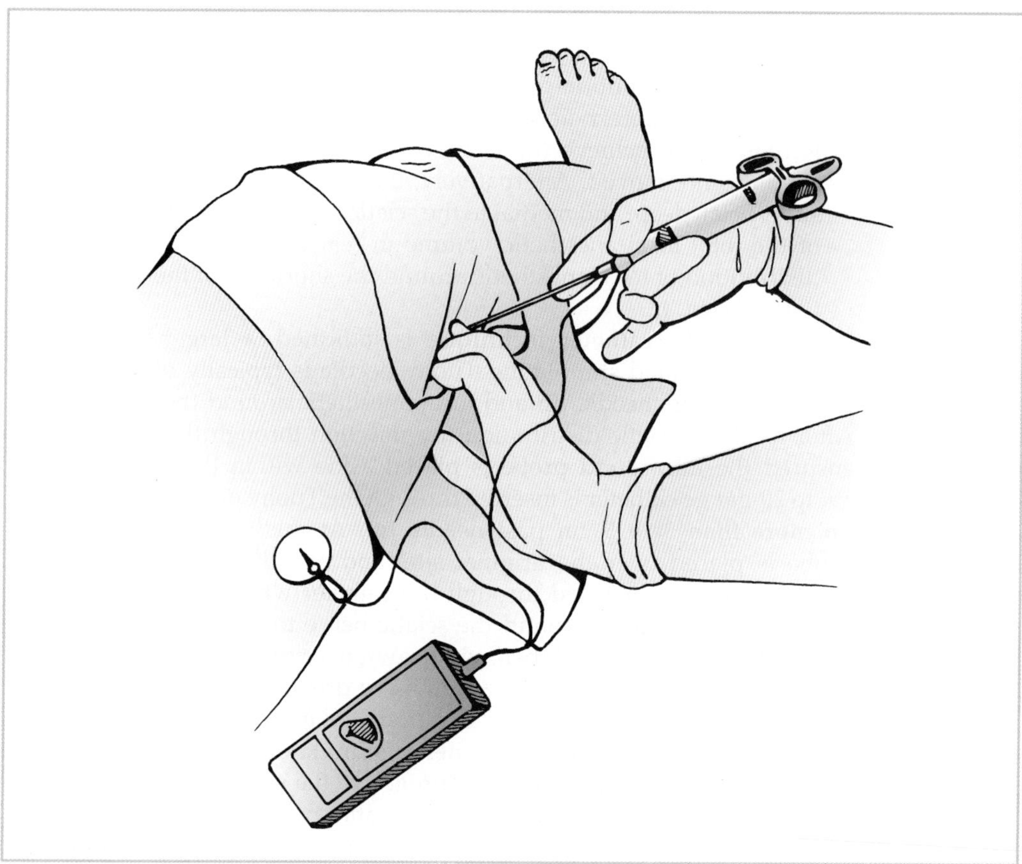

Figure 16.10. Popliteal fossa, lateral nerve stimulator approach, patient position.

provides an estimate of the depth of the sciatic nerve from the lateral thigh (typically 1–2 cm beyond the skin-femur distance), as well as the baseline from which the **needle needs to be redirected posterior** to reach the sciatic nerve (Figure 16.11). After contact with the femur, the needle is withdrawn to just below the skin and redirected **30 degrees posterior** to the angle at which the needle initially contacted the femur. The needle is then slowly advanced until a desired EMR is elicited. Typically, a CPN EMR is obtained first as this nerve is positioned lateral and more superficial than the TN (Figure 16.11). **If the EMR is dorsiflexion**, it is recommended that the tip of the stimulating needle be slightly **readjusted further medial** in order to obtain either inversion or plantar flexion in order to increase the success rate of complete block of the sciatic nerve (21). An alternative approach is to perform a "*double-stimulation*" technique by injection of half of the total local anesthetic volume after first eliciting a CPN EMR, followed by redirection of the needle tip slightly more medial to obtain a TN EMR and injection of the remaining volume of local anesthetic (22). If the initial pass of the stimulating needle does not elicit the desired EMR, the stimulating needle is withdrawn to just below the skin and the needle angle is redirected 5 to 10 degrees further posterior and advanced until the desired sciatic nerve EMR is elicited. This maneuver is repeated with systematic 5- to 10-degree

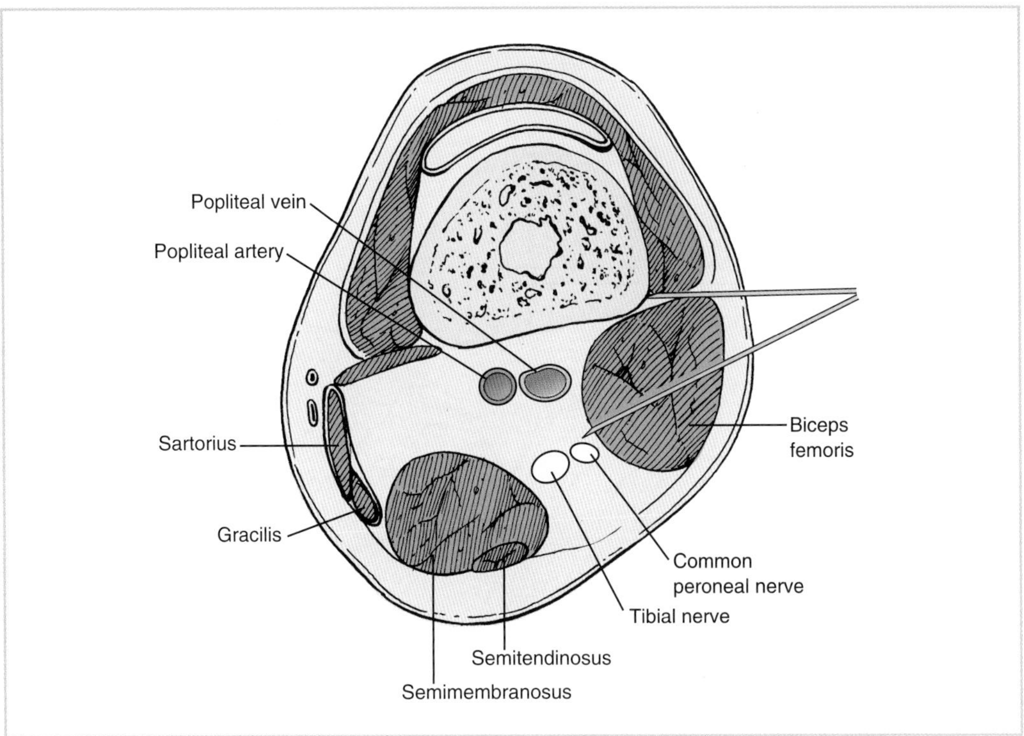

Figure 16.11. Popliteal fossa, nerve anatomy of lateral approach.

further posterior angulation until the needle angle is 60 degrees posterior from the original approach.

5. After the final needle position(s) is (are) obtained and an initial 3-mL test dose to confirm the absence of intravascular location of the local anesthetic injection, **a total of 40 mL** (20 mL at each branch of the sciatic nerve if a double-stimulation technique is utilized) of local anesthetic is incrementally injected with frequent intermittent aspirations to reduce the risk of intravascular injection. Typical onset time for sensory and motor anesthesia is 10 to 25 minutes depending on the total mass of local anesthetic injected, the type and number of EMR elicited.
6. A **continuous catheter technique** may be utilized to provide extended duration analgesia. The initial needle insertion site and approach are the same as the single-injection technique. A larger bore (17- to 18-gauge) insulated stimulating Tuohy needle is typically used to localize the sciatic nerve. After localization of the sciatic nerve and injection of the local anesthetic, the needle is angulated further cephalad to facilitate catheter passage. A 19- to 20-gauge catheter is inserted through the Tuohy needle and advanced no more than 2 to 3 past the needle tip. The needle is then withdrawn over the catheter and the latter fixed in place with a sterile clear adhesive dressing. The proximal end of the catheter is then connected to an automated infusion pump.

I. Popliteal fossa, USG supine lateral approach. The USG technique to the lateral approach offers several advantages compared to the PNS technique. First, the cephalad distance from the popliteal crease where the TN and CPN

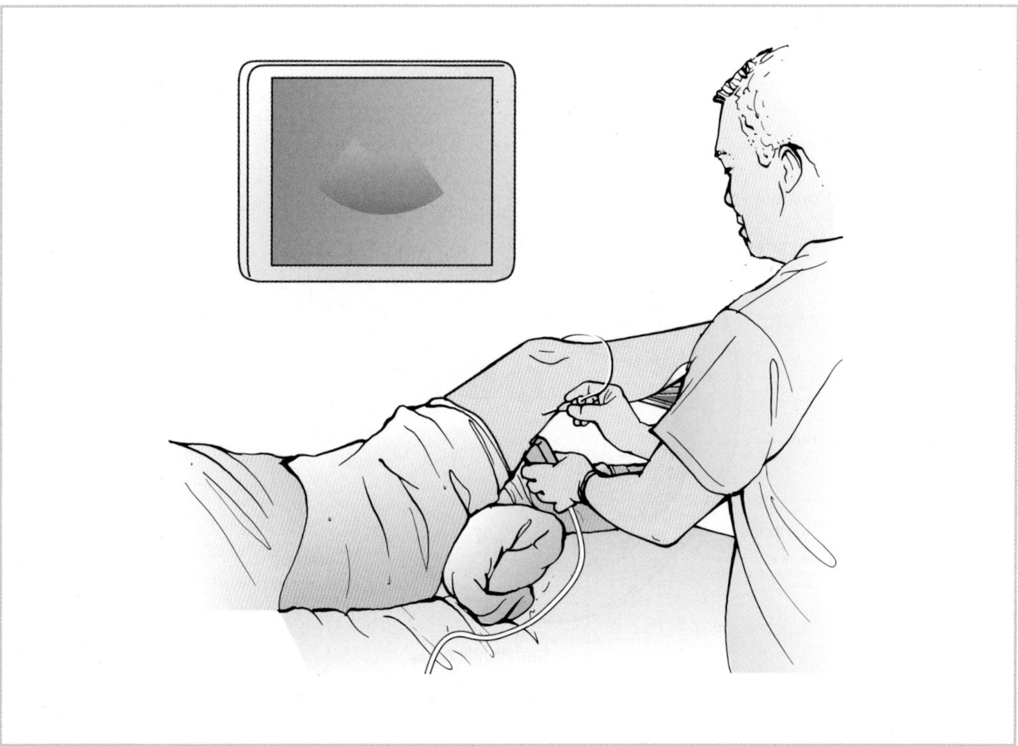

Figure 16.12. Ultrasound-guided sciatic popliteal fossa block, supine-lateral approach. The patient is positioned supine with the lower leg elevated on a Mayo stand to allow the US probe to be placed under the thigh in the popliteal fossa. At the level where the TN and CPN come together as the SN, the needle is introduced from the lateral side between the muscle bodies of the vastus lateralis and biceps femoris and advanced in plane to approach the SN.

come together to form the sciatic nerve can be seen precisely measured. Second, femur contact is avoided as the depth from the skin to the sciatic can be precisely measured. Third, the angle of approach to the sciatic nerve can be adjusted in real time. Therefore, by minimizing the number of needle redirections needed to reach the sciatic nerve, patient comfort is enhanced and time required to perform the block is minimized. Lastly, the needle tip may be adjusted in real time followed by incremental injections of local anesthetic to ensure uniform distribution of local anesthetic around the short axis of the sciatic nerve.

1. **Patient position.** The patient is **supine** and the **leg to be blocked is elevated off the gurney so that an ultrasound probe may be placed in between the posterior popliteal fossa and the surface of the gurney** (Figure 16.12).
2. **Probe selection.** A **high frequency (8–12 MHz) linear array transducer** is typically used for this block. The higher frequency allows for greater resolution, as the sciatic nerve is typically located at a depth of 2 to 4 cm from the skin surface.
3. **Probe placement and sonoanatomy.** The long axis of the ultrasound probe is parallel to the popliteal crease and slowly moved cephalad. The anesthesiologist will need to maintain constant upward pressure on the ultrasound probe to maintain contact with the skin. A simple but important difference

between the USG supine and prone approach is the orientation of the anatomic structures on the screen. Because the transducer probe (and ultrasound beam) is approaching the sciatic nerve from below (in contrast to the approaching the nerve from above with the prone approach), the orientation of the structures appear "inverted" on the screen. This must be appreciated when making needle redirections to reach the sciatic nerve. Alternatively, most ultrasound machines have a control setting to simply invert the screen, so the anesthesiologist can obtain the more familiar "popliteal prone lateral" orientation.

a. At this level, the popliteal **artery is seen as a round, pulsatile hypoechoic** structure in the middle of the screen located superficial to the distal femur. The popliteal vein is typically slightly superficial and lateral to the popliteal artery and may not be seen as the pressure of the ultrasound probe easily compresses it (20).
b. The probe is slowly advanced cephalad observing for the appearance of the TN branch of the sciatic nerve. The **TN should be seen as a hyperechoic structure** that is always **superficial and lateral to the popliteal artery**. The ultrasound probe is slowly advanced further cephalad until the **CPN becomes visible just medial to the biceps femoris muscle and lateral to the TN** (Figure 16.13). At this point, the ultrasound probe is advanced further cephalad until the TN and CPN come together to form the sciatic nerve, and the location of the probe on the posterior thigh is marked. Note the location of the sciatic nerve in between the convergence of the lateral (biceps femoris) and medial (semimembranosus and

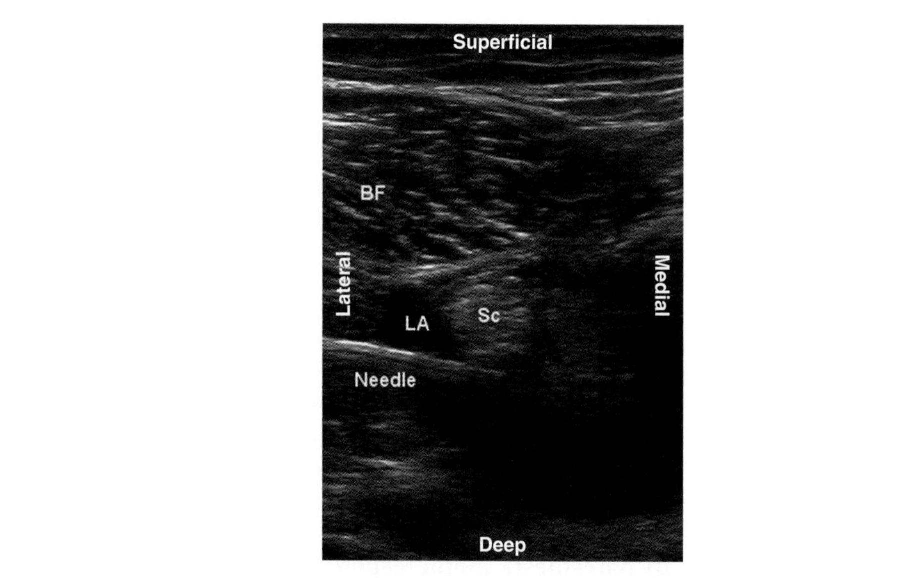

Figure 16.13. Lateral popliteal fossa block with ultrasonography. The needle is advanced under the biceps femoris (*BF*) in plane to approach the nerves (*Sc*), and local anesthetic (*LA*) injected to surround the nerve trunk. Injection in several locations (above and below the nerve) provides the best circumferential coverage.

semitendinosus) hamstring muscles corresponding to the apex of the popliteal fossa.

4. **Needling technique**
   a. After aseptic skin preparation and draping followed by local anesthetic skin infiltration of the proposed needle insertion site, a 50- to 100-mm (2–4 in.), 21- to 22-gauge stimulating needle is attached to a PNS (typical settings of 1.5–2.0 mA, 2 Hz, 100 μs) and a syringe of local anesthetic.
   b. The ultrasound **probe is held against the posterior thigh** with slight upward pressure to maintain contact with the skin of the popliteal fossa and its location is then maintained.
   c. After placing the **target neural structures in the middle of the screen,** the stimulating **needle is inserted in the groove between the vastus lateralis and biceps femoris muscles** parallel to the midpoint of the long axis of the ultrasound probe. The needle is advanced in plane (to the ultrasound beam) at an appropriate angle toward the sciatic nerve (Figure 16.13). The needle tip will approach the sciatic nerve from a lateral to medial direction. As the needle approaches the sciatic nerve, a visible and palpable "pop" occurs as the needle tip penetrates a fascial plane located just superficial to the sciatic nerve.
   d. The **initial target site for needle tip is lateral to the sciatic nerve**. At this point, local anesthetic is slowly injected while observing for the desired local anesthetic distribution as evidenced by the appearance of a **hypoechoic fluid collection around the hyperechoic sciatic nerve.** Typically a **volume of 25 to 40 mL** is required to achieve the desired local anesthetic distribution if the needle is not moved. Alternatively, the needle tip may be repositioned above, below, and medial to the sciatic nerve followed by fractioned injection of the total local anesthetic volume in real time to achieve a uniform distribution of local anesthetic around the short axis of the sciatic nerve (the "donut sign").
5. If **a continuous catheter technique** is indicated, a larger bore (17- to 18-gauge) insulated stimulating Tuohy needle is typically used for initial placement of the needle tip and local anesthetic around the sciatic nerve. After local anesthetic distribution (by injection through the needle tip) is ensured, the ultrasound probe is placed aside within the sterile field. A 19- to 20-gauge catheter is inserted through the Tuohy needle and advanced no more than 3 to 5 cm past the needle tip. At this point, the ultrasound probe is placed over the original site, and an additional 3 to 5 mL of local anesthetic is injected through the catheter while observing for local anesthetic distribution around the sciatic nerve to ensure correct catheter tip position. The needle is then withdrawn over the catheter and the latter fixed in place with a sterile clear adhesive dressing. The proximal end of the catheter is then connected to an automated infusion pump.

j. **Ankle block.** The ankle block technique involves **more injections** and therefore may be more **time consuming,** but it **can be performed without seeking specific nerve localization by paresthesia, motor response, or ultrasonography**. A ring of anesthesia is produced that blocks all **five branches** of the foot (Figure 16.14). Alternatively, for distal operations, local blockade of terminal branches can be performed.

1. **Posterior TN.** This can be performed with the patient in the **prone or supine** position. If the patient is supine, the knee is flexed to bring the

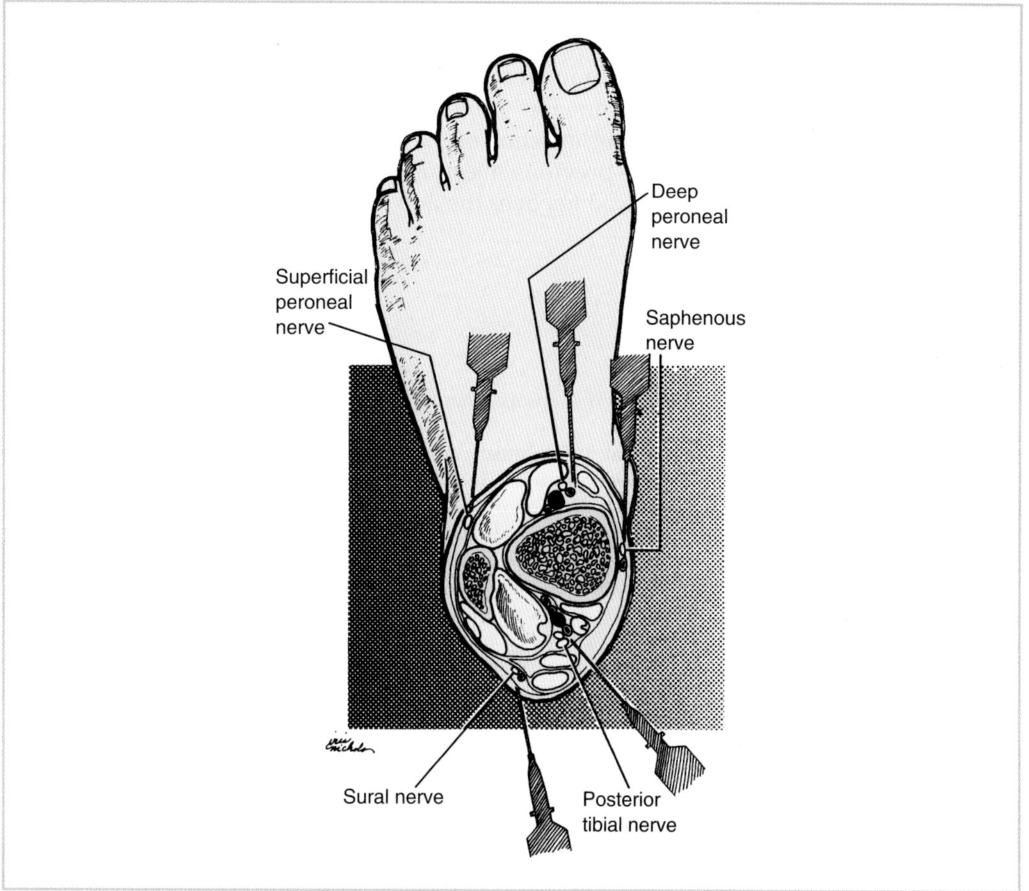

Figure 16.14. Ankle block. Injections are made at five separate nerve locations. The superficial peroneal nerve, the sural nerve, and the saphenous nerve are usually blocked simply by subcutaneous infiltration because they may have already generated many superficial branches as they cross the ankle joint. Paresthesias can be sought in the posterior tibial nerve or the deep peroneal, but the bony landmarks will usually suffice to provide adequate localization for the deeper injections.

sole of the foot flat on the bed surface. A 1.5-in. 23- to 25-gauge needle is introduced at the level of the medial malleolus just behind the **posterior tibial artery** pulsation and is directed **45 degrees anteriorly** to seek a paresthesia in the sole of the foot. Then 5 mL of anesthetic will be sufficient if the nerve is located. If the nerve is not located, 10 mL can be injected in a fan-shaped area in the triangle formed by the tibia, the artery, and the Achilles tendon.

2. **Sural nerve.** With the patient still either prone or supine with the knee flexed, 5 mL more is injected **superficially behind the lateral malleolus** to fill the groove between the malleolus and the calcaneous.
3. **Saphenous nerve.** Next, 5 mL is injected around the saphenous vein at the **level of the medial malleolus between the skin and the bone itself.**
4. **Deep peroneal nerve.** Moving to the front of the ankle, a needle is inserted into the deep planes below the fascia **just lateral to the anterior tibial artery at the level of the skin creases** and 5 mL more is injected. If the artery is

not palpable, the tendon of the extensor hallicus longus can be used as a landmark.

5. **Superficial peroneal branches.** A **subcutaneous ridge of anesthetic** solution is laid down from the anterior tibia around the lateral malleolus (overlying the previous injection of the deep peroneal nerve and continuing laterally to meet the previous injection for the sural nerve). A total of 5 to 10 mL may be required to cover the 2 to 3 in. necessary to catch all of these superficial fibers.

REFERENCES

1 Birnbaum K, Prescher A, Hebler S, et al. The sensory innervation of the hip joint: an anatomical study. *Surg Radiol Anat* 1997;19:371–375.

2 **Sukhani R, Candido KD, Doty R, et al. Infragluteal-parabiceps sciatic nerve block: an evaluation of a novel approach using a single-injection technique. *Anesth Analg* 2003;96:868–873.**

3 **Vloka JD, Hadzic A, April E, et al. The division of the sciatic nerve in the popliteal fossa: anatomical implications for popliteal nerve block. *Anesth Analg* 2001;92:215–217.**

4 Schwemmer U, Markus CK, Greim CA, et al. Sonographic imaging of the sciatic nerve division in the popliteal fossa. *Ultraschall Med* 2005;26:496–500.

5 Taboada Muniz M, Alvarez J, Cortes J, et al. The effects of three different approaches on the onset time of sciatic nerve block with ropivacaine 0.75%. *Anesth Analg* 2004;98:242–247.

6 Taboada Muniz M, Rodriguez J, Valino C, et al. What is the minimum effective volume of local anesthetic required for sciatic nerve block? A prospective randomized comparison between a popliteal and subgluteal approach. *Anesth Analg* 2006;102:593–597.

7 Cappelleri G, Aldegheri G, Ruggieri F, et al. Minimum effective anesthetic concentration (MEAC) for sciatic nerve block: subgluteal and popliteal approaches. *Can J Anaesth* 2007;54:283–289.

8 **Mansour NY. Reevaluating the sciatic nerve block: another landmark for consideration. *Reg Anesth* 1993;18:322–323.**

9 Morris GF, Lang SA, Dust WN, et al. The parasacral sciatic nerve block. *Reg Anesth* 1997;22:223–228.

10 Ho AM, Karmakar MJ. Combined paravertebral lumbar plexus block and parasacral sciatic nerve block for reduction of hip fracture in a patient with aortic stenosis. *Can J Anaesth* 2002;49:946–950.

11 De Visme V, Picart F, LeJouan R, et al. Combined lumbar and sacral plexus block compared with plain bupivacaine spinal anesthesia for hip fractures in the elderly. *Reg Anesth Pain Med* 2000;25:158–162.

12 Ripart J, Cuvillon P, Nouvellon E, et al. Parasacral approach to block the sciatic nerve; a 44-case survey. *Reg Anesth Pain Med* 2005;32:193–197.

13 Hagon BS, Itani O, Bidgoli JH, et al. Parasacral sciatic nerve block: does the elicited motor response predict success rate? *Anesth Analg* 2007;105:263–266.

14 Cuvillon P, Ripart J, Jeannes P, et al. Comparison of the parasacral approach and the posterior approach with the single- and double-injection techniques to block the sciatic nerve. *Anesthesiology* 2003;98:1436–1441.

15 **Karmakar MK, Kwok WH, Ho AM, et al. Ultrasound-guided sciatic nerve block: description of a new approach at the subgluteal level. *Br J Anaesth* 2007;98:390–395.**

16 **Sukhani R, Nader A, Candido KD, et al. Nerve stimulator-assisted evoked motor responses predict the latency and success of a single-injection sciatic nerve block. *Anesth Analg* 2004;99:584–588.**

17 **Chan VW, Nova H, Abbas S, et al. Ultrasound examination and localization of the sciatic nerve: a volunteer study. *Anesthesiology* 2006;104:309–314.**

18 Hadzic A, Vloka VD, Singson R, et al. A comparison of intertendinous and classical approaches to popliteal nerve block using magnetic resonance imaging simulation. *Anesth Analg* 2002;94:1321–1324.

19 Risch M, Blumenthal S, Borgeat A. Is the double-injection technique really needed? *Anesth Analg* 2007;105:285–286.

20 Tsui BC, Finucane BT. The importance of ultrasound landmarks: a "traceback" approach using the popliteal blood vessels for identification of the sciatic nerve. *Reg Anesth Pain* 2006;31:481–482.

21 Taboada Muniz M, Alvarez J, Cortes J, et al. Lateral approach to the sciatic nerve block in the popliteal fossa: correlation between evoked motor response and sensory block. *Reg Anesth Pain Med* 2003;28:450–455.

22 Paqueron X, Bouaziz H, Macalou D, et al. The lateral approach to the sciatic nerve block at the popliteal fossa: one or two injections? *Anesth Analg* 1999;89:1221–1225.

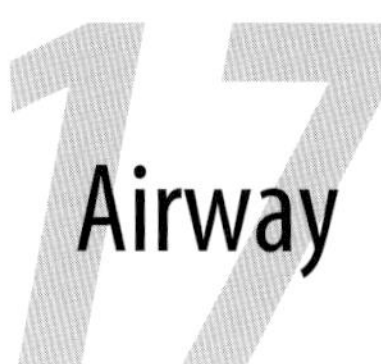

Airway

Michael F. Mulroy

Anesthesiologists frequently intubate patients for whom the routine general anesthetic induction technique is not appropriate. Adequate regional or topical anesthesia of the nasal and pharyngeal airway makes the painless passage of nasal or oral endotracheal tubes or fiberoptic bronchoscopes possible in these patients.

I. Anatomy

A. **Sensory** fibers of the **nasal mucosa** arise from the middle division of the fifth cranial nerve by means of the sphenopalatine ganglion. This major branch lies under the nasal mucosa posterior to the middle turbinate (Figure 17.1). Fibers from this ganglion also provide sensory innervation for the superior portion of the pharynx, uvula, and tonsils. These fibers can be blocked proximally by direct injection of the maxillary branch of the trigeminal nerve, but they are more easily approached by transmucosal topical application of local anesthetic.

B. The **ninth cranial nerve** (glossopharyngeal) provides the sensory innervation of the oral pharynx and supraglottic regions, as well as the posterior portion of the tongue. This nerve can be blocked by direct submucosal injection behind the tonsillar pillar, but it is more easily approached by topical anesthesia of its terminal branches in the mouth and throat.

C. Sensation in the **larynx** itself above the vocal cords is provided by the **superior laryngeal** branch of the vagus. This nerve departs the main vagal trunk in the carotid sheath and courses anteriorly, sending an internal branch that penetrates the thyrohyoid membrane. Behind this membrane, the nerve branches to provide sensory innervation to the cords, epiglottis, and arytenoids.

D. Below the vocal cords, sensory innervation is provided by branches of the **recurrent laryngeal** nerve, which also provides motor fibers to all but one of the intrinsic laryngeal muscles. Sensation in the trachea itself is also a function of the recurrent laryngeal nerve. Although direct blockade of this nerve is possible (and is seen as a side effect of several other regional block techniques in the neck), topical anesthesia is again the simplest approach.

II. Indications

A. In the presence of **facial trauma** or distortion of the upper airway by **abscess** or **malignancy**, it is safer to perform tracheal intubation with the patient awake or lightly sedated. This is also appropriate in the presence of a history of **previously difficult intubation**, cervical radiculopathy, severe respiratory distress, and possibly morbid obesity. Although new techniques such as the intubating laryngeal mask airway (LMA) have reduced the frequency of difficult intubations, familiarity with these techniques is suggested by the American Society of Anesthesiologists (ASA) guidelines for airway management (1,2).

B. Nasal mucosal anesthesia is useful if a **nasal tube** is passed, and is particularly helpful if a vasoconstrictor is used to reduce the chance of mucosal bleeding. Anesthesia of the mouth and oral pharynx will allow introduction of both the **laryngoscope** and the tube down to the level of the epiglottis, and is also

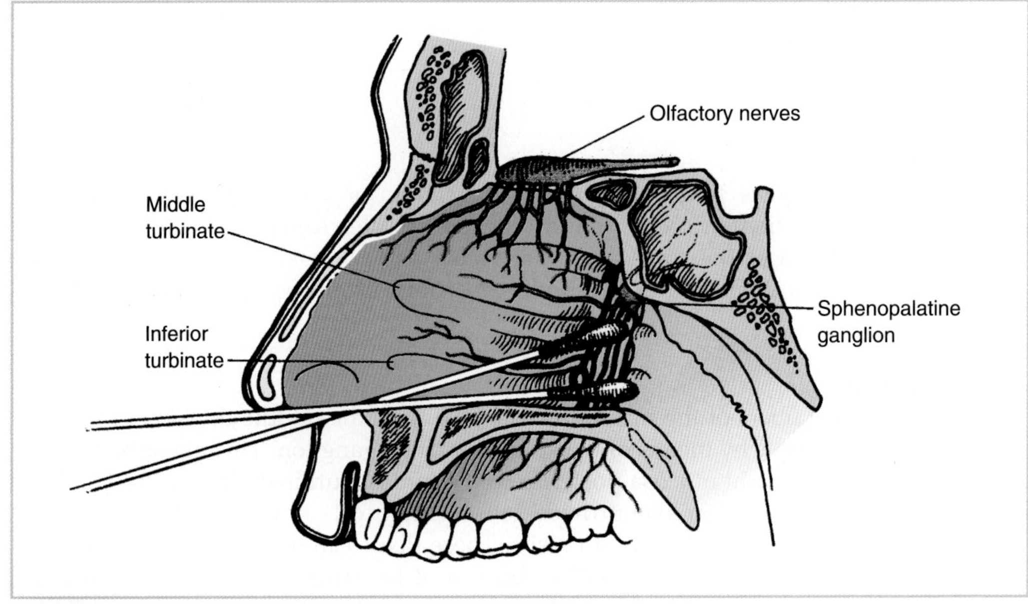

Figure 17.1. Nasal airway anesthesia. Cotton pledgets soaked with anesthetic are inserted along the inferior and middle turbinates to produce anesthesia of the underlying sphenopalatine ganglion by transmembrane diffusion of the solution. Wide pledgets are needed to provide maximal topical anesthesia and vasoconstriction of the nasal mucosa as well.

helpful when **transesophageal echocardiography** is performed on a patient who is awake. Anesthesia of the larynx and trachea themselves (by blockade of the branches of the vagus nerve or by transtracheal injection) allows the patient to tolerate insertion of the tube or **fiberoptic scope** below the cords without coughing or bucking (3), and will reduce the significant cardiovascular responses usually associated with tracheal intubation. Blockade of laryngeal sensation may be contraindicated, however, if there is concern about vomiting and aspiration.

C. Tracheal anesthesia is also unwise if preservation of **active cough reflexes** is desired.

D. Airway anesthesia is also useful in facilitating diagnostic **fiberoptic laryngoscopy**, and may help **agitated intubated patients** in intensive care units tolerate the presence of an endotracheal tube.

III. Drugs

A. Direct blockade of the **superior laryngeal nerves** can be performed by infiltration with local anesthetic agents such as **1% or 1.5% lidocaine**.

B. The other innervation of the airway is just as easily approached by **topical anesthesia**. Higher concentrations of local anesthetics are required for topical application to overcome the usual slow penetrance of the drugs across mucosal membranes. Commercial preparations of local anesthetics (such as 10% flavored lidocaine) are available as oral sprays, but the delivered quantity cannot be measured. A better approach is to **nebulize** a known quantity of anesthetic (such as 10 mL of 4% lidocaine) with an atomizer such as those used in otolaryngology. **Lidocaine 4%** and **tetracaine 0.5%** to 1% are available for transtracheal injection or oral topical application in this manner. These **high concentrations** carry the obvious risk of rapidly exceeding the maximum recommended doses of these agents. This problem is further compounded by the common practice of using unmeasurable quantities of several different drugs for the multiple blocks performed.

C. Nasal anesthesia carries the additional requirement for **vasoconstriction** to reduce the incidence of bleeding from the nasal mucosa. Cocaine 4% has been the traditional agent of choice because it is the only local anesthetic with intrinsic vasoconstrictor properties. Because of cocaine's high toxicity and abuse potential, the use of 3% lidocaine with 0.25% phenylephrine may be a better alternative for nasal topical anesthesia.

IV. Technique

Airway anesthesia can be performed with the patient in the supine position, but it is often more comfortable for the patient if it is done with the head slightly elevated or in the sitting position. If full mental alertness is not required, a mild sedative such as dexmedetomidine (which has minimal respiratory depression) can be used.

A. Nasal mucosa

1. For the nasal mucosa, **cotton pledgets** on long applicators are soaked in 4% cocaine (or a mixture of lidocaine-phenylephrine) and inserted gently into both nares. The first applicator is inserted directly posterior along the inferior turbinate to the posterior pharyngeal wall (Figure 17.1).
2. A second applicator is inserted with a slight cephalad angle to follow the middle turbinate and is again advanced to its full depth until it touches the mucosa over the sphenoid bone.
3. Anesthesia is performed **bilaterally**, because the object is to provide anesthesia of the branches of the sphenopalatine ganglion as well as topical anesthesia of the mucosa itself. Two to 3 minutes of contact time is usually required to provide adequate penetration of the agent into the mucosa. Cotton-tipped applicator sticks are available in most operating rooms, and are tolerated by patients. The more generous sized pledgets used by otolaryngologists are less comfortable, but more effective in providing adequate surface area for delivery of the anesthetic.

B. Superior laryngeal block

1. While the nasal applicators are in place, the **superior laryngeal nerves** are blocked bilaterally. The patient's head is extended, and the thyroid cartilage and hyoid bone are identified. The index finger retracts the skin down over the **superior ala of the thyroid cartilage**, and the skin is wiped with an alcohol swab. A 23- or 25-gauge needle on a 5-mL syringe filled with 1% lidocaine is inserted onto the tip of the cartilage. The index finger then releases the skin traction, and the needle is "walked off" the cartilage superiorly and is inserted just through the firm thyrohyoid membrane. The tip now lies in the loose areolar tissue plane beneath the membrane (Figure 17.2). After aspiration to detect unwanted intravascular placement, 2.5 mL is injected into the plane beneath the membrane. This sequence is repeated on the opposite side.
2. Alternatively, the needle can be inserted onto the posterior (greater) cornu of the hyoid bone and "walked" caudad off the bone onto the membrane.

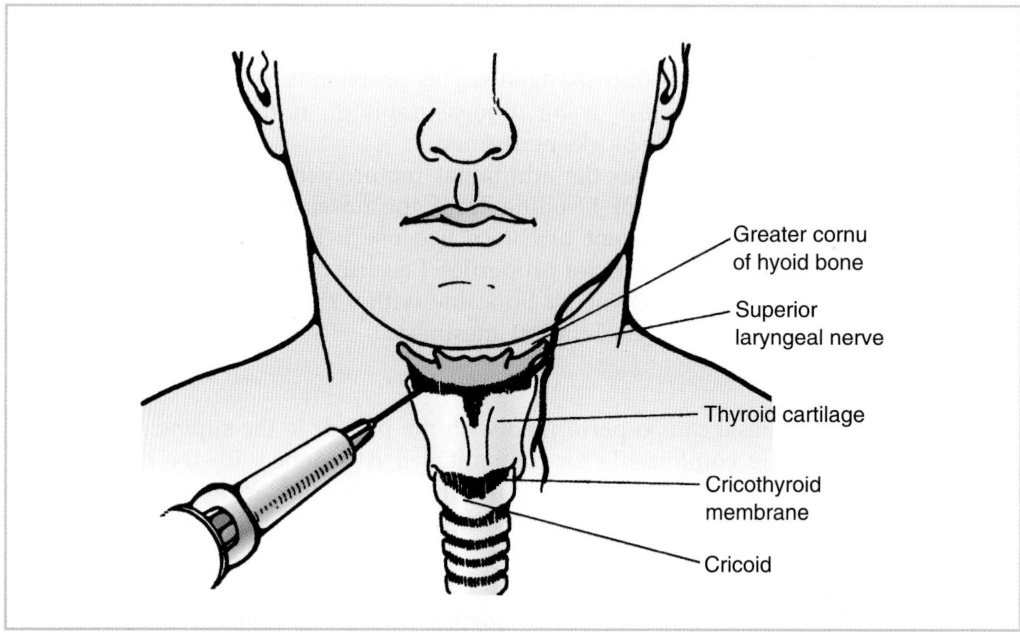

Figure 17.2. Superior laryngeal nerve block. The 23- to 25-gauge needle is introduced onto the superior border of the lateral wing of the thyroid cartilage. It is then gently advanced off the cartilage to drop through the thyrohyoid membrane. After gentle aspiration to exclude intravascular injection, 2 to 3 mL of local anesthetic is injected into the space below the membrane.

3. If a transtracheal injection (step 4) is to be performed, this syringe and needle can be used to inject a final 0.3 mL local anesthetic intradermal wheal over the cricothyroid membrane in the midline of the neck.

C. Mouth and pharynx

1. The mouth and pharynx are anesthetized **topically**. A total of 4 mL 4% lidocaine or 0.5% tetracaine is placed in an atomizer. The tongue is sprayed with local anesthetic, and then the patient is asked to gargle with the residue. Next, the numbed tongue is grasped with a dry gauze sponge and gently held with one hand. The patient is then instructed to pant vigorously ("like a puppy") while the rest of the local anesthetic is sprayed into the posterior pharynx with each inspiration. The anesthesia provided by the superior laryngeal block should allow the patient to aspirate the nebulized anesthetic without gagging and will provide some tracheal anesthesia.
2. Direct **submucosal injection** into the base of the anterior tonsillar pillar will produce denser anesthesia and gag suppression (2). After initial topical anesthesia, the tongue is retracted medially with a tongue depressor, revealing the inferior curve of the anterior tonsillar pillar (Figure 17.3). A 25-gauge spinal needle is used to inject 2 mL of 1% lidocaine 0.5 cm below the mucosa at a point 0.5 cm lateral to the base of the tongue itself. The longer length of the spinal needle will allow easier control by permitting the syringe itself to remain outside the mouth. **Aspiration** is performed before injection to detect intravascular placement or advancement of the needle through the posterior border of the pillar. Bilateral injection is needed to block both lingual branches of the glossopharyngeal nerve. The risks of intravascular

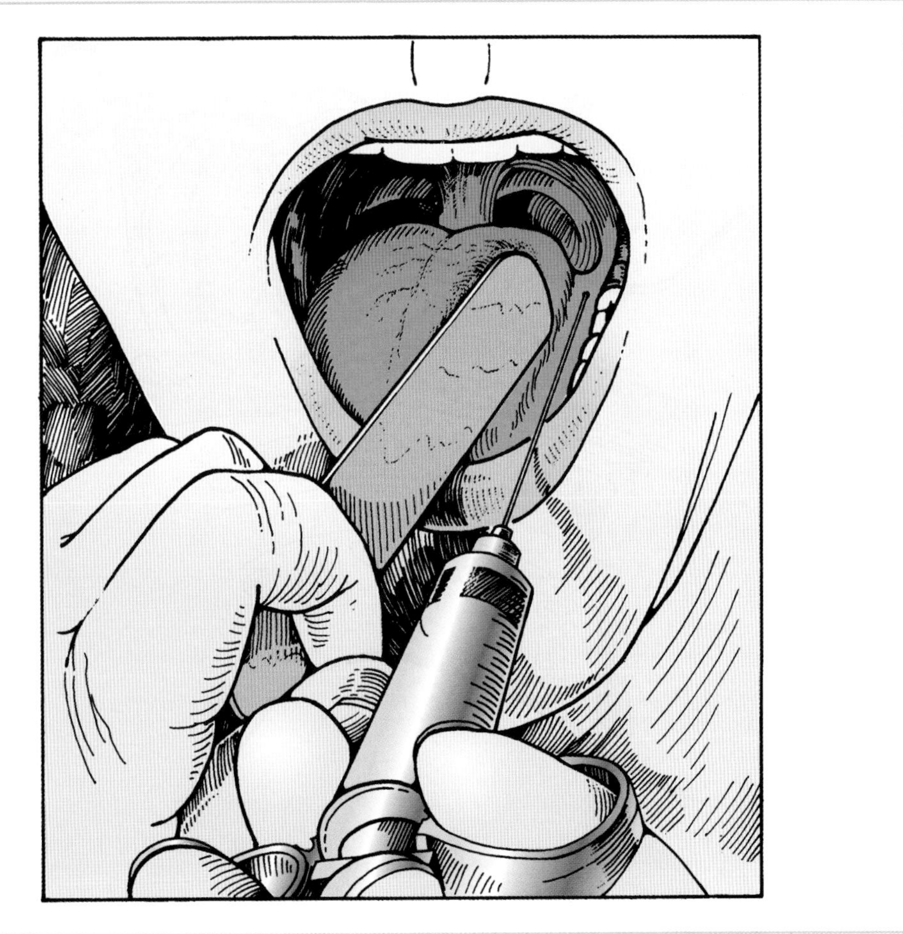

Figure 17.3. Glossopharyngeal nerve (lingual branch) block. The tongue is pushed medially with a tongue depressor, and a spinal needle is inserted into the base of the anterior tonsillar pillar 0.5 cm lateral to the base of the tongue and advanced 0.5 cm deep. After aspiration of the needle, 2 mL of local anesthetic is injected. Both sides need to be injected for adequate block of the gag reflex. A three-ring syringe makes aspiration easier, and the use of a 3-in. (spinal) needle allows better visualization of the injection site while the hand remains outside the mouth.

injection and the greater discomfort make simple topical anesthesia a better choice for most patients.

C. **Transtracheal injection.** Finally, the **trachea** is topically anesthetized by **transtracheal injection**. A 20-gauge plastic intravenous catheter with a metal stylet is introduced through the cricothyroid membrane through the previously injected skin wheal (Figure 17.4). Entry into the trachea is confirmed by aspiration of air. The metal stylet is removed, and a syringe with 4 mL 4% lidocaine is attached to the plastic cannula remaining in the trachea. The lidocaine is injected as the patient inspires; the spray will produce a cough that will spread the solution up the trachea to the level of the cords.

D. **Final steps**

1. As an optional addition to the topical anesthesia of the nasal passages, the applicators can be removed and a **soft rubber nasal airway** coated

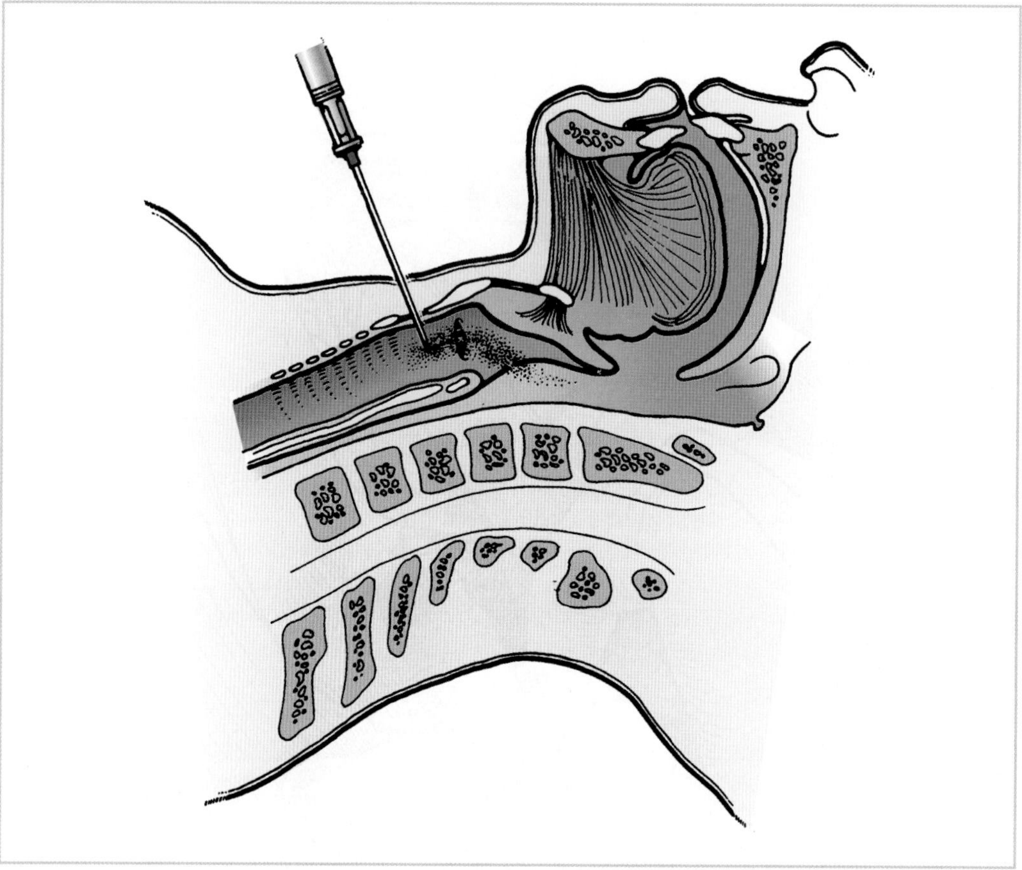

Figure 17.4. Transtracheal injection. A 20-gauge intravenous catheter is introduced through the cricoid membrane. After tracheal entry is confirmed by air aspiration, the metal introducer is removed, and a syringe is attached to the plastic needle, which is left in place. Four milliliters of topical anesthetic is injected as the patient inspires; the inward air flow will carry the solution down the trachea, and the usual reflex cough will spread it up to the undersurface of the vocal cords.

with lidocaine cream can be inserted. If a series of these nasal airways are introduced in sequentially larger sizes, they will dilate the nasal passages and will help lubricate them for eventual passage of an endotracheal tube. With a large airway in place, a final spray of nebulized lidocaine by this route will be delivered almost directly to the vocal cords.

2. If the nasal airways are not used, the nasal applicators are removed and endotracheal tube insertion is begun. The interval required for the other blocks is usually sufficient to allow development of nasal and oral anesthesia. If the trachea itself was not anesthetized, the anesthesiologist must be ready to administer rapidly acting intravenous sedation or anesthesia to blunt the cardiovascular and coughing reflexes that will occur when the tube passes below the cords.

V. Complications

A. Systemic toxicity is the most likely adverse outcome, owing to absorption rather than intravascular injection. Although not all the local anesthetic is

Table 17.1 Common dosages used for airway anesthesia

Drug	Amount (mL)	Concentration	Total milligrams	Percentage of maximum recommended dose
Cocaine	3	4%	120	60
Tetracaine	5	1%	50	25
Lidocaine	5	1%	50	12
Lidocaine	4	4%	160	40

absorbed, the total quantities used as shown in Table 17.1 are significant. Resuscitation equipment should be at hand, and the patient must be observed closely during the block and for at least 20 minutes after completion of the block.

B. Epistaxis may occur even with the use of a vasoconstrictor in the nose. Gentle insertion and generous lubrication of the tube will reduce this possibility, whereas the presence of a deformity or coagulopathy will increase the risk.

C. Aspiration of gastric contents may occur if anesthesia of the cords and trachea is created in the presence of reflux or active vomiting. These techniques should be used with caution (or not at all) if there is significant risk of aspiration.

REFERENCES

1 American Society of Anesthesiologists Task Force on Management of the Difficult Airway. Practice guidelines for management of the difficult airway: an updated report by the American Society of Anesthesiologists Task Force on Management of the Difficult Airway. *Anesthesiology* 2003;98:1269–1277.

2 **Benumof JL. Management of the difficult adult airway. With special emphasis on awake tracheal intubation. *Anesthesiology* 1991;75:1087.**

3 Graham DR, Hay JG, Clague J, et al. Comparison of three different methods used to achieve local anesthesia for fiberoptic bronchoscopy. *Chest* 1992;102:704.

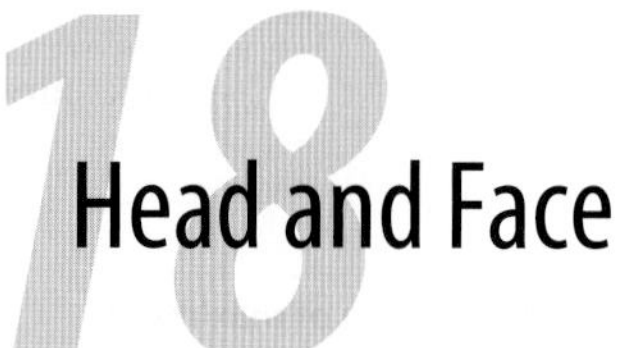

18 Head and Face

Christopher M. Bernards

I. **Introduction.** Surgery of the head is rarely performed with regional anesthesia alone but these blocks can still be useful for a number of indications, for example, analgesia for awake neurosurgical procedures or for "sewing-up" lacerations. In addition, they are useful in many diagnostic and therapeutic pain procedures. This chapter describes the extraoral approach to blocking facial innervation. For a discussion of intraoral approaches the reader is referred to any comprehensive textbook of dentistry.

II. **Anatomy**

A. **Head**

1. **Occipital nerves.** The occipital nerves innervate the back of the head, the posterior third of the top of the head and the side of the head to just behind the ear (Figure 18.1).

a. **Greater occipital nerves.** These paired nerves arise from the dorsal rami of the second cervical nerves and course posteriorly and superiorly through the paraspinal muscles to become superficial at the level where the trapezius muscles insert on the skull base (superior nuchal line), just lateral to the occipital protuberance and immediately adjacent to the occipital artery (Figure 18.1). The greater occipital nerves provide innervation to the head from about the superior nuchal line to the vertex.

b. **Lesser occipital nerves.** This nerve also arises from the dorsal rami of C2 and forms part of the superficial cervical plexus. It emerges to become superficial at approximately the middle or superior third of the posterior border of the sternocleidomastoid muscle. The nerve then courses superiorly to provide innervation to the skin of the back of the ear and the skin behind the ear (Figure 18.1).

c. **Great auricular nerve.** The great auricular nerve arises from the dorsal rami of C2 and C3 and is also part of the superficial cervical plexus. It emerges at the posterior border of the sternocleidomastoid muscle inferior to the lesser occipital nerves. The great auricular nerve courses superiorly across the surface of the sternocleidomastoid muscle to innervate the anterior skin of the ear and the skin overlying the posterior third of the mandible and the parotid gland (Figure 18.1).

B. **Face.** The face, the forehead, and the anterior two-thirds of the top of the head are innervated by the three branches of the **trigeminal** (cranial nerve V) nerve (Figure 18.2). The neurons comprising the trigeminal nerve originate in several brainstem nuclei and converge in the **trigeminal** (Gasserian, semilunar) **ganglion**. The ganglion is an intracranial structure located at the medial end of the petrous temporal bone just lateral to the cavernous sinus and the internal carotid artery (Figure 18.2). The ganglion gives rise to the three nerves that provide sensory innervation to the face, oral cavity, and nasal cavity: ophthalmic (V1), maxillary (V2), and mandibular (V3).

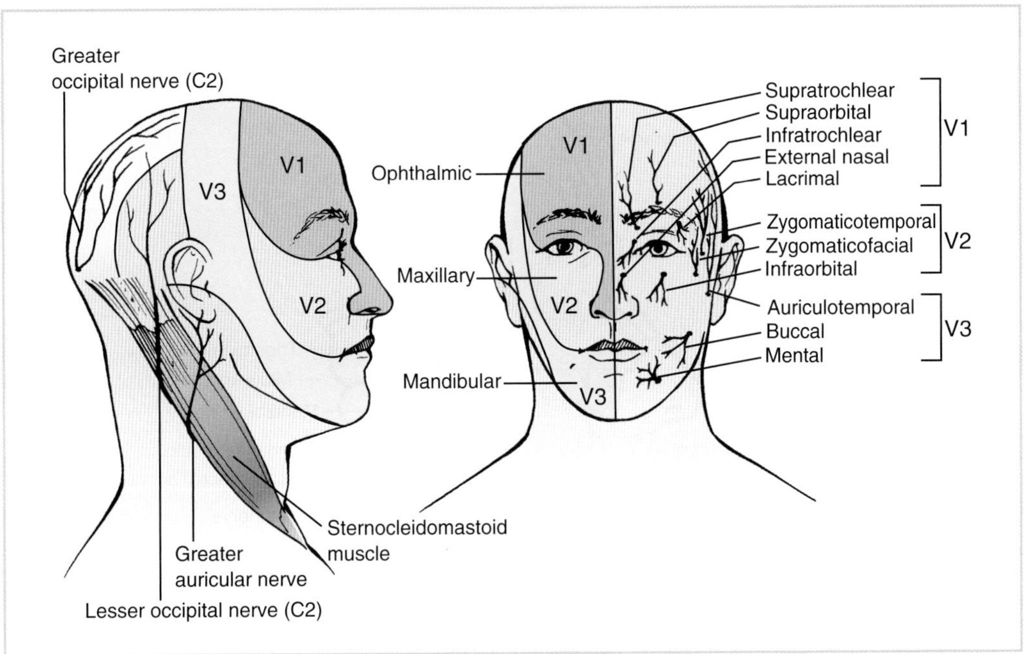

Figure 18.1. Cutaneous innervation of the head and face. The posterior half of the head is innervated by branches from the dorsal rami of the *C2* spinal nerves. The face and anterior half of the head are innervated by divisions of the fifth cranial nerve (*V1, V2, V3*). Terminal cutaneous branches of V1 include supratrochlear, supraorbital, infratrochlear, external nasal, and lacrimal. Terminal cutaneous branches of V2 include zygomaticotemporal, zygomaticofacial, auriculotemporal, and infraorbital. Terminal cutaneous branches of V3 include mental and buccal (generally blocked intraorally).

1. **Ophthalmic nerve** (V1). The ophthalmic nerve is the smallest and most superior of the three trigeminal divisions. Its branches enter the orbit to supply a variety of **intraorbital** and **extraorbital** structures associated with the eye. The only branches that have a significant extraorbital course, and are therefore readily amenable to nerve block, are the supraorbital and supratrochlear branches.
    a. **Supraorbital nerve.** The supraorbital nerve exits the orbit through the supraorbital notch, which is located near the middle of the supraorbital rim directly above the pupil when looking straight ahead (Figure 18.3). The supraorbital nerve supplies the upper eyelid, forehead, and scalp to the vertex (Figures 18.1, 18.2, and 18.3).
    b. **Supratrochlear nerve.** The supratrochlear nerve emerges from the upper, medial quadrant of the orbit and courses superiorly across the orbital rim. The supratrochlear nerve innervates the medial portion of the upper lid and the medial portion of the lower forehead (Figures 18.1, 18.2, and 18.3).
2. **Maxillary nerve** (V2). The maxillary nerve exits the cranial vault through the foramen rotundum to cross through the pterygopalatine fossa, which lies between the pterygoid plate and the posterior border of the maxilla (Figures 18.2 and 18.4). Within the fossa, the maxillary nerve gives off several branches that provide sensory innervation to the maxilla, maxillary sinus, nasal canal, palate, and the skin over the temple and zygomatic arch.

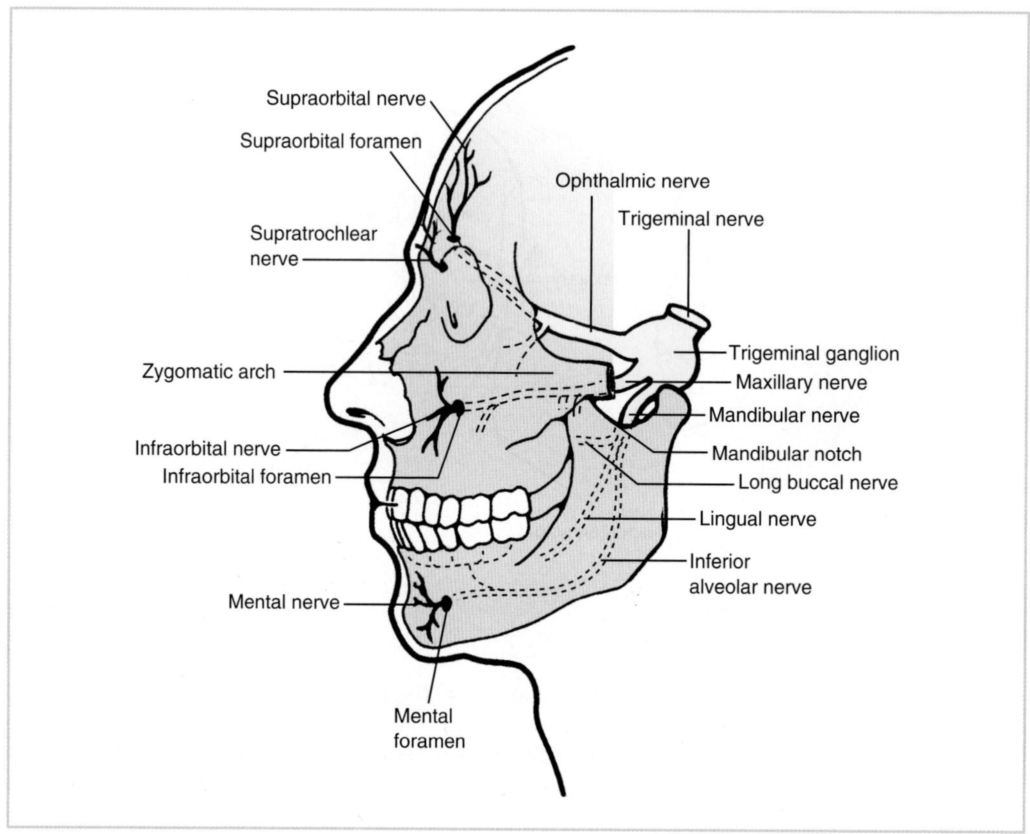

Figure 18.2. Anatomy of the trigeminal nerve, trigeminal ganglion, and primary divisions of the trigeminal nerve. Only the terminal branches of the ophthalmic nerve are accessible for extracranial blockade. In contrast, the maxillary and mandibular nerves can be blocked at multiple points along their course from the lateral pterygoid plate to the terminal branches exiting the infraorbital and mental foramina.

The nerve continues forward and enters the orbit through the infraorbital canal, pierces the orbital floor to traverse the maxillary sinus (this is why maxillary sinusitis can present as cheek pain) and exits the maxilla as the infraorbital nerve.

a. **Infraorbital nerve.** The infraorbital nerve exits the maxilla through the infraorbital foramen, which lies just below the infraorbital rim in line with the pupil when looking straight ahead (Figure 18.3). The infraorbital nerve provides sensory innervation to the cheek, the lower eyelid, the nasal ala, and the upper lip.
b. **Zygomatic nerve.** The skin over the zygomatic arch and the temple are innervated by the zygomatic and zygomaticotemporal nerves, respectively. These branches of the maxillary nerve arise in the pterygopalatine fossa (Figure 18.4); consequently, block of the infraorbital and supraorbital nerves will leave this area of the facial skin unblocked (compare Figures 18.1 and 18.3).

3. **Mandibular nerve.** The mandibular nerve is the largest of the three trigeminal branches and is the only one with **motor fibers**. It exits the cranial vault through the foramen ovale, which lies in the sphenoid bone

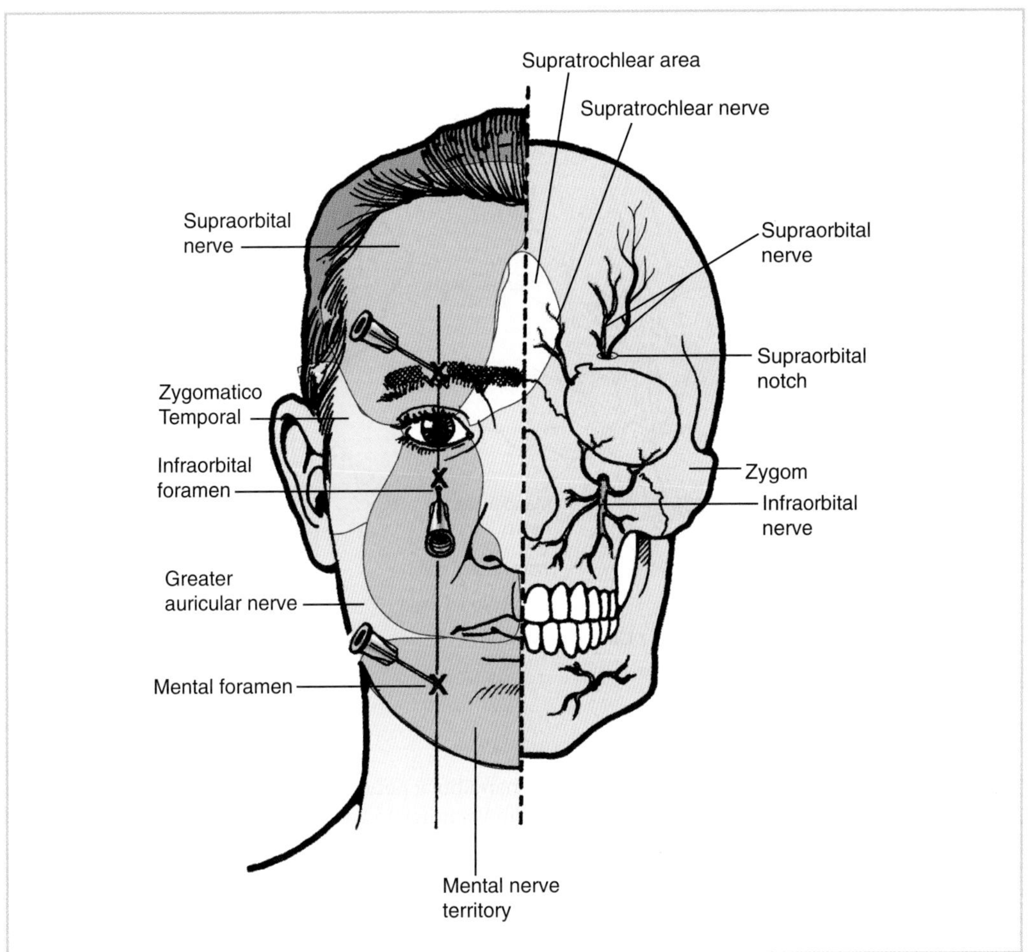

Figure 18.3. Cutaneous innervation of the face. Most of the face and forehead are innervated by the terminal branches of the ophthalmic (supraorbital, supratrochlear), maxillary (infraorbital), and mandibular (mental) nerves. The foramina through which the supraorbital, infraorbital, and mental nerves emerge lie along a straight line passing through the pupil when the subject looks straight ahead.

just posterior to the origin of the pterygoid plate (Figure 18.4). After exiting the foramen ovale, the mandibular nerve gives several branches to muscles in the pterygoid fossa and muscles of mastication (masseter, temporalis). Sensory fibers include:

a. **Auriculotemporal nerve.** The auriculotemporal nerve courses medial to the condylar process of the mandible and turns superiorly at the posterior border of the process becoming superficial near the posterior part of the zygomatic arch (Figure 18.4). It runs superiorly providing sensory innervation to the anterior half of the ear, the skin anterior to the ear and the skin over temporalis muscle.

b. **Inferior alveolar nerve.** As the mandibular nerve courses inferiorly within the pterygopalatine fossa it divides into two main branches–inferior alveolar and lingual (Figure 18.4). The inferior alveolar nerve descends parallel to the ramus of the mandible to enter the mandible

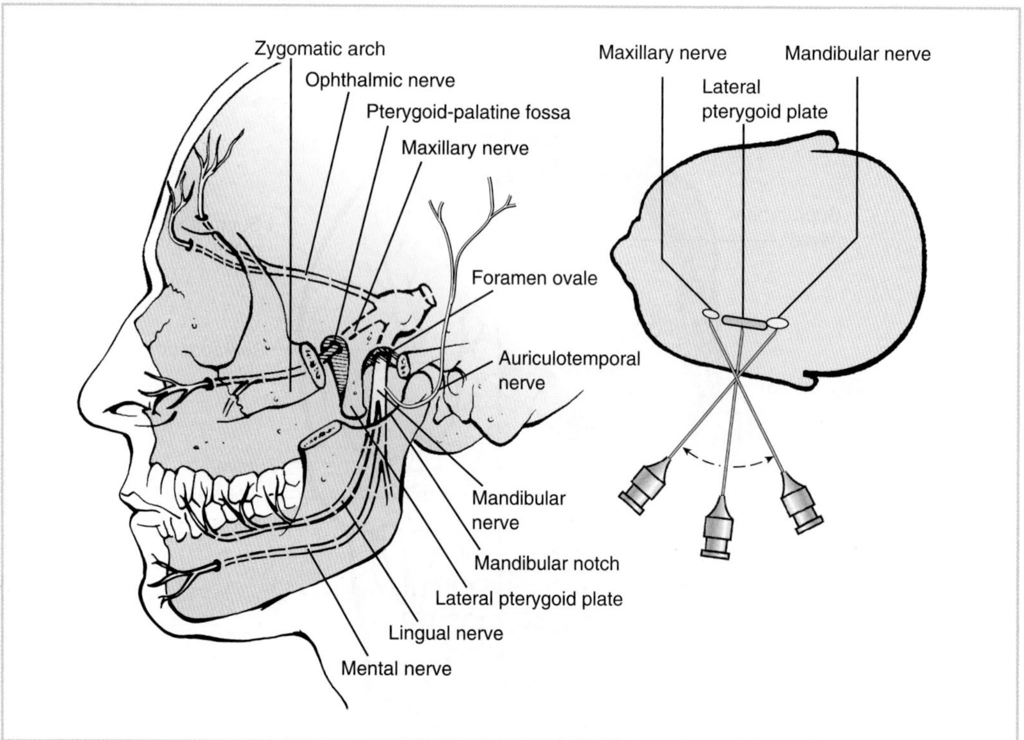

Figure 18.4. Lateral approach to the maxillary and mandibular nerves. For both mandibular and maxillary nerve blocks the needle is inserted through the mandibular notch to contact the lateral pterygoid plate. For maxillary nerve block, the needle is walked anteriorly off the pterygoid plate and into the pterygopalatine fosse where 5 mL local anesthetic is injected. For mandibular nerve block the needle is walked posteriorly off the lateral pterygoid plate. See text for details.

through the mandibular foramen, which lies at approximately the center of the ramus (Figure 18.2). The inferior alveolar nerve provides innervation to the buccal gingiva, mandible, and lower teeth.

(1) Mental nerve. The mental nerve is the terminal sensory branch of the inferior alveolar nerve. It exits the mandible through the mental foramen, which lies in line with the pupil when looking forward and approximately midway between the alveolar and inferior borders of the mandible (Figure 18.3). The mental nerve innervates the lower lip and chin.

c. Lingual nerve. The lingual nerve courses anterior to approximately parallel to the inferior alveolar nerve (Figure 18.2 and 18.4). It reaches the medial surface of the mandible near the junction of the vertical and horizontal portions of the mandible. At the level of the third molar the nerve courses anteromedially beneath the sublingual salivary gland to the tongue. The lingual nerve innervates the anterior two-thirds of the tongue, the lingual gingival, and the floor of the mouth.

III. Drugs

A. Local anesthetics. All local anesthetics used for peripheral nerve block are appropriate for nerve blocks in the head and face. Because many of the nerves to be blocked are only sensory, **less concentrated solutions** are effective (e.g., 1% lidocaine, 0.25% bupivacaine).

1. Because facial nerves course among numerous blood vessels, great care (repeated aspiration, epinephrine-containing test doses, incremental injection with constant vigilance and reassessment) must be taken when administering local anesthetics to avoid intravenous injection.
2. When cranial nerves are blocked near the foramina through which they exit from the cranial vault (e.g., foramen rotundum, foramen ovale), the potential for the drug to reach the cranial subarachnoid space through the foramina must be kept in mind. Because the brainstem is very near these foramina, respiratory arrest, "coma" and profound vasodilatation and bradycardia can occur. This has occurred with volumes as small as 0.25 mL 1% lidocaine injected through the foramen ovale in an effort to block the trigeminal ganglion.

B. Neurolytic drugs. Neurolytic ablation of cranial nerves to treat pain has largely been abandoned in favor of more precise surgical or radiofrequency destruction. Both techniques have better safety records than do alcohol or phenol injections. However, in circumstances where neurolytic block may be the best option for a particular patient, radiologic guidance (e.g., computed tomographic [CT] scan), nerve stimulation/paresthesia and local anesthetic test injections should be used.

IV. Techniques

A. Greater and lesser occipital nerves and great auricular nerve. Because these three nerves become superficial along a line from the greater occipital protuberance to the mastoid process they can be readily blocked by subcutaneous infiltration along this line (Figure 18.1).

1. After appropriate skin preparation (alcohol will not leave a sticky residue in the hair-like chlorhexidine or Betadine will), raise a local anesthetic skin wheal at the occipital protuberance.
2. Insert a 25-gauge spinal needle subcutaneously at a shallow angle directed toward the mastoid process. A flexible spinal needle can generally be "curved" around the base of the head by applying pressure just *behind* the tip as the needle advances (keep the finger behind the advancing needle tip less the needle pierce the skin and enter your finger). Although not necessary for successful block, this approach avoids the need to withdraw and reinsert the needle multiple times along the intended path.
3. Local anesthetic is injected as the needle is slowly directed through the subcutaneous tissue; 10 mL is generally sufficient.

B. Greater occipital nerve. The greater occipital nerve can also be blocked by identifying the occipital artery at a point 2 to 3 cm (1 in.) lateral to the occipital protuberance along the line connecting the protuberance to the mastoid process. Infiltrating 3 to 5 mL around the artery will block the nerve.

C. Superficial cervical plexus. The lesser occipital nerve and the great auricular nerve are part of the superficial cervical plexus and can be blocked here as well.

1. Place the patient supine with the head turned away from the side to be blocked.
2. Identify the posterior border of the sternocleidomastoid muscle and mark the midpoint between the mastoid process and the clavicle. Having the patient raise the head may facilitate identification of the muscle.

3. After appropriate sterile preparation, raise a skin wheal at the mark. Insert a 4 to 6 cm, (1.5–2.5 in.) 22-gauge (or smaller) needle subcutaneously at the edge of the muscle and inject 3 to 5 mL local anesthetic.
4. Redirect the needle cephalad and caudad in the subcutaneous tissue adjacent to the edge of the muscle. Infiltrate 5 mL local anesthetic in each direction.
   a. Note: The accessory nerve lies near the middle of the superficial cervical plexus but is just deep to the fascial layer beneath the subcutaneous tissue. If the fascia is pierced and local anesthetic deposited there, the accessory nerve may be blocked resulting in paralysis of the ipsilateral trapezius muscle.

D. **Supraorbital, supratrochlear, infraorbital, and mental nerves.** The three terminal branches of the trigeminal nerve provide cutaneous innervation of the face and can all be blocked where they exit their respective foramina (Figure 18.3).
1. Position the patient supine with the head comfortably supported. Consider asking the patient to close the eyes to reduce the psychological discomfort of seeing a needle directed toward the eye (supraorbital, supratrochlear, and infraorbital nerves).
2. Palpate and mark the foramina of the nerve(s) to be blocked.
   a. **Supraorbital foramen.** Have the patient look straight ahead. The supraorbital notch can be palpated along the supraorbital rim directly above the pupil.
   b. **Infraorbital foramen.** With the patient looking straight ahead, the infraorbital foramen lies just below the orbital rim.
   c. **Mental nerve.** With the patient looking straight ahead, the mental foramen can be palpated in line with the pupil at a point midway between the upper and lower borders of the mandible.
3. Aseptically prepare the skin. Because alcohol is highly volatile, it can irritate the eyes if used near them.
4. **Supraorbital nerve.** Insert a 22-gauge or smaller needle at the supraorbital foramen (not into it) and inject 2 mL local anesthetic.
5. **Supratrochlear nerve.** Infiltrate 5 mL local anesthetic along the supraorbital rim from the supraorbital notch to just across the midline.
6. **Infraorbital nerve.** Raise a skin wheal approximately 0.5 cm (0.25 in.) below the infraorbital foramen and insert a 22-gauge or smaller needle directed cephalad toward the foramen (the foramen angles cephalad). Inject 2 mL local anesthetic at the foramen.
7. **Mental nerve.** A 22-gauge or smaller needle is appropriate. The canal of the mental nerve angles medially and inferiorly so it is more easily approached by entering the skin approximately 0.5 cm (0.25 in.) lateral and superior and angling the needle toward the foramen. Two milliliters of local anesthetic applied at the foramen is generally sufficient.

E. **Maxillary nerve.** The maxillary nerve is blocked where it comes from behind the lateral pterygoid plate to cross the pterygopalatine fossa (Figure 18.4).
1. Place the patient supine with the head turned slightly away from the side to be blocked.
2. Feel for the mandibular notch by having the patient open and close the mouth while palpating the upper border of the mandibular ramus. The notch will be felt moving up and down as the mouth is opened and closed. Mark an "X" over the notch at its deepest point.

3. Aseptically prepare the skin and raise a skin wheal at the "X" overlying the mandibular notch.
4. Insert an 8- to 10-cm (3.5–4 in.) 22-gauge needle through the "X" directed toward the rear of the ipsilateral eyeball (approximately 45 degrees cephalad and slightly anterior). The advancing needle will contact the pterygoid plate at a depth of 4 to 5 cm (1.5–2 in.) (1); note the actual depth.
5. Withdraw and redirect the needle more anteriorly and walk off the pterygoid plate and into the pterygopalatine fossa. On average, the pterygopalatine fossa lies 0.22 cm (0.1 in.) deeper than the pterygoid plate (1). Do not insert the needle more than 0.5 cm (0.25 in.) deeper than the depth at which the pterygoid plate was contacted. "Spontaneous" paresthesias to the nasal cavity and upper teeth occur approximately 60% of the time and are helpful to confirm correct needle location, but are not necessary unless performing neurolytic block. The maxillary nerve does not have a motor component so nerve stimulation will not produce a motor response, but can be used to elicit sensory paresthesias.
6. After careful aspiration, incrementally inject 5 mL local anesthetic (1 mL alcohol for neurolytic block).
7. **Complications**
   a. If the needle is not directed anteriorly enough it may miss the pterygoid plate and enter the nasopharynx.
   b. If the needle is directed too cephalad and not anteriorly it may enter the foramen ovale or foramen lacerum.
   c. If not angled anteriorly enough the carotid artery may be punctured.
   d. With an appropriately placed needle, drug may enter the orbit through the nearby infraorbital fissure and affect vision.

F. Mandibular nerve (Figure 18.4)

1. Positioning and landmarks are the same as for the maxillary nerve.
2. Unlike the maxillary nerve, the mandibular nerve has a motor component (muscles of mastication), therefore a nerve stimulator can be used to facilitate identification of the nerve.
3. Insert the needle through the mandibular notch perpendicular to the skin in all planes. The lateral pterygoid plate should be contacted at a depth of 4 to 5 cm (1.5–2 in.).
4. Walk the needle slightly posteriorly off the pterygoid plate. The mandibular nerve lies approximately 0.5 cm (0.25 in.) deep to the posterior edge of the pterygoid plate. Paresthesias to the jaw or lower teeth confirm correct needle placement. Paresthesias are not required for local anesthetic block, but as with other blocks they increase the confidence in the location of the needle. Paresthesias or radiographic confirmation are important for neurolytic blocks.
5. Following careful aspiration, incrementally inject 5 to 10 mL local anesthetic in volumes of 1 or 2 mL while observing for signs of systemic toxicity or misplaced local anesthetic.

REFERENCES

1 Singh B, Srivastava SK, Dang R. Anatomic considerations in relation to the maxillary nerve block. *Reg Anesth Pain Med* 2001;26(6):507–511.

19 Cervical Plexus Blocks

Michael F. Mulroy

The nerve roots of the second, third, and fourth cervical vertebrae supply sensory and motor fibers to the neck and posterior scalp. Direct plexus anesthesia provides the usual motor and sensory anesthesia to its distribution. The anatomy of the superficial plexus allows blockade of just the sensory fibers.

I. Anatomy

A. The cervical vertebrae are unusual in that their elongated transverse processes include a medial passage for the ascent of the vertebral artery and a well-formed **trough** (sulcus) for the emergence of their respective nerve roots lateral to the artery (Figure 19.1). Each sulcus has a **posterior and anterior tubercle**, which can often be palpated easily in the neck. The anterior divisions of the second through fourth roots form an extensive plexus that provides motor innervation for the muscles of the neck and sensation for the occipital region, the neck below the mandible, and the shoulder above the clavicle. The most significant motor fibers are the contributions of the third, fourth, and fifth roots to the **phrenic nerve**.

B. All of the fibers emerge (like the brachial plexus) between the anterior and middle scalene muscles. The anterior scalenes are attenuated at this level but still form a landmark for the cervical plexus, as they do for the brachial plexus.

1. The cervical **motor** branches curl around the lateral border of the anterior scalene muscle and proceed caudad and medially toward the muscles of the neck, giving anterior branches to the sternocleidomastoid (SCM) muscle as they pass behind it.
2. The **sensory** fibers also emerge from behind the scalene, but they continue laterally and emerge superficially under the posterior border of the SCM to ramify to both the anterior and posterior skin of the neck.

II. Indications

A. Superficial cervical plexus anesthesia provides sensory anesthesia to the skin of the neck and shoulder above the clavicle and is useful for providing superficial anesthesia for **thyroidectomy** or **tracheostomy** incisions. If motor relaxation is desired, deep cervical plexus blockade is required. Even with deep plexus anesthesia, the surgeon may occasionally need to supplement the block with local anesthesia, particularly around the upper pole of the thyroid, which has some sensory innervation from cranial nerves. Cervical plexus blockade provides good postoperative **analgesia** (1). It is also possible to perform **carotid** surgery with this block, although some local infiltration of the glossopharyngeal branches around the carotid sinus may be required. Superficial plexus block alone appears to be sufficient for this surgery **(2)**. Cervical plexus block can be combined with thoracic epidural anesthesia for breast surgery.

B. Shoulder anesthesia can be obtained with deep cervical plexus anesthesia, but is usually provided by the interscalene approach to the brachial plexus, which inevitably blocks the lower cervical fibers. The latter approach may even be preferable in shoulder surgery patients owing to the motor relaxation of the arm.

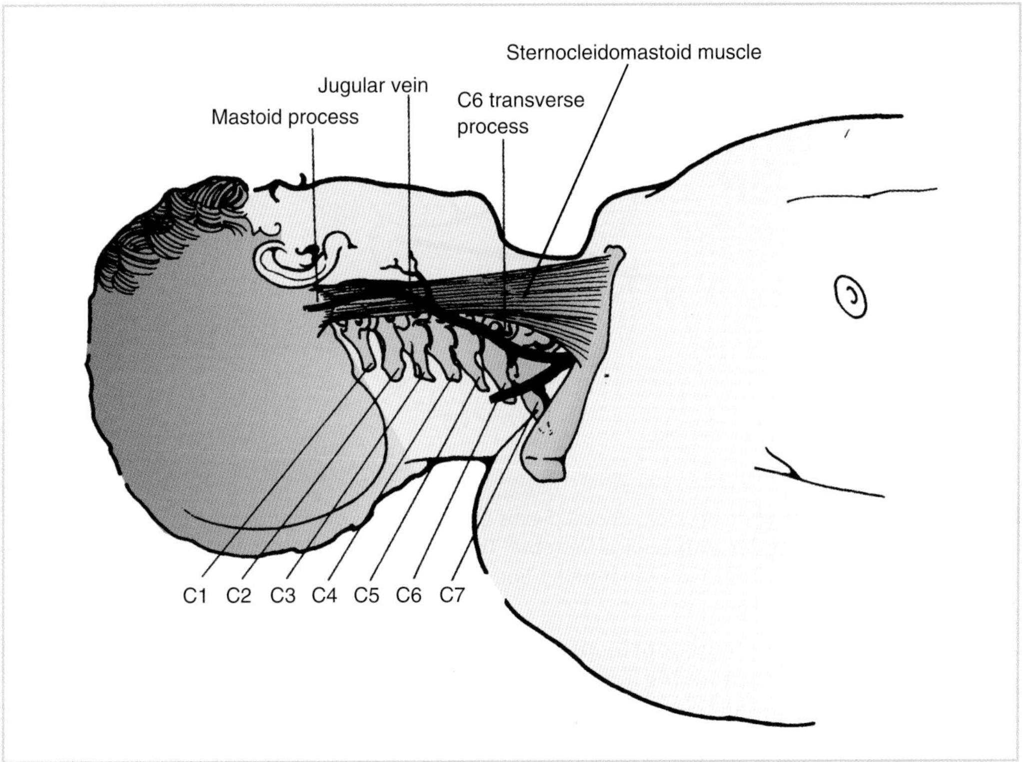

Figure 19.1. Anatomy of deep cervical plexus block. The transverse processes lie under the lateral border of the sternocleidomastoid muscle, each with a distal trough or sulcus that defines the path of nerve exit.

III. Drugs

For surgery, any of the intermediate- or long-acting aminoamides are appropriate. Lower concentrations are sufficient for the superficial (sensory) block, but higher concentrations such as 1.5% lidocaine or 0.5% bupivacaine (or ropivacaine) will give better motor anesthesia with deep plexus block. All of the drugs will demonstrate a slightly shortened duration in the neck compared to other peripheral areas because of the generous blood supply of the region.

IV. Techniques

For both deep and superficial blocks, the patient is placed supine with a small towel under the occiput and the head turned to the side opposite the one to be blocked.

A. Deep cervical plexus anesthesia

1. The **mastoid process** is identified and marked, as is the **transverse process of the sixth cervical vertebra**. This is the most prominent tubercle in the neck, and it lies at the level of the cricoid cartilage.
2. A line is drawn between these two points, indicating the plane of the transverse processes of the cervical vertebrae (Figure 19.2). The lateral border of the SCM muscle is also marked.
3. Starting 1.5 cm below the mastoid, gentle palpation is used to identify the **tubercle of the second vertebra** just posterior (approximately 0.5 cm) to the first line. An "X" is placed over this process.

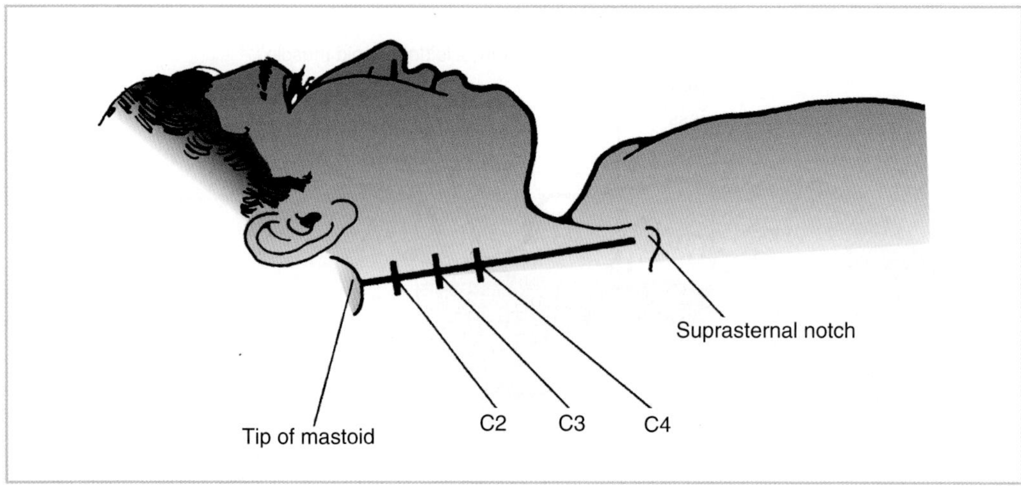

Figure 19.2. Superficial landmarks for cervical plexus block. A line is drawn from the mastoid process to the prominent tubercle of the sixth cervical vertebra. The transverse processes of the second, third, and fourth cervical vertebrae lie 0.5 cm posterior to this line, and at 1.5-cm intervals below the mastoid.

4. The third and fourth processes are identified and marked in the same manner by moving 1.5 cm caudad for each level. The third mark should fall approximately at the level of the junction of the external jugular vein and the SCM muscle.
5. After aseptic preparation, a skin wheal is raised at each of the three "X" marks.
6. A 3.5-cm (1.5-in.) 22-gauge needle is introduced perpendicular to the skin and is directed posterior and slightly caudad at each "X" until it rests on the transverse process. A palpating finger of the opposite hand helps in guiding the placement.
7. Placement on the transverse process is confirmed by "walking" the needle caudad and cephalad; it should slip off the bone of the process rather than continuing to contact bone, as it would if on the vertebral body (Figure 19.1). The latter situation is undesirable because the needle is not near the nerve, but is more likely to produce intravascular or subarachnoid injection.
8. A syringe is attached to each needle in turn while it is securely held in place just above the transverse process. Then 3 to 5 mL of anesthetic solution is injected in small increments with frequent aspiration and assessment of the patient's mental status.
9. Onset of anesthesia should occur within 5 minutes.
10. An alternative is to use a variation of the interscalene technique with a **peripheral nerve stimulator**. A single stimulating needle is introduced into the groove between the muscles at the C4-5 level (at the upper border of the thyroid cartilage). Stimulation of the levator scapulae muscle produces elevation and internal rotation of the scapula, and injection of a single bolus of 40 mL of anesthetic produces plexus blockade. Local anesthetic can be shown to spread in a hemicylindrical column from approximately the C1 to the C7 level (3,4).

B. **Superficial cervical plexus anesthesia** is performed with the patient in the same position as for deep plexus anesthesia.

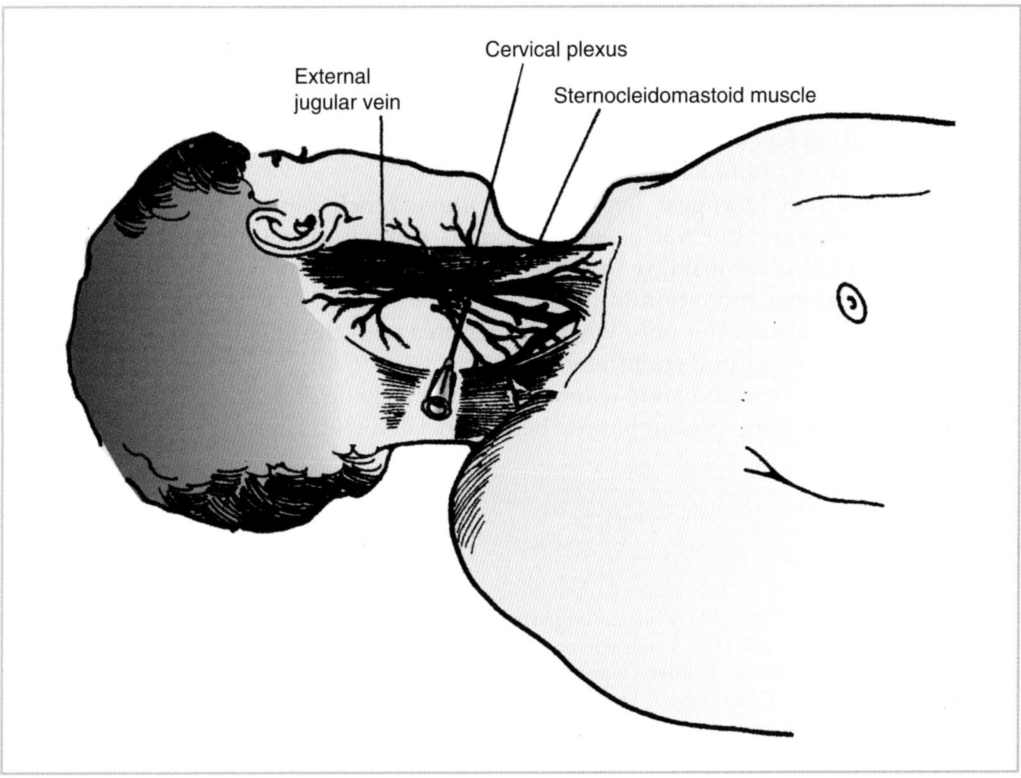

Figure 19.3. Superficial cervical plexus block. The sensory fibers of the plexus all emerge from behind the lateral border of the sternocleidomastoid muscle. A needle inserted at its midpoint, usually where the external jugular vein crosses the muscle, can be directed superiorly and inferiorly to block all of these terminal branches.

1. An "X" is made at the level of the transverse process of the fourth cervical vertebra, as described, or simply at the junction of the external jugular vein with the posterior border of the SCM muscle.
2. After aseptic preparation, a skin wheal is made at the "X."
3. A 5-cm (2-in.) needle is introduced through the wheal, and local infiltration is performed along the posterior border of the SCM muscle 4 cm (1.5 in.) above and below the level of the "X" (Figure 19.3). This may require 10 mL of anesthetic solution to block all of the superficial sensory fibers.

V. **Complications**

A. **Central nervous system toxicity** is the most serious consequence of deep cervical plexus block, owing to the proximity of the vertebral artery to the injection site. Multiple careful aspirations are required, and injections should be in small increments (1.0–1.5 mL), with careful monitoring of the patient's mental status.

B. **Spinal anesthesia** is also potentially produced because the cervical roots carry long sleeves of dura through their intervertebral foramina. These may be entered easily if the needle is directed cephalad in the sulcus. Maintaining a caudad direction helps prevent entry of the needle too far medially. Again, careful aspiration and incremental injection are appropriate.

C. **Phrenic nerve block** is inevitable, and deep cervical plexus block should be used with caution in any patient who is dependent on the diaphragm for ventilation. Fortunately, most patients have adequate tidal ventilation from their intercostal muscles, and many phrenic nerve blocks are simply undetected. Bilateral blockade obviously increases the possibility that this complication may become symptomatic.

D. **Recurrent laryngeal nerve–vagus nerve block** can occur and, again, is a troublesome but not usually a serious complication (5). The only potential problem is the inability to assess laryngeal function following thyroidectomy.

E. **Hematoma formation** in the neck also can occur if a major vessel is entered. This is distressing only when it interferes with the anticipated surgery, as in the case of carotid endarterectomy.

F. Altered **hemodynamic response** due to blockade of the carotid baroreceptors is a possibility (6), but has not been associated with clinical problems.

REFERENCES

1 Dieudonne N, Gomola A, Bonnichon P, et al. Prevention of postoperative pain after thyroid surgery: a double-blind randomized study of bilateral superficial cervical plexus blocks. *Anesth Analg* 2001;92:1538.

2 **Pandit JJ, Bree S, Dillon P, et al. A comparison of superficial versus combined (superficial and deep) cervical plexus block for carotid endarterectomy: a prospective, randomized study. *Anesth Analg* 2000;91:781.**

3 **Merle JC, Mazoit JX, Desgranges P, et al. A comparison of two techniques for cervical plexus blockade: evaluation of efficacy and systemic toxicity. *Anesth Analg* 1999;89:1366.**

4 Dhonneur G, Saidi NE, Merle JC, et al. Demonstration of the spread of injectate with deep cervical plexus block: a case series. *Reg Anesth Pain Med* 2007;32:116–119.

5 Weiss A, Isselhorst C, Gahlen J, et al. Acute respiratory failure after deep cervical plexus block for carotid endarterectomy as a result of bilateral recurrent laryngeal nerve paralysis. *Acta Anaesthesiol Scand* 2005;49:715–719.

6 Kim YK, Hwang GS, Huh IY, et al. Altered autonomic cardiovascular regulation after combined deep and superficial cervical plexus blockade for carotid endarterectomy. *Anesth Analg* 2006;103:533–539.

20 Ophthalmic Anesthesia

Susan B. McDonald

Surgery of the eye is frequently performed with regional anesthesia, though topical anesthesia for simple cataract extraction with smaller flexible lenses has increased in popularity. Ophthalmology patients are frequently older and more likely to have systemic diseases, and are most likely to profit from regional blockade without heavy systemic sedation or general anesthesia.

I. **Anatomy**

   A. **The extraocular muscles form a cone** about the globe, with the apex at the optic foramen. Passing through this foramen are the ophthalmic artery, ciliary ganglion, ophthalmic division of the trigeminal nerve, cranial nerves supplying the extraocular muscles (III, IV, and VI) and the optic nerve.

   B. **Sensory innervation**

      1. Sensation in the eye is transmitted through afferent fibers from the cornea and conjunctiva.
      2. These fibers pass through the **ciliary ganglion** in the retrobulbar space to the first branch (ophthalmic division) of cranial nerve V.

   C. **Motor innervation**

      1. The motor fibers of the extraocular muscles arise from the cranial nerves.
         a. **Cranial nerve VI (abducens)** innervates the lateral rectus muscle.
         b. **Cranial nerve IV (trochlear)** innervates the superior oblique muscle.
         c. **Cranial nerve III (oculomotor)** innervates all of the other muscles of the eye.
      2. The oculomotor and abducens motor nerve fibers pass through the muscle cone in the retrobulbar space with the ciliary ganglion. The trochlear nerve lies outside the cone on the superior medial side of the orbit.
      3. The motor fibers of the **cranial nerve VII (facial)** control contraction of the orbicularis oculi muscles. These fibers emerge from the base of the skull near the mastoid process and travel anteriorly from the tragus of the ear to ramify into the muscles surrounding the orbit.

II. **Indications**

   A. The anesthesiologist can provide regional anesthesia for ophthalmic surgery by a combination of **local infiltration of the facial nerve** and blockade of the motor and sensory branches of the posterior orbit by means of a **peribulbar** or **retrobulbar block**.

      1. **Facial nerve block** will produce both sensory anesthesia of the periorbital area and motor block of the lid.
      2. **Bulbar block creates the akinesia** needed for cataract extraction, enucleation, and other superficial ophthalmic procedures, **as well as sensory anesthesia** of the terminal branches of the trigeminal nerve in the ciliary ganglion.

   B. Peribulbar or retrobulbar blocks are performed for a variety of ophthalmic surgeries, most commonly cataract extraction and intraocular lens implantation, but **are not suitable for open globe surgeries.**

C. With the increasing use of smaller incisions for cataract surgery, the use of simple topical anesthesia is growing in popularity, and is considered advantageous in avoiding the risk of globe perforation associated with the more invasive injection techniques described here.

III. Drugs

A. Local anesthetic

1. For facial nerve blockade, **lidocaine or mepivacaine in 1% concentrations** is adequate.
2. For the retrobulbar and peribulbar blocks, higher concentrations are used to provide adequate muscular block. Lidocaine 2% is adequate for short cases, but **0.75% bupivacaine or ropivacaine** (either alone or mixed with 2% lidocaine) will provide good akinesis and longer analgesia. The potential advantages of dense motor block must be weighed against the risk of intravascular injection in this area.

B. Additives

1. **Hyaluronidase** (7.5 units/mL) has been added to retrobulbar injections to promote spread of the anesthetic through the muscle cone (1). Postoperative diplopia after peribulbar block has been blamed on the lack of hyaluronidase presumably caused by the lack of local anesthetic spread causing focal myotoxicity (2).
2. **Epinephrine** 1:200,000 may be added, but does not appear to provide any advantage with bupivacaine. It may also increase the risk of retinal artery vasoconstriction.
3. The adjustment of the pH with **sodium bicarbonate** has been shown to speed the onset of bupivacaine and reduce the need for supplemental blocks with the peribulbar technique (3).
4. The addition of nondepolarizing muscle relaxants such as **atracurium** to peribulbar blocks has been described in an attempt to decrease the onset time of motor block (4).
5. Some have advocated adding **clonidine** to provide longer analgesia and akinesia. Side effects of hypotension, sedation, and dizziness limit the dose, but 1.0 μg/kg mixed in a lidocaine-hyaluronidase solution may offer prolonged analgesia with limited side effects (5,6). The need for such duration is offset by the usually short duration of cataract surgery.

IV. Technique

A. Sedation and monitors. For bulbar blocks, intravenous sedation is useful to provide analgesia, amnesia, and patient cooperation, which is an important factor in reducing the chance of globe injury. Many drugs have been employed, but the shortest duration of sedation (such as a small propofol bolus) is ideal in this population. With the high frequency of associated disease and age in these patients, monitoring and supplemental oxygen are advisable if sedation is used. Once the block is injected, these patients generally do not require further sedation during the procedure.

B. Facial nerve blockade. The facial nerve can be blocked at any point from the terminal fibers near the eye to its exit from the cranium at the base of the skull. The choice is usually based on the perceived frequency and comfort level for the side effects (facial droop, ecchymosis).

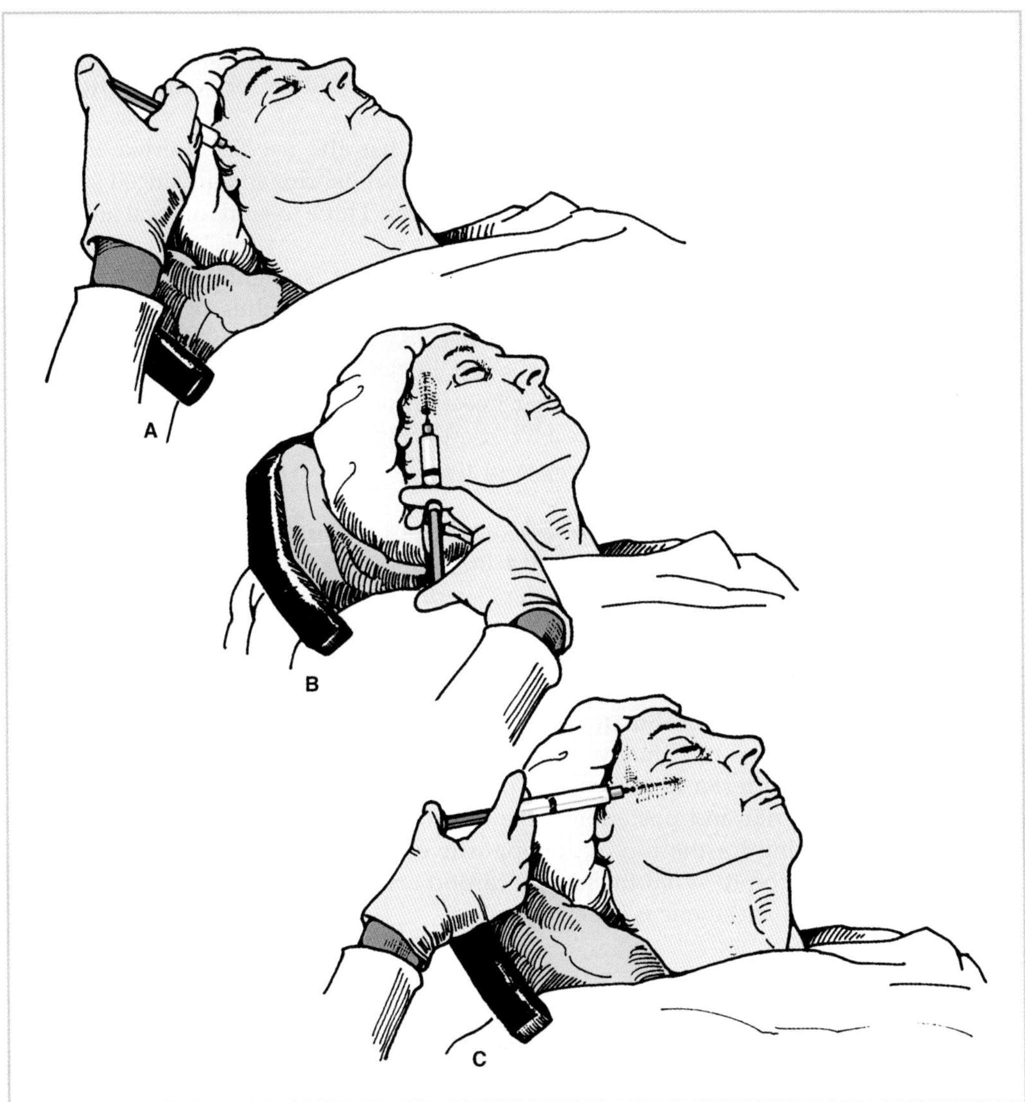

Figure 20.1. Modified Atkinson approach to facial nerve block. The needle is inserted 2 cm lateral to the lateral border of the orbit, which is usually 2 to 3 cm further lateral than the van Lint approach. Infiltration is first performed with 2 or 3 mL as the needle is withdrawn up from its first contact with the bone (**A**). Local anesthetic is then injected superiorly (**B**) and inferiorly (**C**) from this point to catch the spreading fibers of the facial nerve as they surround the eye.

1. A **modified Atkinson approach** (Figure 20.1) is a simple technique to block the terminal branches of the facial nerve. A 38-mm (1.5-in.) needle is inserted through a skin wheal 2 cm (0.8 in.) lateral to the orbital rim. The needle is advanced first superior toward the upper orbital rim, and 3 to 4 mL of anesthetic injected as it is withdrawn to the insertion point. It is then redirected toward the inferior orbital rim, and a repeat injection is made. Sensory blockade of the lid is achieved by a subcutaneous injection of 1% lidocaine or mepivacaine through this single skin puncture. This approach

has less chance of producing periorbital ecchymosis than the classic van Lint approach, and it is less likely to produce a total facial paralysis as would be obtained with a more proximal (such as O'Brien or Nadbath-Rehman) approach.

2. The approach described by **Atkinson** has the needle inserted over the zygomatic arch at the level of the lateral orbital rim and advanced subcutaneously upward toward the top of the ear. Three to 4 mL of local anesthetic is injected as the needle is withdrawn.
3. The **classic van Lint approach** (Figure 20.2) is slightly more medial, at a point 2 cm (0.8 in.) posterior to the lateral canthus of the eye. Three milliliters of local anesthetic is injected as the needle is withdrawn to the entry point. The needle is left in the skin and redirected inferiorly and anteriorly, with a similar injection of 3 mL on withdrawal. The two injections should produce a ''V'' bordering the eye. An additional 2 mL can be injected deeper at the apex of the ''V'' to provide anesthesia of deeper fibers.
4. **O'Brien** described a more proximal block of the facial nerve (near the ear). A needle is inserted 1 cm (0.4 in.) anterior to the tragus of the ear, and 2 mL of local anesthetic is deposited subcutaneously. The advantages of this block include producing paresis of the orbicularis oculi and having a less likelihood of producing periorbital ecchymoses, which are disturbing to the patient and family.
5. The **Nadbath-Rehman block** (Figure 20.3) anesthetizes the facial nerve even more proximally. It is performed by inserting a 16-mm (5/8-in.) needle anterior to the mastoid process at the base of the skull, and directing it superior and posterior in the direction of the stylomastoid foramen (as if aiming for the top of the opposite ear through the skull). After careful aspiration to avoid the nearby carotid artery, the needle is fixed and 3 mL of local anesthetic is injected.

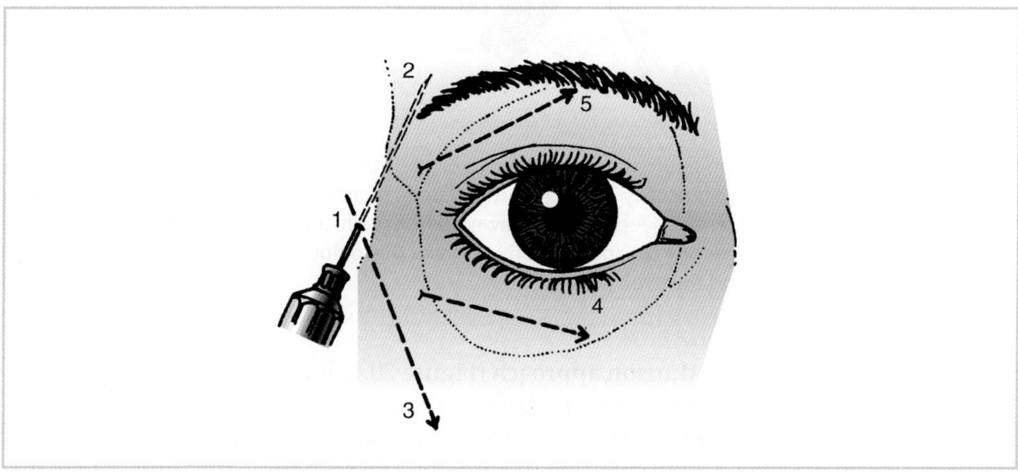

Figure 20.2. Classic van Lint approach to facial blockade. The needle is inserted 2 cm laterally to the lateral canthus of the eye and subcutaneous injection is performed in the superior and inferior borders of the orbit. (From Hersh PS. *Ophthalmic surgical procedures*. Boston: Little, Brown and Company, 1988:17, with permission.)

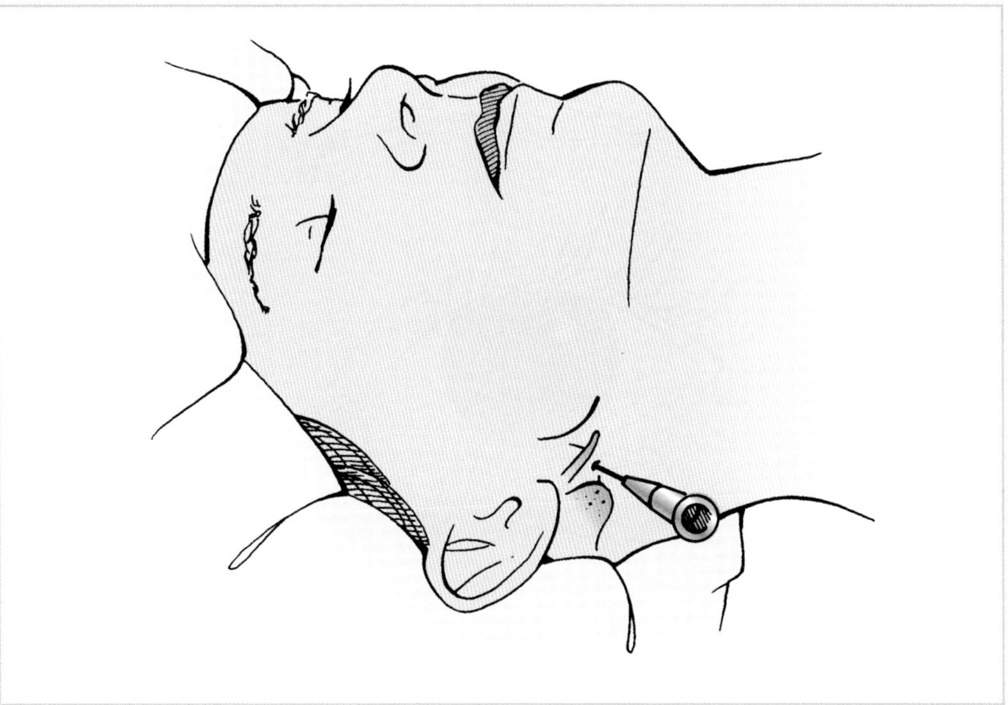

Figure 20.3. Nadbath-Rehman facial nerve block. As most proximal block of the facial nerve, there is often disconcerting facial drooping as a consequence of unneeded sensory and motor blockade of the lower face.

6. **Side effects**
   a. O'Brien and Nadbath techniques produce unneeded sensory and motor blockade of the lower face. The resulting **facial drooping** may be disconcerting to the patient and family.
   b. The more distal techniques, however, carry the risk of **ecchymosis** (black eye).
   c. The choice of injection site is a compromise between these side effects. An alternative is to avoid facial nerve injection by using large volumes of anesthetic with the peribulbar technique.

C. **Retrobulbar block** is a regional anesthetic technique for ophthalmic surgery that is more commonly practiced by ophthalmologists than anesthesiologists. Placement of the local anesthetic **within the muscular cone of the eye** can provide **faster onset, denser block, and require less anesthetic** than other regional techniques such as peribulbar or sub-Tenon blocks.

1. Instillation of **topical local anesthetic to the conjunctiva** is usually performed as an associated step. Tetracaine 1% or other ophthalmologic preparations are all adequate.
2. The **inferior border of the orbital rim** is located at a point approximately one-third of the distance from the lateral to the medial canthus. This point is usually directly inferior to the lateral border of the dilated pupil (Figure 20.4). The eye is held in neutral forward gaze; upward medial deviation may rotate the optic nerve and vessels into the intended path of the needle **(7)**.

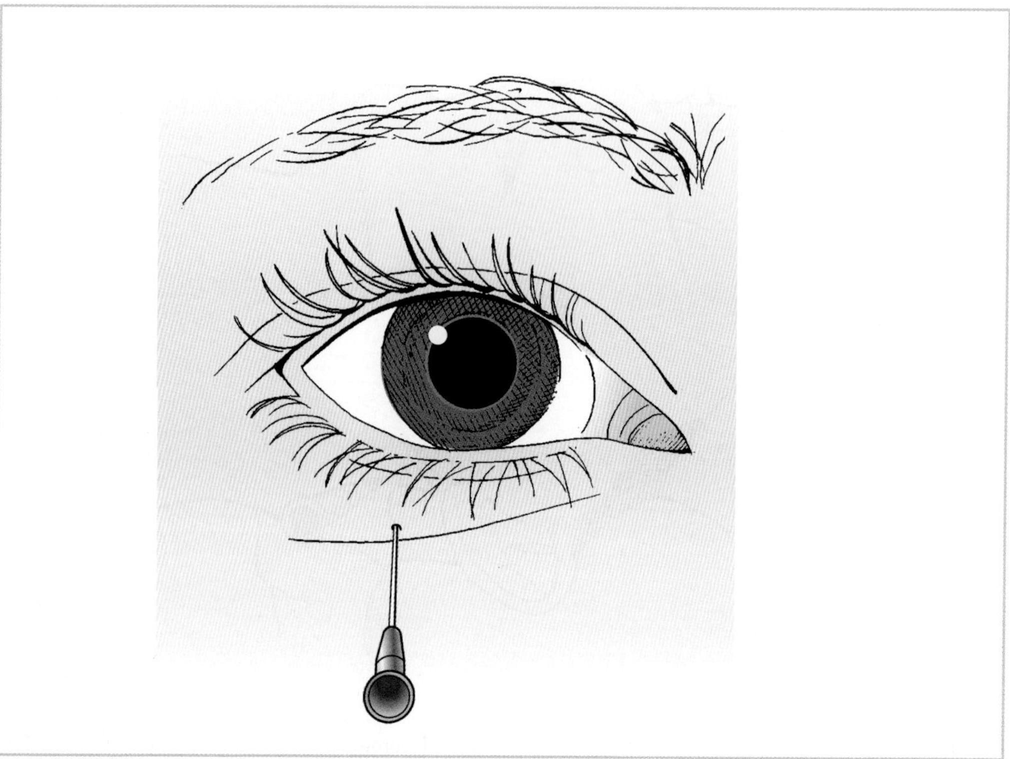

Figure 20.4. Needle placement for retrobulbar block.

3. A 38-mm (1.5-in.) 23-gauge blunt-tipped needle is **introduced perpendicularly into the skin and advanced directly posterior parallel to the floor of the orbit** (Figures 20.5A and 20.6).
4. **After the needle is advanced past the equator of the globe, it is angled superonasally at approximately a 45-degree angle to pass into the muscular cone (Figure 20.5B).** Entry into the muscle body will cause the globe to rotate inferiorly, rotating the eye down 15 to 30 degrees. Once the needle passes through the muscle body into the cone, there is an **abrupt release of this traction**, and the globe springs back to a neutral position (Figure 20.5C). If this release is not obtained, the needle is withdrawn and reinserted.
5. After careful aspiration, 3 to 4 mL of anesthetic is injected slowly. There should be no resistance to injection if the needle is in the cone. **Resistance might indicate undesirable intramuscular placement, or entry into the globe**, and the needle should be repositioned if it is felt.
6. **Scleral perforation should be suspected if the patient complains of pain on injection.** Many blocks are performed with sedation, which may mask this sign. Other indications are continued movement of the globe with needle movement once the muscle body is penetrated. Special blunt-tipped needles, which are designed to reduce the chance of perforation of the globe, are available for retrobulbar block, but the best protection is to **avoid too shallow an angle when advancing the needle**. The greatest risk exists with the myopic patient with an elongated globe. The axial length should be evaluated in all of these patients, and a **steeper angle maintained in**

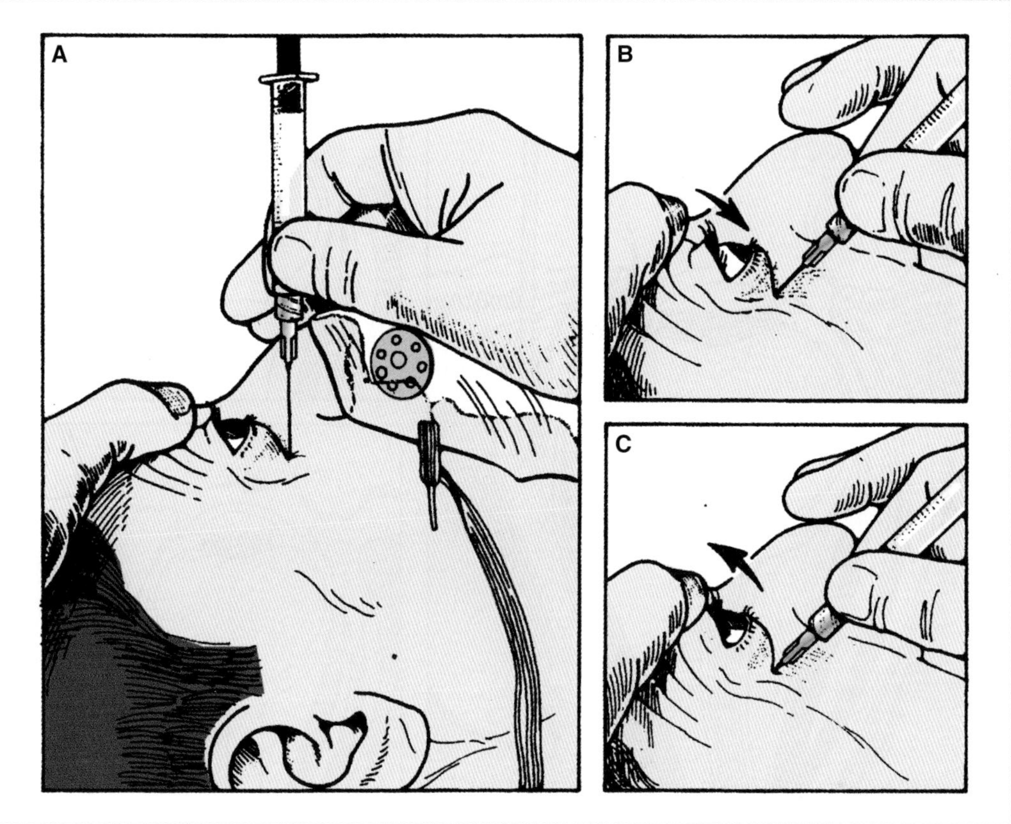

Figure 20.5. Retrobulbar block. **A:** The needle is inserted perpendicular to the skin at the lateral border of the dilated pupil just above the inferior orbital rim. **B:** Once the skin is penetrated, the angle of the needle is changed to approximately 45 degrees cephalad and advanced until the globe rotates down as the needle tip enters the muscle cone. **C:** When the tip penetrates into the central cone, the globe will dramatically rotate back to the neutral position. At this point, 3 mL of the local anesthetic mixture is injected into the retrobulbar area.

any patient whose axial length exceeds 25 mm (1 in.). Alternatively, a peribulbar block may reduce the chance of perforation in these patients.

7. Gentle pressure is applied to the globe for 5 minutes to facilitate spread of the solution, but it is released every 30 seconds to preserve retinal blood flow.
8. A slightly larger volume of anesthesia will produce more reliable block of the trochlear nerve (motor innervation of the superior oblique muscle), which lies outside the muscle cone containing the other motor nerves and the ciliary ganglion. Sparing of this muscle is not usually a problem because of its limited motion. If troublesome intorsion of the eye persists after classic retrobulbar block, the trochlear nerve can be blocked by injection of an additional 1 mL of anesthetic above the globe near the superior oblique muscle.

D. **Peribulbar block may reduce the risk of retrobulbar hemorrhage and globe perforation** associated with the classic retrobulbar approach. Anatomic studies suggest that the cone of muscles is not a closed space with dense septae, but

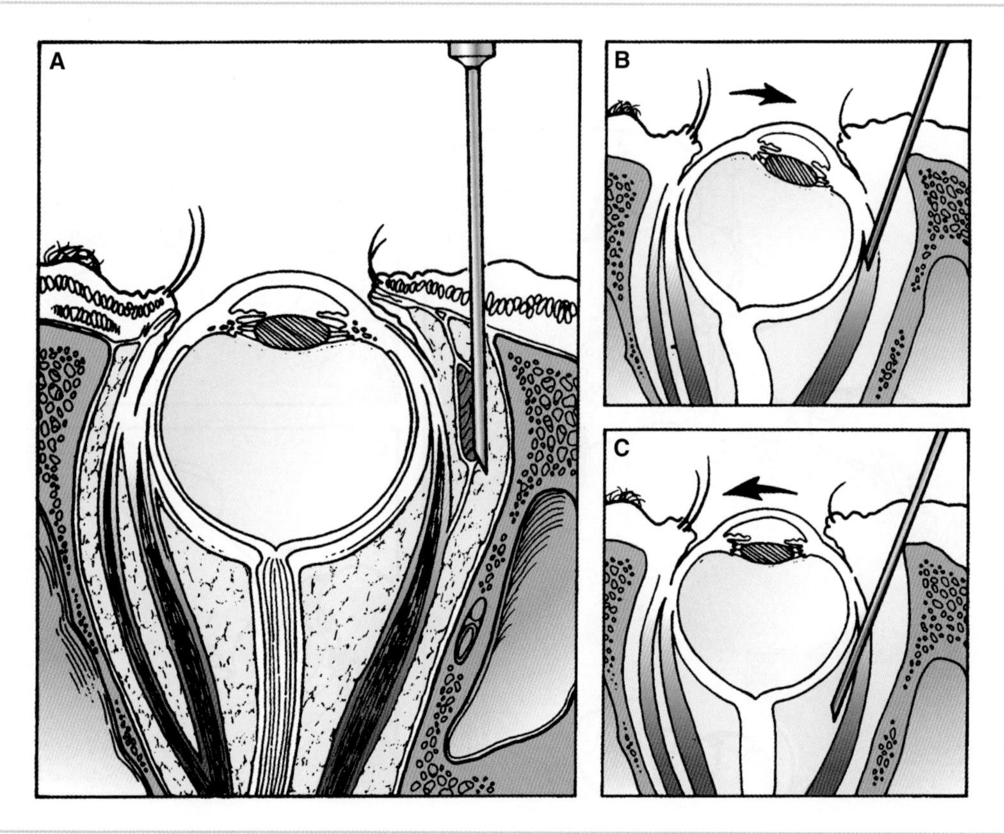

Figure 20.6. Needle direction associated with retrobulbar injection. The three positions **(A, B, and C)** correspond to the stages in Figure 20.5.

that there is easy access to the ciliary ganglion from outside the muscles **(8)**. The peribulbar needle **does not enter the muscle cone**, so theoretically this approach reduces the chance of complications. This presumed reduction of risks is balanced by a **slower onset of anesthesia and a need for reinjection** of 25% to 35% of these patients (7, 9, **10**) compared with 10% with retrobulbar injections.

1. **Topical anesthesia** is produced as for retrobulbar injection.
2. A 38-mm (1.5-in.) 25-gauge needle is inserted through the conjunctiva **at the inferior temporal area** above the inferior orbital rim (Figure 20.7). The needle is advanced in a slight upward direction (parallel to the rising orbital floor at this level) **without any attempt to enter the cone**, and 4 to 5 mL of local anesthetic is injected.
3. The needle is reinserted **in the superior nasal area** just below and medial to the supratrochlear notch, and an additional 4 to 5 mL is injected. Again, insertion is basically tangential to the globe without any attempt to enter the cone. **With both injections, the needle is advanced only 25 mm (1 in.) into the orbit.** This is generally sufficient to reach behind the equator of the globe, but the insertions are both tangential to the globe and are unlikely to enter the cone.

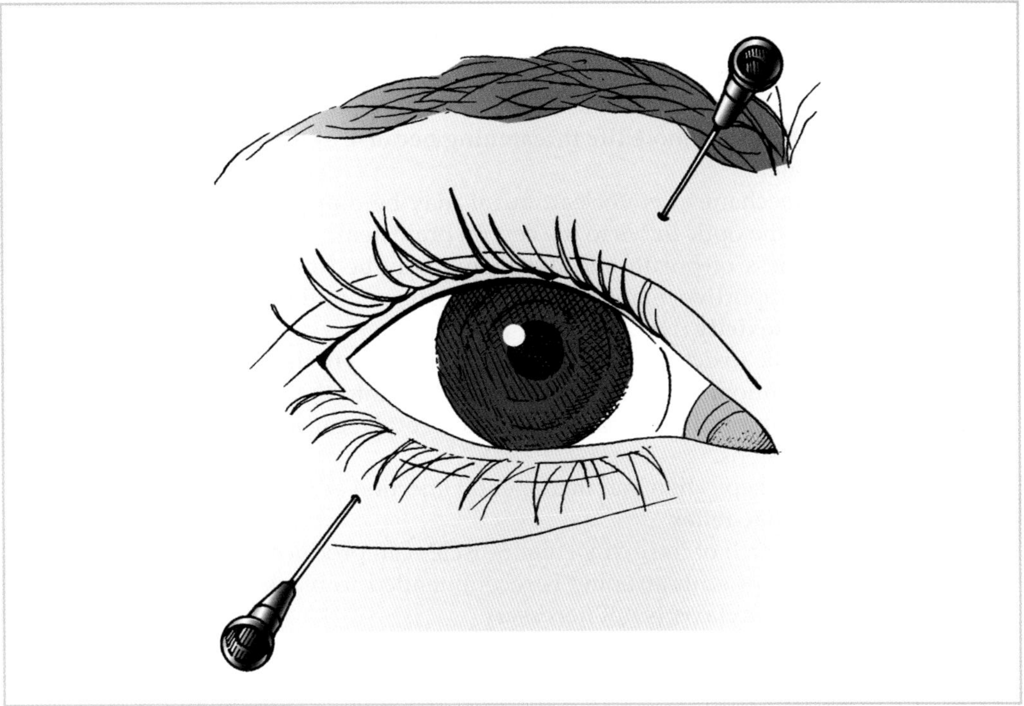

Figure 20.7. Needle entry sites for peribulbar block. Performed at two positions, inferotemporal and superonasal, the needle never enters the muscle cone of the eye and therefore larger volumes of local anesthetic are required.

4. The onset of anesthesia is slower, and the **block needs to be assessed at 10 minutes** for potential supplemental injection. Loss of vision does not always occur with this approach, but seventh nerve anesthesia is often obtained by diffusion of the anesthetic into the subcutaneous tissues of the upper lid without the need for separate injection.

E. A sub-Tenon block has been introduced as another alternative method to reduce the chance of globe injury. It is a more complex approach, involving a medial incision in the conjunctiva and Tenon capsule and insertion of a blunt-tipped catheter (11).

V. Complications

A. Retrobulbar hematoma formation

1. **Hemorrhage is the most frequent complication** of retrobulbar blockade and occurs as often as 1% of cases in some reported series, although it appears to be less frequent in larger series **(10)**.
2. Easily reversible defects of coagulation mechanisms should be reversed before retrobulbar injection.
3. **Retrobulbar hemorrhage during ophthalmic anesthesia is a serious complication, which may interfere with retinal blood supply if excessive pressure develops.** Signs include immediate proptosis, increased pressure in the globe, and appearance of subconjunctival blood. Monitoring of retinal pulsations and postponement of surgery are warranted, and

drainage through lateral canthotomy by the surgeon may be needed to relieve pressure.

B. **Brainstem anesthesia**
   1. Spread of the anesthetic to the brainstem area is less common (less than 0.5%), but it is more **life threatening because of the potential development of apnea**.
   2. The mechanism is unclear, but it may be due to the spread of anesthetic along the optic nerve to the central brainstem.
   3. Shortness of breath and dysphagia may be presenting signs. Ventilation and supportive therapy will usually suffice until the symptoms resolve.

C. **Systemic toxicity**
   1. Systemic toxicity is possible because of **the proximity of the retinal artery**. Unintentional injections under pressure into the arterial circulation of the head can produce rapid high intracerebral local anesthetic blood levels and convulsions.
   2. Careful aspiration and incremental injection are needed.

D. **Oculocardiac reflex**
   1. Any stretch of the extraocular muscles can produce **reflex bradycardia**.
   2. Treatment with atropine is recommended to block the vagal component, but **prophylaxis is not necessary**.

E. **Perforation of the globe**
   1. Perforation of the globe can occur, even with blunt-tipped needles and even with the peribulbar technique, but is generally less than 0.1% in frequency.
   2. **Risk factors also include elongated globe, multiple injections, previous scleral buckling, and the use of long-beveled needles (7).**
   3. It can be recognized by movement of the globe when the needle is moved before injection. Perforation will also usually produce pain and restlessness. Surgery should be canceled and appropriate ophthalmologic care rendered.

F. **Intramuscular injection.** Direct injection of the local anesthetic into the muscle body can produce **muscle destruction and ultimate paresis (10)**. Fortunately, this is rare and can be **avoided by halting any injection that meets resistance**.

REFERENCES

1 Kallio H, Paloheimo M, Maunuksela EL. Hyaluronidase as an adjuvant in bupivacaine-lidocaine mixture for retrobulbar/peribulbar block. *Anesth Analg* 2000;91(4):934–937.

2 Troll G, Borodic G. Diplopia after cataract surgery using 4% lidocaine in the absence of Wydase (sodium hyaluronidase). *J Clin Anesth* 1999;11(7):615–616.

3 Zahl K, Jordan A, McGroarty J, et al. Peribulbar anesthesia. Effect of bicarbonate on mixtures of lidocaine, bupivacaine, and hyaluronidase with or without epinephrine. *Ophthalmology* 1991;98(2):239–242.

4 Kucukyavuz Z, Arici MK. Effects of atracurium added to local anesthetics on akinesia in peribulbar block. *Reg Anesth Pain Med* 2002;27(5):487–490.

5 Mjahed K, el Harrar N, Hamdani M, et al. Lidocaine-clonidine retrobulbar block for cataract surgery in the elderly. *Reg Anesth* 1996;21(6):569–575.

6 Madan R, Bharti N, Shende D, et al. A dose response study of clonidine with local anesthetic mixture for peribulbar block: a comparison of three doses. *Anesth Analg* 2001;93(6):1593–1597.

7 Wong DH. Regional anaesthesia for intraocular surgery. *Can J Anaesth* 1993;40:635.

8 Ripart J, Lefrant JY, de La Coussaye JE, et al. Peribulbar versus retrobulbar anesthesia for ophthalmic surgery: an anatomical comparison of extraconal and intraconal injections. *Anesthesiology* 2001;94:56.

9 Ali-Melkkila TM, Virkkila M, Jyrkkio H. Regional anesthesia for cataract surgery: comparison of retrobulbar and peribulbar techniques. *Reg Anesth* 1992;17:219.

10 Hamilton RC, Gimbel HV, Strunin L. Regional anaesthesia for 12,000 cataract extraction and intraocular lens implantation procedures. *Can J Anaesth* 1988;35:615.

11 Guise PA. Sub-tenon anesthesia: a prospective study of 6,000 blocks. *Anesthesiology* 2003;98:964–968.

21 Pediatric Regional Anesthesia

Kathleen L. Larkin

The use of regional anesthesia has increased dramatically over the years. However in children, these same blocks tend to be underutilized. This is often due to fear of neurologic complications, lack of experience, or lack of appropriate pediatric-sized equipment. In pediatrics, it is standard to do a regional technique while under a general anesthetic. A large French prospective study demonstrated no increased incidence of complications with regional anesthesia done under general anesthesia **(1)**. The undisputed advantage of a successful regional technique added to a general anesthetic is that the child wakes up more comfortably. This may minimize complications from opioids and would be especially helpful in more vulnerable pediatric populations (neonates, expreemies, and children with cystic fibrosis).

Although regional techniques have similar advantages in pediatric patients as in adults, the methods used for performing these techniques in adults must be modified. The key to success of regional anesthesia in children is proper knowledge of anatomy, pharmacology, equipment, and preblock sedation or anesthesia. Because sedation is often required, two individuals are helpful; one to place the block and the other to monitor the child. All techniques, whether regional or general, have risks, and these risks must be weighed against the potential benefits of employing these techniques in anesthetized children, just as in adults. This chapter has a primary emphasis on how regional techniques performed in children differ from the previously described adult techniques. There are many excellent reviews of pediatric regional anesthetic techniques for those who wish to pursue these techniques in more detail (2–5).

I. Topical blocks

A. Topical local anesthesia can be utilized for the skin to **diminish needle pain** during intravenous (IV) catheter insertion or during regional techniques (6). Local anesthetics pose a somewhat increased risk of systemic toxicity in infants due to decreased plasma protein concentration, higher free fraction, slower hepatic metabolism, slightly reduced plasma pseudocholinesterase activity, and decreased methemoglobin-reductase activity (7).

1. The most commonly applied topical cream is **eutectic mixture of local anesthetics (EMLA) cream** (eutectic mixture of 2.5% lidocaine and 2.5% prilocaine). It is effective for anesthetizing the dermis to a depth of 5 mm. EMLA can cause the unwanted side effect of vasoconstriction. The benefit of decreasing a child's distress usually outweighs the disadvantage of vasoconstriction. It is recommended to apply EMLA cream a minimum of 45 minutes before needle insertion, but the longer it is on, the better the anesthesia. Because of this time constraint, EMLA may be underutilized. Some advocate giving parents a tube for application at home before bringing the child to the hospital for morning surgery.
2. **ELA-Max** (4% liposomal lidocaine) is a rapidly acting topical agent for intact skin that works by way of a liposomal delivery system. Studies demonstrate that a 30-minute application of ELA-Max is as safe and as effective as a

60-minute application of the EMLA (8). Additionally, ELA-Max is reported to cause less blanching of the skin.

3. Another alternative is **J-Tip**, a needleless injection system that can be used for delivery of local anesthetic. Eighty-four percent of pediatric patients reported no pain at the time of J-Tip lidocaine application compared to 61% in the EMLA group at the time of dressing removal (9).
4. **Numby stuff** is a device that allows iontophoresis of lidocaine 2% and epinephrine providing similar anesthesia of intact skin approximately 20 minutes after application. This device employs a small electric current to provide the iontophoresis that some younger children find objectionable.
5. All topical local anesthetic preparations have the limitation that they must be placed over the area to be anesthetized, and they take varying amounts of time to become effective. If the anesthesiologist misses the vein and has to go elsewhere, the skin at the new location will not be anesthetized.

B. Topical local anesthetics have also been successfully employed to provide surgical anesthesia for exposed **mucous membranes**.

1. Oral mucous membranes can be anesthetized to allow earlier placement of oral airways or laryngoscopy in infants and children with potentially difficult airways.
2. Topical intratracheal lidocaine (1–2 mg/kg) is often employed following induction of general anesthesia in infants who require diagnostic direct laryngoscopy in order for the otolaryngologist to view vocal cord movement.
3. EMLA has been employed for anesthesia for newborn **circumcisions** because it can penetrate the intact foreskin. Topical 0.5% lidocaine or 0.25% to 0.5% bupivacaine has been utilized to provide effective postoperative analgesia as well (10). Application of these local anesthetics must be done following amputation of the foreskin in order to expose the mucous membranes that will absorb these preparations. Because this is a topical technique, only enough local anesthetic is required to contact all of the "target" mucous membrane. If jelly or ointment is employed, parents need to be reassured regarding the appearance of the wound because the sight of the dried local anesthetic mixed with a tinge of blood may be unsettling. Repeated administration of the local anesthetic every 6 hours for 2 days will provide effective postoperative analgesia (11).

C. Topical local anesthetics have also been employed to provide effective **postoperative analgesia** for children undergoing **hernia or hydrocele repair**. Here, 0.25% to 0.5% bupivacaine or ropivacaine 0.2% to 0.5% in enough volume to fill the wound is instilled at the end of surgical dissection, just before wound closure, and is left in contact with the exposed ilioinguinal nerve and surrounding muscle tissue for 1 minute (12). The resulting analgesia is equivalent to a more formal block of the ilioinguinal nerve.

II. Spinal anesthesia

This technique is rarely used outside the neonatal period, but has an important role in decreasing postoperative apnea in neonates after herniorrhaphy. This is especially useful in the premature neonate who is at risk of periodic breathing, apnea, and bradycardia following general anesthesia. The techniques are the same as in adults, although with a short small gauge needle. Lower insertion levels (L4-5, L5-S1) are used in consideration of the lower level of the spinal cord terminus in the neonate. In contrast to other pediatric regional techniques, spinal blockade is usually performed without sedation or general anesthesia.

III. Caudal block

In the older and larger children, neuraxial blockade is usually performed following general anesthesia. Epidural anesthesia can be delivered by the thoracic, lumbar, or caudal route. As paresthesias cannot be detected in the anesthetized child, less experienced providers prefer approaching the epidural space caudally. The single-injection caudal block is one of the most popular and versatile pediatric regional anesthetic techniques. Placement of a catheter allows continuous infusion of local anesthetic or local anesthetic and opioid mixture. A combination of caudal blockade supplemented with light general anesthesia allows for a quicker wake up due to less volatile anesthetic agent required.

A. Anatomy. Caudal blocks are **technically easier** to perform in children than in adults. The poorly developed gluteal musculature and limited amount of subcutaneous fat means that landmarks defining the sacral hiatus are not obscured. There is less fusion in the region of the sacral hiatus, and less distortion of the bony landmarks in infants and children, who have not developed the gluteal fat pad that is common after puberty.

1. The fifth sacral cornua are very prominent, lying well above the gluteal cleft.
2. The sacrococcygeal ligament is not calcified in the infant or child; indeed, the distinct "pop" one encounters is quite similar to the tactile sensation experienced when entering a peripheral vein with an 18-gauge IV catheter in an adult.
3. The **dural sac** ends between the second and third sacral vertebrae (Table 21.1), whereas the length of the sacrum is reduced in proportion to the overall size of the child. It is possible to pierce the fragile sacrum or perform a dural puncture in an infant. Most catastrophic complications of caudal block have occurred in infants less than 10 kg in weight. Meticulous attention to technique is vital in these small patients (13).

B. Indications

1. A caudal block combined with a light general anesthetic provides excellent perioperative **analgesia** for children undergoing sacral segment surgery as well as most other surgeries below the diaphragm. This includes commonly performed groin surgeries, such as **herniorrhaphy**, **orchidopexy**, and **hydrocele** repair. Children undergoing lower-extremity **orthopedic** procedures (e.g., club foot) or **urologic** procedures also enjoy profound postoperative analgesia provided by a caudal block.
2. Caudal blocks are usually placed following induction of general anesthesia, and placement of an IV catheter. Only a very light plane of general anesthesia is required once the block has taken effect. The time spent placing the block

Table 21.1 Caudal anatomy in infants

	Dural sac ends at	Conus medularis ends at
Infant	S2	L2
Adult	S1	L1

before the beginning of surgery is recovered at the end of surgery because the child usually awakens quicker.

C. **Drugs.** In children, most local anesthetics should be dosed in milliliter per kilogram to avoid toxicity associated with larger volumes used in adult blocks.

1. **Bupivacaine.** A dose of 0.25% provides minimal motor blockade with adequate sensory blockade. An easy approximation of caudal dose is 1 mL/kg of 0.25% bupivacaine. The total dose of bupivacaine should not exceed 3 mg/kg. In the epidural space, it lasts 4 to 6 hours. Fifty percent of children will have analgesia for up to 12 hours if adequate doses are employed.
2. **Ropivacaine** 0.2%, in doses that do not exceed 2 mg/kg, has also been employed (14).
3. An easy calculation of volume is that employed by Armitage **(15)**. A dose of 0.5 mL/kg for sacral blockade, 0.75 mL/kg for lower thoracic segments, and 1.25 mL/kg for upper thoracic levels of blockade (Table 21.2).
4. The rate of **uptake** of local anesthetic is usually more rapid in children than adults. Using a **vasoconstrictor** can reduce the rate of uptake and prolong the duration of the block.
5. Neonates may have a **higher free drug level** and be more susceptible to the toxic effects of local anesthetics. The bolus dose and infusion should be reduced by 30% for infants younger than 6 months to decrease the risk of toxicity. This would result in an hourly maximal rate of 0.25 mg/kg of bupivacaine (16)

D. **Technique.** The block is usually performed following the induction of general anesthesia and IV placement.

1. The patient is turned into the lateral position, and the hips and knees are flexed similar to the position that would be appropriate for performance of a lumbar puncture (Figure 21.1).
2. The cornua of the sacral hiatus are the most easily palpated as two bony ridges at the beginning crease of the buttocks. It can be useful to identify the **equilateral triangle** between the two posterior superior iliac spines and the hiatus (see Figure 8.2).
3. A *"no-touch"* technique or sterile gloves may be used after aseptic preparation of the area. Start by breaking the skin with an 18-gauge needle to avoid tracking an epidermal plug into the epidural space. Then insert a 22-gauge IV catheter into the sacrococcygeal ligament at a 60-degree angle to the skin. The bevel should be maintained in a ventral position to avoid puncture of the anterior wall of the sacrum. If bone is encountered, the needle is withdrawn several millimeters and the angle with the skin is decreased before advancing again. A distinct "pop" will be felt as the needle punctures the membrane; the needle and catheter are then dropped into a plane parallel

Table 21.2 Block volumes

Block height	Volume (mL/kg)
Sacral	0.5
Lower thoracic	0.75
Upper thoracic	1.25

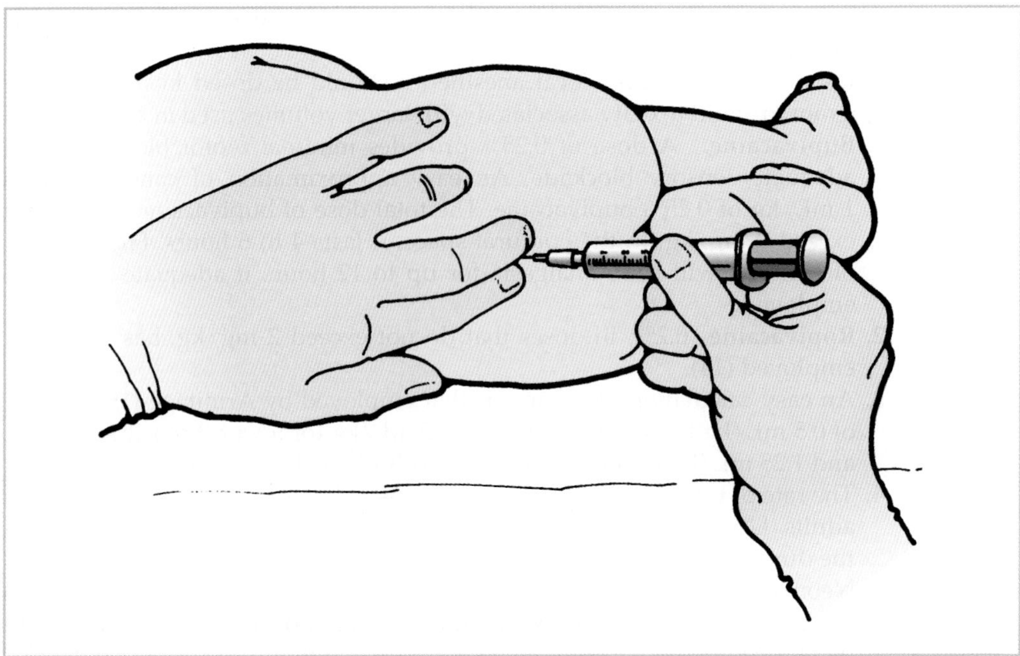

Figure 21.1. Pediatric caudal anesthesia, lateral position. This technique is performed following the induction of general anesthesia and placement of an intravenous catheter. It is easily done in children in either the lateral or the prone position. The sacrococcygeal membrane is easily identified with the characteristic "pop," and the injection is made after advancing the needle 1 to 2 mm.

to the spinal axis, and the needle shaft is advanced an additional 2 mm to be certain that the entire bevel of the needle is in the caudal space. Then the IV catheter is advanced gently into the caudal space, taking care not to puncture the dural sac.

4. **Test dose.** After negative aspiration for blood and cerebrospinal fluid (CSF), a test dose of the local anesthetic solution with epinephrine is injected (0.5 μg/kg) **(17)**. Attention should be paid to the heart rate and ECG tracing for 1 minute. An increase of 10 beats/min suggests intravascular injection. The sensitivity of the test dose is diminished in the anesthetized patient. A transient elevation of the T waves, especially in V5, can also alert the provider to an intravascular injection of bupivacaine. The noninjecting hand can be placed superior to the injection site to detect any crepitance that occurs when the injection is subcutaneous rather than epidural.
5. Frequent **aspiration** and **fractionated injection** of local anesthetic is the best safeguard against undetected intravascular injection because test doses can be unreliable in children (13,18,19). Intraosseous injections into the marrow have rapid uptake similar to intravascular injections.
6. **Caudal catheter.** A 22-gauge catheter can be threaded through the 18-gauge IV to allow repeated boluses of local anesthetics in longer cases or for postoperative infusions. Before placement, the catheter should be measured to determine length from sacral hiatus to the desired dermatome. Catheter tip site can be confirmed with fluoroscopy or ultrasonography. A test dose should be done through the catheter before dosing it. In patients younger

than 5 years, the catheter can usually be advanced to the thoracic level easily. Care should be taken with the dressing to minimize fecal soiling. A recommended infusion maximum of bupivacaine is 0.4 mg/kg/h, with even less in infants.

E. **Complications**

1. **Dural puncture** with resultant total spinal anesthesia is possible. Careful stabilization of the needle, careful advancement of the catheter, and frequent gentle aspiration will assist in avoiding this complication. A sacral dimple may be associated with spina bifida occulta and the risk of dural puncture may therefore be quite high.
2. Injection of local anesthetic **intravascularly** or **intraosseous** may lead to toxicity. Bupivacaine cardiac toxicity in children may be increased by the concomitant use of volatile anesthetics. The central nervous system (CNS) effect of the general anesthetic may obscure any signs of neurotoxicity until devastating cardiovascular effects are apparent. Dysrhythmias and cardiac arrest have occurred, usually in infants less than 10 kg. Extensive experience in older children before using this technique in infants is recommended.
3. Infection is possible but uncommon as most indwelling caudal catheters are removed within 2 to 3 days.

IV. Peripheral nerve blocks

The use of peripheral nerve blocks in children is growing with the increased manufacturing of pediatric-sized needles, catheters, and ultrasound probes.

A. **Techniques**

1. **Nerve stimulator.** Like in adults, a nerve stimulator is very helpful in placing these blocks. It is crucial to remember to avoid muscle relaxants before placing a block with a nerve stimulator in the anesthetized child.
2. **Ultrasound** -guided nerve blocks have increased in popularity in adult anesthesia. This device can be very helpful in nerve localization as well as visualizing the spread of local anesthetic in the desired tissue plane. It is increasingly being studied in children **(20)**, but the technology requires significant training to master. Smaller "hockey-stick" probes are available that are more suited to the smaller anatomic relationships in children. Additional advantages of ultrasound-guided nerve blocks include requiring less volume of local anesthetic for an adequate block and potentially decreasing intravascular or intraneuronal injections.

B. **Head and neck blocks.** The use of nerve blocks for head and neck procedures is on the rise in pediatrics. Most are field blocks of sensory nerves with easily identified landmarks that can significantly improve postoperative pain management.

1. **Supraorbital and supratrochlear** nerve block
   a. **Anatomy.** These are the end branches of the ophthalmic division (V1) of the trigeminal nerve. The supraorbital nerve exits the supraorbital foramen. The supratrochlear nerve exits 1 cm medially to the supraorbital nerve.
   b. **Indications.** This block can be useful in frontal craniotomies, ventriculoperitoneal shunt revisions, and scalp nevus excision.
   c. **Technique.** With the patient supine, palpate the supraorbital notch along the medial eyebrow in line with the midline pupil. Sterilely prepare the site. A 27-gauge needle is inserted just superior to the notch

so as to avoid the artery that travels through it. Aspirate before placing 1mL of 0.25% bupivacaine. The needle is then withdrawn to skin level, redirected medially, and advanced several millimeters. Another 1 mL of bupivacaine is injected to block the supratrochlear nerve.

d. **Complications.** The vascular periorbital tissue has the potential for hematomas. Pressure applied to the injection site can minimize this.

2. **Infraorbital nerve block.** This simple block provides profound pain relief for 12 to 18 hours in children undergoing cleft lip or palate repair or other surgery on the anterior hard palate, lower eyelid, side of nose, or upper lip (21). Local anesthetic injected directly into the surgical site by the surgeon does not last as long as with this peripheral nerve block.

   a. **Anatomy.** The infraorbital notch lies on a line connecting the supraorbital and mental foramina and the pupil of the eye (Figure 18.3).

   b. **Technique.** There are two techniques for blocking this nerve, intraoral and extraoral. Both are field blocks and are not intended to be injected in the notch or in the nerve.

      (1) **Extraoral.** First locate the infraorbital foramen with the index finger of the nondominant hand—approximately 0.5 cm from the midpoint of lower orbital margin. A 27-gauge needle is inserted at a 45-degree angle to the notch until touching bone. The needle is then withdrawn slightly so that the injection is not intraosseous, and 0.25 to 0.5 mL of local anesthetic is injected. A small skin wheal should be visible.

      (2) **Intraoral.** The second technique is transoral and will leave no mark on the face. Again the infraorbital foramen is palpated with the nondominant hand. The superior lip is elevated and a 1.5-in. 25-gauge needle is inserted parallel to the upper incisor and guided toward the nondominant index finger palpating the notch. Inject 0.5 to 1.5 mL of local anesthetic. If this technique is planned, it should be performed before the surgery so that there is no risk of disruption of the surgery by the manipulation of the upper lip.

C. Rectus sheath block

1. **Indications.** This block can be used commonly in pediatrics, especially for surgeries around the umbilicus. It blocks the 10th intercostal nerves from both sides as they become the anterior cutaneous branch. The nerve passes between the transverse abdominus muscle and the internal oblique muscle, between the sheath and the posterior wall of the rectus abdominus muscle.
2. **Technique.** A 23-gauge needle is perpendicularly inserted above or below the umbilicus 0.5 cm medial to the linea semilunaris. The anterior rectus sheath can be appreciated by "scratching" the needle back and forth on it. Pass the needle through the anterior sheath and the muscle belly. Again the posterior sheath should be identified by a sensation of scratching on the sheath with the needle tip. Local anesthetic is deposited anterior to this posterior sheath to avoid intraperitoneal injection. The needle depth is usually 0.5 to 1.5 cm. Block placement can be facilitated by ultrasonography (22).
3. **Drug.** After negative aspiration, 0.25% bupivacaine can be injected, 0.2 mL/kg on each side.
4. **Complications.** Injection can be too superficial in the belly of the muscle and not spread posteriorly to the nerve, resulting in a failed block. Then also, an intravascular injection is possible in the belly of the muscle.

D. Ilioinguinal and iliohypogastric nerve block. This block provides analgesia equivalent to that of caudal blockade for children undergoing **inguinal hernia, hydrocele, or orchidopexy repair**. If there is a contraindication to a caudal, such as a sacral dimple, or the child is old enough to be disconcerted about the loss of leg strength postoperatively, this block is advantageous.

1. **Technique.** These nerves can be blocked by topical anesthetic into the wound, as described in the preceding text. A formal block of the nerves can be performed following induction of general anesthesia and before surgery as described in Figure 21.2 (23). An alternative technique, where the surgeon infiltrates the wound edges at the end of dissection (which also instills local anesthetic into the wound) is more effective than when the surgeon infiltrates the skin edges before closing the skin. This block can also be performed with ultrasound guidance (24).
2. **Dose.** Bupivacaine 0.25% is most often employed, in a dose of 5 to 10 mL depending on patient size. Ropivacaine 0.5% has also been used in children for this block.
3. **Complications.** Three percent to 5% of children receiving this block by techniques other than application of topical anesthesia may demonstrate transient blockade of the femoral nerve, with temporary inability to stand due to loss of quadriceps strength.

E. Penile blocks. This block is useful for perioperative analgesia for boys undergoing **circumcision or hypospadias repair**. Although the American Academy

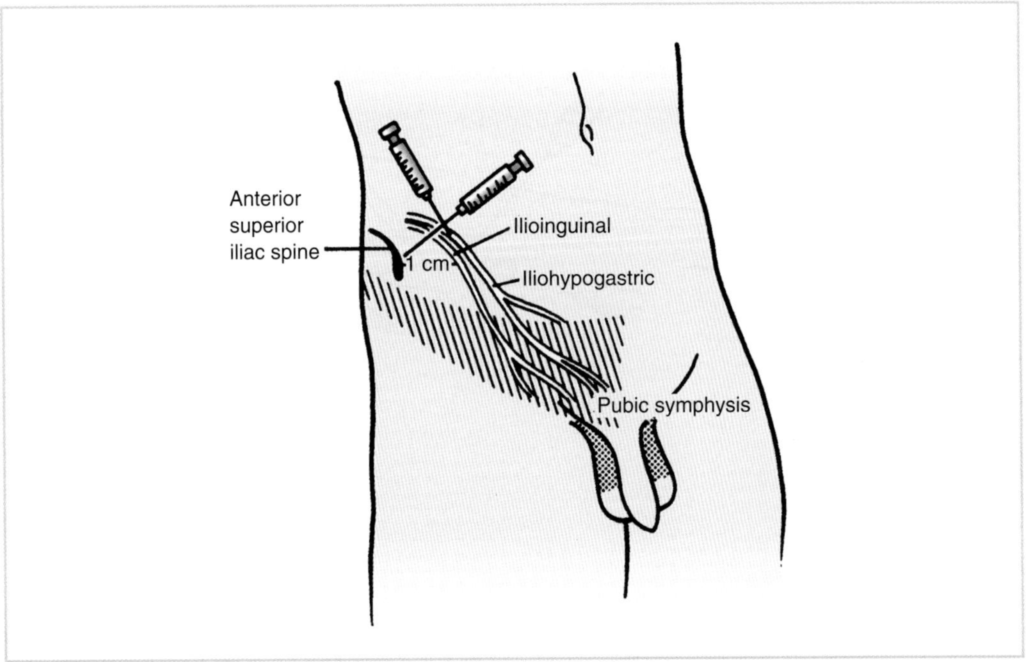

Figure 21.2. Ilioinguinal and iliohypogastric block. A 23- to 25-gauge needle is inserted 1 cm medial to the anterior superior iliac spine, and a wall of anesthesia is created by injecting in a fan-like manner along the muscle wall from the ilium to the border of the rectus. A total of 5 to 10 mL of 0.25% bupivacaine will provide anesthesia for the ilioinguinal (crosshatched) and the iliohypogastric (stippled) innervation. (Adapted from Yaster M, Maxwell LG. Pediatric regional anesthesia. *Anesthesiology* 1989;70:324, with permission.)

of Pediatrics does not endorse circumcision, it does endorse the use of local anesthetics if the family desires a circumcision in the neonatal period. Both the topical application of EMLA cream and the ring block of the penis are simple and have minimal risk to the newborn.

1. **Technique.** Two approaches are commonly used.
   a. **Ring block.** The simplest way to block the dorsal penile nerves is to place a subcutaneous wheal of 0.25% to 0.5% bupivacaine **without** epinephrine that rings the base of the penis (25). This subcutaneous block places local anesthetic just superficial to the tough Buck fascia that surrounds the corpora, and the dorsal nerve, arteries, and veins of the penis. The local anesthetic diffuses across this fascia to provide anesthesia.
   b. **Dorsal penile nerve block.** Another technique involves blockade of the dorsal penile nerves in the subpubic area (Figure 21.3) (3). This involves downward traction on the penis, and the injection of local anesthetic under Scarpa fascia (which is continuous with Buck fascia in the shaft of the penis). Two injections are made 0.5 to 1 cm lateral to the midline below the symphysis pubis. A 23- to 25-gauge needle is inserted slightly medially and caudally until the characteristic "pop" is felt as the needle traverses Scarpa fascia just below the pubis and 2 to 5 mL of local anesthetic is injected.
2. **Complications.** There have been no complications observed with the ring technique. Blockade of the dorsal penile nerve deep to Buck fascia in the shaft of the penis has been associated with decreased perfusion to the tip of the glans penis.

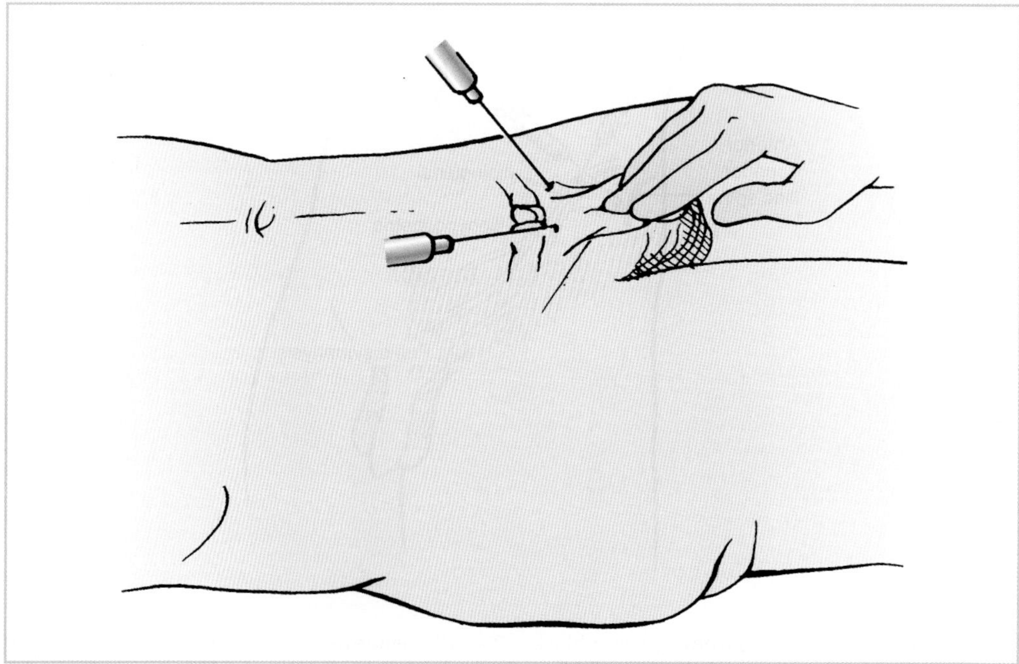

Figure 21.3. Suprapubic penile block. The penis is retracted downward and injections are made on each side of the base, 0.5 to 1 cm lateral to the midline and below the symphysis pubis. The needle is inserted slightly medially and caudally to pierce Scarpa fascia.

F. Extremity blocks The basic techniques of extremity blockade in infants and children are similar to those used in adults, with the exception that these blocks are placed once the child is anesthetized. Therefore, a nerve stimulator or ultrasound is important in neural blockade in infants and children. The principles of use of both of these are detailed in Chapter 5.

1. **Indications**
   a. **Upper extremity blocks** can provide muscle relaxation and analgesia for the reduction of fractures as well as in the immediate perioperative period following an open procedure.
   b. A **femoral nerve block**, alone or in conjunction with a lateral femoral cutaneous nerve block, or a "three-in-one" block can provide anesthesia for muscle biopsy. Femoral nerve blockade also provides excellent analgesia and muscle relaxation for children with femur fractures, especially if the fracture is in the middle third of the femoral shaft.
   c. With the addition of a **sciatic block**, all lower extremity surgery is possible. Usually, however, caudal blockade with its single needle is preferred for lower extremity surgery in the pediatric population before they are school aged.
2. **Drugs.** The longer-acting agents, bupivacaine and ropivacaine with epinephrine 1:200,000, provide effective anesthesia and analgesia for up to 12 hours. It must be remembered that toxicities are additive when compounding local anesthetics (Table 21.3). Ropivacaine has been widely studied in caudals but there is little research on its use in extremity blocks for pediatric patients (23).
3. **Techniques**
   a. **Brachial plexus block**
      (1) The most common approach to the brachial plexus in children is the axillary or infraclavicular approach, as compared to the interscalene approach in adults. The placement of these blocks is the same as in adults (see Chapter 12).
      (2) For an **axillary block**, the nerve stimulation approach is preferred to the transarterial approach as there is a higher incidence of vessel

Table 21.3 Drug doses and volumes for pediatric regional techniques

Agent	Maximum doses (mg/kg) with added epinephrine 1:200,000
Lidocaine	7–10
Bupivacaine	2–3
Compound	
Lidocaine	5
Tetracaine	2
Peripheral nerve block	**Volume (mL/kg)[a]**
Axillary	0.33
Interscalene	0.25
Inguinal paravascular	0.50
Sciatic	0.20

[a]Volume of 0.25% bupivacaine or lidocaine–tetracaine.

spasm in children than adults, causing limb jeopardy. A nerve stimulator is useful, but simple infiltration on either side of the easily palpable artery will usually produce adequate anesthesia. Appropriate volumes of local anesthetics are noted in Table 21.3; these volumes usually include blockade of the musculocutaneous nerve.

(3) The infraclavicular approach is the other popular alternative in children, and is performed essentially as described for adults in Chapter 12. In children, ultrasound guidance with this block is more comfortable and produces faster onset and longer duration of blockade (26).

(4) **Dosing.** Children younger than 6 to 7 years should have no more than 0.3 to 0.5 mL/kg of 0.25% bupivacaine or 0.2% ropivacaine. Older children may have more milligrams per kilogram, and therefore 0.5% bupivacaine or ropivacaine may be used at 0.3 to 0.5 mL/kg, with a maximum of 20 mL. Epinephrine 1:200,000 should be added to increase duration of the block and to detect intravascular placement.

b. Lower extremity blocks

(1) The **femoral nerve block** is described in Chapter 15; few modifications are required for pediatric patients. This is the most common lower extremity block in children and can be quite useful in femur fractures or muscle biopsies. A nerve stimulator is useful, but simple infiltration lateral to the artery is effective. A volume of 0.2 to 0.4 mL/kg is injected with epinephrine to detect intravascular placement.

(2) The **sciatic nerve** is easily blocked more peripherally than in the classic Labat description. Children rarely have the gluteal fat pad that develops at puberty and one can frequently see their sciatic groove. Place the child in the lateral (Sims) position; the ankle of the upper leg is placed on the knee of the lower leg. The child can also be supine with the leg elevated. Locate and mark the greater trochanter and the ischial tuberosity of the upper leg. A 22-gauge needle (3.5-in. spinal needle, if the child is big enough) is connected to a nerve stimulator, and inserted midway between the two landmarks until dorsiflexion or plantar flexion of the foot is noted. All flexion should be abolished with 1 mL of local anesthetic solution if the needle is in the proper place. Motor activity above the knee is most likely due to direct muscle stimulation and is not a reliable indicator that the needle is in the proper position. A total of 0.5 mL/kg to a maximum of 20 mL should be injected.

(3) The use of **ultrasound** guidance for both these techniques can allow for lower doses (because the injection is done under direct imaging of the nerves) and results in a longer duration of blockade (27).

(4) The **popliteal fossa** can be the ideal location for blocking the sciatic nerve (28). A more distal approach allows smaller volumes to be used without diminishing efficacy. Children are usually anesthetized and supine, so the lateral approach would be advantageous. However, most providers prefer the posterior approach, and in small children the leg can be lifted with ease to expose the popliteal fossa.

This block is described in Chapter 16. Nerve localization can be achieved with nerve stimulator or ultrasound guidance. In children the volume injected should be 0.2 to 0.3 mL/kg.

(5) Dosing. Because of the complex nerve supply from two plexuses, anesthetizing the leg requires more volume of local anesthetic than upper extremity blocks. If multiple blocks are planned, remember that doses are additive toward toxicity.

4. Continuous catheters

a. There are many reports of improved postoperative pain management in children with continuous infusion of local anesthetics through a peripheral nerve catheter, both in the upper and lower extremities (29). Even patient-controlled analgesia (PCA) has been used with a peripheral nerve catheter in children (30). Continuously infusing catheters serve to eliminate the pain crisis that sometimes occurs the first night when the original local anesthetic wears off. Catheter sets are now available in pediatric sizes.

b. Dose. For postoperative analgesia through a continuous catheter, the suggested starting dose of local anesthetic is 0.1 mL/kg/h of bupivacaine 0.25% or ropivacaine 0.2%, not to exceed 10 mL/h. The maximum dose is 0.4 mg/kg/h. These doses should be reduced in newborns and infants.

V. Summary

The role of regional anesthesia in pediatrics is established and growing. Despite their many advantages, peripheral nerve blocks are currently underutilized in children. Although these techniques are very safe, they are not without risk **(1,31)**. The use of ultrasonography should decrease some of these risks. Thoughtful consideration of the risk and benefits of any technique are the responsibility of all caregivers.Optimal analgesia is achieved by a multimodal approach to pain. Preoperative administration of acetaminophen or nonsteroidal anti-inflammatory drugs, followed by appropriate regional analgesia, will be helpful.

Clear postoperative instructions must be given to the parents about the block wearing off and the timing of oral analgesics. Regular dosing of acetaminophen and opioids can minimize a pain crisis when the block wears off. Explain to the parents the importance of treating pain early and staying ahead of the pain with oral analgesics and of encouraging children to report sensations of discomfort early. Children can potentially benefit from the opioid-sparing benefits of regional anesthesia like adults, as long as the provider is capable of placing these blocks safely.

REFERENCES

1 **Giaufre E, Dalens B, Gombert A. Epidemiology and morbidity of regional anesthesia in children: a one-year prospective study of the French-Language Society of Pediatric Anesthesiologists. *Anesthesiology* 1996;83:904.**

2 Broadman LM, Rice LJ. Neural blockade for pediatric surgery. In: Cousins MJ, Bridenbaugh PO, eds. *Neural blockade in clinical anesthesia and management of pain*, 3rd ed. Philadelphia: Lippincott Williams & Wilkins, 1998.

3 Dalens BJ. Regional anesthesia in children. In: Miller RDM, ed. *Anesthesia*, 5th ed. New York: Churchill Livingstone, 2000.

4 Rice LJ. Regional anesthesia. In: Motoyama E, Davis P, eds. *Smith's anesthesia for infants and children*, 6th ed. St. Louis: Mosby, 1995.

5 Sethna NF, Berde CB. Pediatric regional anesthesia. In: Gregory GA, ed. *Pediatric anesthesia.* New York: Churchill Livingstone, 1994.
6 Squire SJ, Kirchhoff KI, Hissong K. Comparing two methods of topical anesthesia used before intravenous cannulation in pediatric patients. *J Pediatr Health Care* 2000;14:68.
7 Carceles MD. Amethocaine-lidocaine cream, a new topical formulation for preventing venopuncture-induced pain in children. *Reg Anesth Pain Med* 2002;27(3):289–295.
8 Eichenfield LF. A clinical study to evaluate the efficacy of ELA-Max (4% liposomal lidocaine) as compared with eutectic mixture of local anesthetics cream for pain reduction of venipuncture in children. *Pediatrics* 2002;109(6):1093–1099.
9 Jimenez N. A comparison of a needle-free injection system for local anesthesia versus EMLA for intravenous catheter insertion in the pediatric patient. *Anesth Analg* 2006;102(2):411–414.
10 Andersen KH. A new method of analgesia for relief of circumcision pain. *Anaesthesia* 1989;44:118.
11 Tree-Trakarn T, Pirayavaraporn S, Lertakyamanee J. Topical analgesia for relief of post-circumcision pain. *Anesthesiology* 1987;67:395.
12 Casey WF, Rice LJ. A comparison between bupivacaine instillation versus ilioinguinal/iliohypogastric nerve block for postoperative analgesia following inguinal herniorrhaphy in children. *Anesthesiology* 1990;72:636.
13 Veyckemans F, Van Obbergh LJ, Gouverneur JM. Lessons from 1100 pediatric caudal blocks in a teaching hospital. *Reg Anesth* 1992;17:119.
14 Koinig H, Krenn CG, Glaser C, et al. The dose response of caudal ropivacaine in children. *Anesthesiology* 1999;90:1339.
15 Armitage EN. Local anesthetic techniques for prevention of postoperative pain. *Br J Anesth* 1986;58:790.
16 Berde CB. Convulsions associated with pediatric regional anesthesia. *Anesth Analg* 1992;75:164–166.
17 Tobias JD. Caudal epidural block: a review of test dosing and recognition of systemic injection in children. *Anesth Analg* 2001;93:1156–1161.
18 Brendel JK, Yemen TA, Berry FA. Intravenous injection of local anesthetic: identification with isoproterenol and epinephrine in children during halothane anesthesia. *Reg Anesth* 1993;18:49.
19 Freid EB, Bailey AG, Valley RD. Electrocardiographic and hemodynamic changes associated with unintentional intravascular injection of bupivacaine with epinephrine in infants. *Anesthesiology* 1993;79:394.
20 Marhofer P, Willschke H, Kettner S. Imaging techniques for regional nerve blockade and vascular cannulation in children. *Curr Opin Anaesthesiol* 2006;19:293–30020.
21 Ahuja A, Datta A, Krishna A, et al. Infraorbital block for relief of postoperative pain following cleft lip surgery in infants. *Anaesthesia* 1993;49:441.
22 Willschke H, Bosenberg A, Marhofer P, et al. Ultrasonography-guided rectus sheath block in paediatric anaesthesia—a new approach to an old technique. *Br J Anaesth* 2006;97:244–249.
23 Langer JC, Shandling B, Rosenberg M. Intraoperative bupivacaine during outpatient hernia repair in children: a randomized double blind trial. *J Pediatr Surg* 1987;22:267.
24 Willschke H, Bosenberg A, Marhofer P, et al. Ultrasonographic-guided ilioinguinal/iliohypogastric nerve block in pediatric anesthesia: what is the optimal volume? *Anesth Analg* 2006;102:1680–1684.
25 Broadman LM, Hannallah RS, Belman B, et al. Post-circumcision analgesia—a prospective evaluation of subcutaneous ring block of the penis. *Anesthesiology* 1987;67:399.
26 Marhofer P, Sitzwohl C, Greher M, et al. Ultrasound guidance for infraclavicular brachial plexus anaesthesia in children. *Anaesthesia* 2004;59:642–646.
27 Oberndorfer U, Marhofer P, Bosenberg A, et al. Ultrasonographic guidance for sciatic and femoral nerve blocks in children. *Br J Anaesth* 2007;98:797–801.
28 Fernandez-Guisasola J. A comparison of 0.5% ropivacaine and 1% mepivacaine for sciatic nerve block in the popliteal fossa. *Acta Anaesthesiol Scand* 2001;45:967–970.
29 Dadure C. Perioperative pain management of a complex orthopedic surgical procedure with double continuous nerve blocks in a burned child. *Anesth Analg* 2004;98:1653–1655.
30 Duflo F. Patient-controlled regional analgesia is effective in children: a preliminary report. *Can J Anesth* 2004;51:928–930.
31 Krane EJ, Dalens BJ, Murat I, et al. The safety of epidurals placed during general anesthesia. *Reg Anesth* 1998;23:433.

22 Ambulatory Surgery

Michael F. Mulroy

I. Introduction

Ambulatory surgery had grown to 65% of surgical practice in the United States. Anesthesia in this setting must provide a rapid recovery, early ambulation, and freedom from pain and nausea. Regional techniques should be ideal in this situation. Meta-analysis of published studies has confirmed **lower pain scores** and **less nausea and vomiting** following outpatient surgery, but suggests that there is additional **time** required to perform regional blocks, and (in the case of neuraxial blockade) a potential **prolonged discharge** time **(1)**. Although many of the techniques in this handbook are suitable for the outpatient setting, careful attention to choice of the drugs and performance of the blocks is necessary to make regional techniques effective in ambulatory surgery. Specific challenges include:

A. Time requirement. Regional techniques frequently require more time to perform than general endotracheal anesthesia, and the onset surgical anesthesia can be delayed, especially with long-acting drugs. These challenges are reduced by the following ways:

1. Using an **induction room** setup. Several studies have shown that performance on the block outside the operating room can make the time difference competitive with general anesthesia (2–5) and in some circumstances produce shorter turnover times. The faster emergence from a procedure performed by regional block alone is the reward, as the patient is usually ready to go immediately to the postanesthetic care unit (PACU), and more frequently to the phase 2 or discharge area.
2. The use of simple regional techniques such as spinal anesthesia and intravenous regional techniques (3).
3. **Short-acting rapid-onset** drugs, such as chloroprocaine and lidocaine, also eliminate time delays, allowing rapid onset, usually in the time required for positioning, surgical preparation, and draping.

B. Success rate has also been a challenge for acceptance for regional techniques in the outpatient setting. Reliance on simple techniques, such as intravenous regional anesthesia or spinal anesthesia, improves efficiency and reliability of these blocks. The use of ultrasound-guided peripheral nerve block techniques may ultimately shorten the time for performance of blocks and increase the reliability, but this issue is unclear at the current time.

II. Neuraxial blockade.

II. Neuraxial blockade. Central blocks should be the most reliable and effective, but require a careful choice of drugs. Another issue is that full-block resolution is required before discharge, again mandating a careful choice of local anesthetic and dosage.

A. Spinal anesthesia is the easiest to perform and most reliable technique for outpatients. It is suitable for lower extremity surgeries such as knee and ankle arthroscopy and foot surgery, as well as hernia repair, perineal, and perirectal procedures. Low-dose hypobaric spinal anesthesia has even been used for outpatient laparoscopy (6).

1. Performance **time** in experienced hands is competitive with general endotracheal anesthesia. The block can be performed with any of the techniques described earlier (see Chapter 6), including a hypobaric injection in the jackknife position for rectal surgery (7).
2. **Drug selection** is critical.
   a. **Bupivacaine** is rarely indicated because of its long duration, especially because of its wide variability in duration of blockade. Clinical studies describe an average duration and discharge time of approximately 2 hours, but with a standard deviation of almost an hour (8,9). This drug should be reserved for longer procedures and should be used in small doses such as 5 or 6 mg (8).
   b. **Lidocaine** has been the traditional drug for outpatients, especially for procedures of 60- to 90-minute duration when the lithotomy position or knee arthroscopy are not involved. The unfortunate association of lidocaine with transient neurologic symptom (TNS) has led many to search for alternatives (see Chapter 3). Nevertheless, it is an appropriate choice for selected short procedures.
   c. **2-Chloroprocaine** has seen resurgence in interest as a short-acting drug, now that preservative-free preparations are available. Preliminary studies show duration of approximately 60 minutes of surgical anesthesia following 40 mg, with resolution of block in 2 hours (Figure 22.1) (10,11). The incidence of TNS appears to be rare. Discharge times are competitive with even the fast-acting general anesthetics. Fentanyl can be added to provide some increased duration, but epinephrine needs to be avoided with this drug (see Chapter 2). The question of neurotoxicity with 2-chloroprocaine remains because of previous problems with preservative-containing solutions (12). Use at this time should be limited to preservative-free preparations.

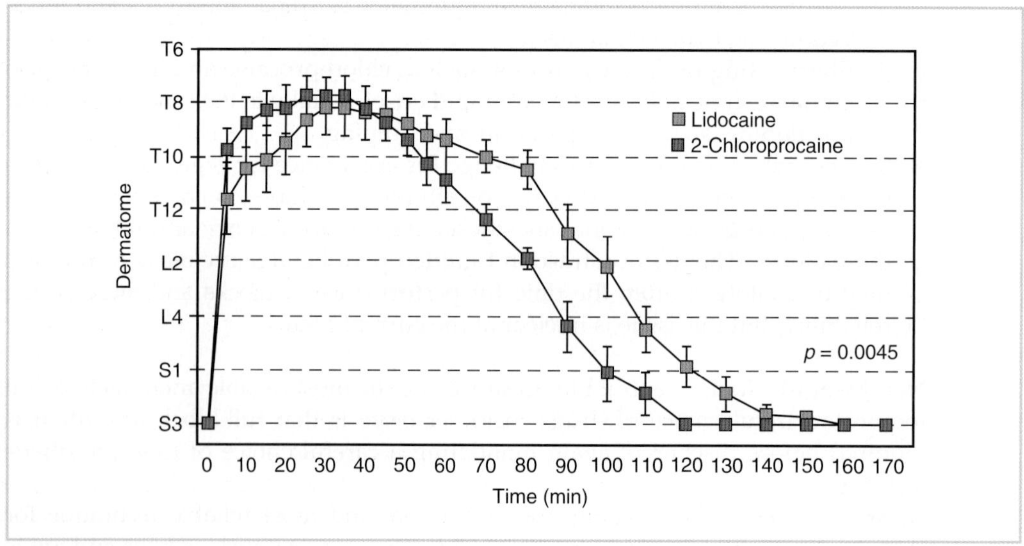

Figure 22.1. Extent and duration of subarachnoid anesthesia with 40 mg lidocaine or 2-chloroprocaine in volunteers. (Adapted from Kouri ME, Kopacz DJ. Spinal 2-chloroprocaine: a comparison with lidocaine in volunteers. *Anesth Analg* 2004;98:75–80.)

3. *Unilateral* **spinal block** has also been advocated for outpatient procedures, particularly of the foot or knee. This requires maintaining the patient in a lateral position for 5 to 15 minutes to allow concentration of a hyperbaric solution in the dependent leg (13,14). This technique allows use of a lower dose of drug, but does not appear to provide faster recovery despite reduced pain and nausea in PACU. Its use may be limited to patients at high risk for nausea, and to where the block can be performed in an induction area.
4. **Complications** are the same in outpatients, but specific considerations may limit spinal anesthesia for outpatients.
   a. **Postspinal headache.** The use of small round beveled needles has significantly reduced this complication, but it is still a potential, particularly in the younger patient group. Careful selection should be used, and the smallest diameter needle, consistent with easy performance of the block, should be used, usually 25 gauge or smaller. Patients must always be given appropriate contact information for follow-up in case symptoms develop. A mechanism for providing treatment should be in place.
   b. **Urinary retention** is traditionally associated with spinal blockade, but usually with longer-duration blocks. Retention is also higher in older men, and perineal procedures such as hernia repair and anal surgery. Experience with short-acting spinal anesthesia (2-chloroprocaine, procaine, lidocaine, small dose bupivacaine) for low-risk surgery shows that the risk of urinary retention is no greater than that with general anesthesia **(15)**.
   c. **TNS.** This syndrome has occurred in association with every local anesthetic, and is particularly a concern in the outpatient because the onset usually occurs after discharge. Patients should be advised of the potential and assured that it is temporary, but a follow-up phone call is advisable to discover its occurrence and give reassurance to the patient if it occurs.

B. **Epidural block.** Spinal anesthesia is limited to a single-injection technique, requiring a single estimate of appropriate drug and dose to accommodate the surgical procedure, yet not to prolong discharge. In situations where surgical duration is unclear, epidural anesthesia, especially with a catheter, provides a reasonable alternative. Epidural injection is also less likely to produce a postdural puncture headache; however, it is technically more difficult to perform and requires more time, and the onset of blockade is longer.

1. **Drug choices.** Performance of epidural block aid in induction room with **2-chloroprocaine** will provide adequate sensory anesthesia by the time the patient is moved to the operating room and surgical preparation and draping completed. The use of epidurals with 2-chloroprocaine for knee arthroscopy (16) or extracorporeal shock wave lithotripsy (ESWL) (Figure 7.4 of Chapter 7) (17) is competitive with general anesthesia discharge times with propofol. **Lidocaine** may be acceptable for longer procedures, such as anterior cruciate ligament (ACL) repair, where a 60- to 90-minute duration can be anticipated. If longer duration is required, it is wiser to use a continuous technique with a short-duration drug and supplement as necessary. The resolution times required for mepivacaine or bupivacaine are unacceptable in most outpatient units.
2. **Postoperative analgesia.** With both epidural and spinal injections, block resolution (as required for discharge) is also associated with loss of any

analgesic effect. Supplemental local anesthetic blockade of the incision performed by the surgeon should be encouraged, including local anesthetic in the joint in case of arthroscopy procedures (18). Supplemental peripheral nerve block of the extremities is useful (19). Patients should be treated with a multimodal analgesic regimen, which should include nonsteroidal analgesics (20,21), as well as small doses of oral opioids before discharge. Excessive opioids negate the advantages of avoiding nausea. Other nonopioids such as gabapentin, clonidine, and magnesium have been shown to be useful (see Chapter 23).

C. **Combined spinal-epidural** anesthesia has also been used in the outpatient, especially when rapid onset of sacral and lumbar anesthesia is needed, but the required duration is unclear. Specific examples include knee arthroscopy (22) and ESWL. A small dose of a short-acting drug can be used in this situation without anxiety of the procedure outlasting the anesthetic. Although this technique requires a somewhat longer time to place, it does provide the rapid onset that can overcome some of the objections to regional anesthesia for outpatients.

III. Peripheral nerve blockade

Unlike neuraxial techniques, peripheral blocks can be performed with long-acting drugs to provide both surgical anesthesia and **prolonged analgesia** even after discharge, and therefore, may help avoid the problems of nausea and vomiting associated with opioid analgesia. With a numb extremity, however, it is critical to provide ambulation aids for the patient and careful dressing of the involved extremity to avoid injury during the period of numbness, but this practice has been shown to be safe in several studies (23).

A. Upper extremity block

1. **Shoulder** surgeries are frequently performed on an outpatient basis. They are ideal candidates for regional anesthesia.
   a. **Interscalene** blockade provides excellent anesthesia for the shoulder itself and is sufficient for simple shoulder arthroscopy, particularly if painful bone procedures are not involved. In those situations, a longer-acting local anesthetic or continuous catheter technique (see subsequent text) may be more appropriate. Performance of this block has been shown to reduce discharge time for outpatients, reduce postoperative pain and analgesic requirements, increase the frequency of phase 1 bypass, and reduce overnight admission (4,24–26). When the block is performed in an induction area, the surgical starting time is competitive with general anesthesia (4,27).
      (1) **Lidocaine** or **mepivacaine** will give 6 to 8 hours of analgesia after an hour of surgical anesthesia.
      (2) **Bupivacaine** 0.25% can provide 12 to 18 hours of analgesia, often sufficient to provide overnight pain relief for procedures such as rotator cuff repairs.
      (3) **Ropivacaine** in 0.25% or 0.5% concentration will provide approximately 10 hours of analgesia in most patients (28).
   b. If general anesthesia is chosen instead, a suprascapular nerve block provides some supplemental analgesia (1), but is not as effective as the interscalene (29).

2. **Hand or upper arm surgery.** Several techniques are available.
   a. **Intravenous regional anesthesia** is an excellent choice for peripheral surgery if a tourniquet is to be used and the surgery is relatively minor (3,30). The rapid return of function facilitates discharge and this technique has been shown to be less costly than general anesthesia (2,31). Lidocaine is an excellent choice, but provides little postoperative analgesia.
   b. **Supraclavicular block** provides the simplest and most reliable blockade of the brachial plexus below the clavicle, but is avoided in most outpatient units because of the associated risk of pneumothorax. The use of ultrasound guidance may reduce this risk and restore the popularity of this block for outpatients.
   c. **Infraclavicular block** has been used extensively, and, like interscalene, produces less pain, less analgesia requirements, more PACU bypass, and faster discharge (31), and (although it may require two injections) may be more comfortable for the patients than axillary blockade (32).
   d. **Axillary blockade** remains the most popular in outpatient settings because of the minimal risk of pneumothorax (compared to more central blocks). It does require **multiple injections,** especially if the upper arm or forearm require anesthesia (see Chapter 12), but has rapid onset and provides earlier discharge than general anesthesia (33) and several hours of analgesia. Any of the many techniques described in Chapter 12 are useful.

B. **Lower extremity blockade.** Spinal and epidural anesthesia work well for the lower extremity, but do not provide analgesia as discussed in the preceding text. Peripheral nerve block requires more time, and generally several injections, but can provide excellent discharge analgesia.

1. **Knee arthroscopy.** Femoral nerve block supplemented with local injection of the portal sites can provide good operating conditions. A combined femoral (or lumbar plexus) and sciatic block is needed if total anesthesia is planned and postoperative analgesia is required. This technique provides faster discharge and more PACU bypass than general anesthesia (34). A supplemental obturator block may be needed for analgesia in some patients. With these blocks, loss of quadriceps function will occur, and patients will need to ambulate with crutches, as is often required after the surgery anyway.
2. **ACL repair.** For longer procedures, such as ACL repair, combined peripheral nerve blocks can be useful. In particular, a long-acting femoral nerve block provides comfort for 18 to 24 hours after surgery, especially if a patellar tendon graft is taken (35). If such blocks are placed in an induction room, the "anesthesia controlled time" in the operating room can actually be reduced compared to general anesthesia for the same procedure (5).
3. **Foot Surgery.** For surgery that is painful in the foot, block of the branches of the sciatic nerve in the popliteal fossa provides excellent anesthesia and analgesia, earlier discharge, and prolonged pain relief (36). A supplemental injection of the femoral branches along the medial side of the knee may be needed if the dorsum of the foot is involved. More proximal block is not needed and may limit ambulation.

C. **Truncal procedures**

1. **Breast surgery** can be performed with paravertebral blocks and light sedation. Again, the use of longer-acting local anesthetics will also provide

prolonged analgesia and facilitate discharge. Patient satisfaction is good, but the potential complications of this application suggest it may not be the best choice for minor breast surgery (37) despite its advantages for larger operations.

2. **Hernia repair** is an ideal situation for regional techniques because of the significant postoperative discomfort. Neuraxial blockade supplemented by local infiltration by the surgeon works well (as does local anesthesia alone). Postoperative analgesia can also be provided by supplemental ilioinguinal and iliohypogastric blocks (38). Good operating conditions and analgesia are produced by paravertebral blocks, which can provide postoperative analgesia because they do not interfere with ambulation or discharge (39,40).

IV. **Continuous catheter techniques**

This is the area of greatest advance in the application of regional techniques. The use of catheters can provide 72 to 96 hours of analgesia after discharge and allows patients to avoid the frequent side effects of oral opioid analgesics after discharge (41). Experience with these catheters has been extensive in research centers **(42)**. Complications are rare **(43)**. In addition to superior analgesia and reduced side effects, catheter use provides great patient satisfaction (44) and improves return to daily function for outpatients after painful surgery **(45)**.

A. **Upper extremity**

1. Painful shoulder surgery is well managed with continuous techniques. **Interscalene catheters** provide excellent pain relief for as long as 72 hours with lower visual analog scale (VAS) scores, decreased opioid consumption, and better sleep pattern (Figure 22.2) (46–48). The catheters are challenging to maintain because movement of the neck tends to dislodge the catheter. Secure dressings are important, and tunneling under the skin may be useful.
2. **Infraclavicular catheters** are useful for hand and upper arm surgeries. Again, they provide several days of improved analgesia compared to oral analgesics, with better sleep patterns (49), and may be easier to fix securely to the skin.
3. **Axillary catheters** have been placed, but are more difficult to maintain because of movement of the insertion site.

B. **Lower extremity**

1. Continuous **femoral nerve catheters** provide better pain relief than oral opioids or single injection techniques, and can maintain VAS scores and opioid consumption at significantly lower levels for several days (Figure 22.3) **(50)**. A sciatic nerve catheter can be added for severe discomfort, but the dual catheters may produce an unwieldy and unmanageable extremity for most patients at home, and a single femoral infusion appears to provide adequate analgesia when supplemented with minimal oral analgesics, especially if a multimodal regimen is used.
2. **Popliteal fossa catheters** are appropriate for foot procedures and again provide significant improvement over oral analgesics alone (51–54). They can be inserted from the lateral approach, but may be easier to secure to the back of the leg using the posterior approach.

C. **Management issues.** The benefits of continuous catheters are impressive. Nevertheless, there is hesitation to use them because of additional time and equipment required as well as concern over potential and theoretical complications. They undeniably require more effort at follow-up and the provision of

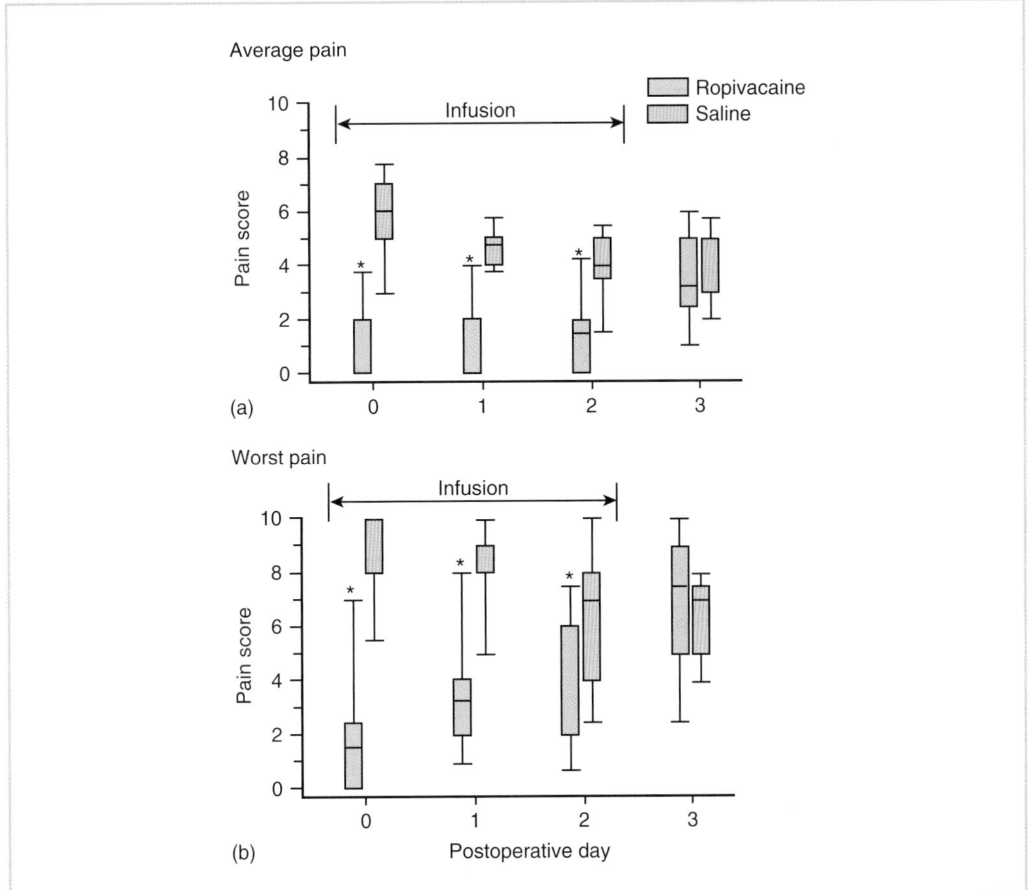

Figure 22.2. Pain scores on a 0 to 10 visual analog scale (VAS) at home with 72-hour continuous interscalene infusion of ropivacaine compared to saline infusion after shoulder surgery. (Adapted from Ilfeld BM, Morey TE, Wright TW et al. Continuous interscalene brachial plexus block for postoperative pain control at home: a randomized, double-blinded, placebo-controlled study. *Anesth Analg* 2003;96:1089–1095.)

a 24-hour resource person for the patients managing these infusions at home. Experience has shown that the problems are infrequent and the equipment reliable (43).

1. **Equipment.** As outlined in Chapter 5, many options are available.
   a. **Catheters.** Most catheters are epidural infusion catheters simply applied to peripheral nerves. As such they are subject to the same challenges of potential kinking and premature withdrawal. The one exception is the use of a stimulating catheter, which may improve nerve localization with a peripheral nerve stimulator. Taping to the skin should allow flexibility to reduce kinking, but securing (through tunneling or strong adhesive) to prevent movement. Care must be taken not to insert an excessive length, so that knotting or kinking under the skin is unlikely, and removal (usually by the patient at home) is not difficult.
   b. **Insertion kits** are available from a number of manufacturers and the choice is based on personal preference. Specialized kits for peripheral nerve stimulator blocks are produced, containing stimulating Tuohy

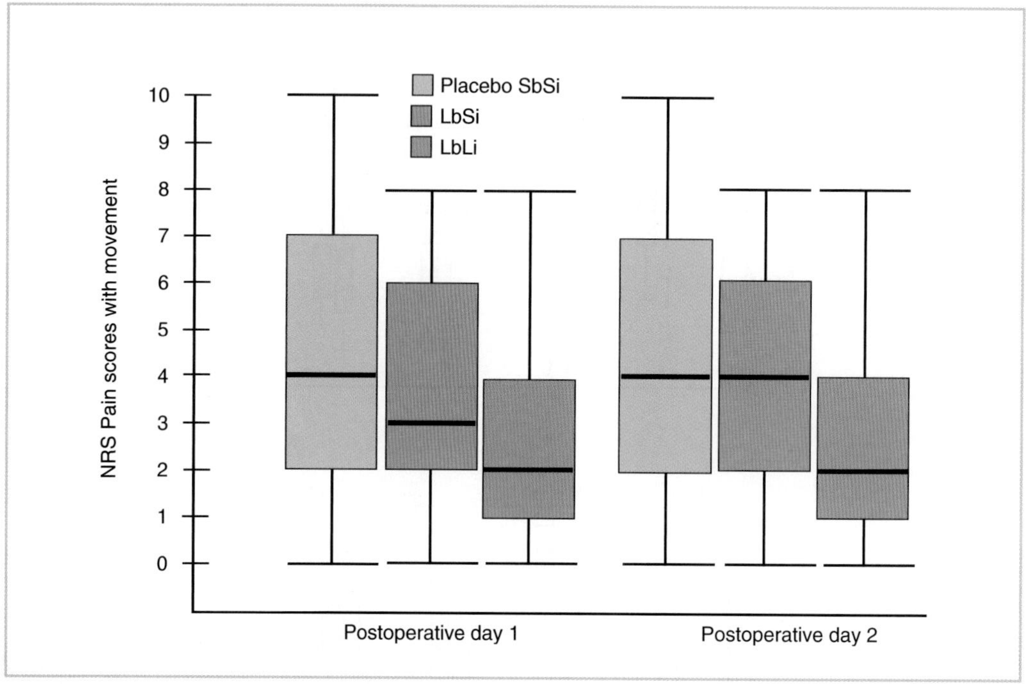

Figure 22.3. Pain scores (on a 0–10 numeric rating scale [NRS]) after anterior cruciate ligament (ACL) repair with placebo injection and infusion (placebo SbSi), single-shot femoral nerve block plus saline infusion (LbSi), or continuous infusion with levobupivacaine (LbLi). (Adapted from Williams BA, Kentor ML, Vogt MT, et al. Reduction of verbal pain scores after anterior cruciate ligament reconstruction with 2-day continuous femoral nerve block: a randomized clinical trial. *Anesthesiology* 2006;104:315–327.)

needles that will allow location of nerves and passage of catheters. With ultrasound guidance, a simple epidural kit contains the large needle and catheter that are sufficient.

c. **Pumps.** A multitude of pumps are also available. They include mechanical and battery-driven devices, and a large variety of potential volumes and refilling options. They appear to be reliable over the standard range of infusion rates, although accuracy may decline as the volume declines in some models (55,56). The choice is usually made on the basis of volume available to deliver and cost. The more complex pumps have a supplemental bolus delivery capability, and the higher-end electronic pumps have adjustable programming. Another desirable feature for the outpatient is a sling or pouch that facilitates carrying the pump around the house.

2. **Solutions.** The most frequent choices are dilute solutions of **bupivacaine** and **ropivacaine,** both of which provide good sensory analgesia in low concentrations (0.125%–0.2%) with minimal motor block. Infusion rates of 4 to 6 mL/h are usually sufficient to provide analgesia, but a "bolus dose" function on a pump allows more flexibility. Ropivacaine may have a slightly greater appearance of separation of motor and sensory block because of its lower potency, and may have a potential advantage in its lower cardiotoxicity (see Chapter 3), although the concentrations and volumes used

for peripheral nerve infusions are unlikely to produce toxicity even if the catheter migrates into a vein.

3. **Communication.** Clear instructions and available support are essential for a successful outpatient catheter service. Patients with impediments to understanding instructions (education or language barriers) are not ideal candidates for these techniques. Preoperative instruction is helpful, but postoperative detailed review of the pump and the process is essential. Most patients undergoing outpatient surgery are overwhelmed with instruction and concerns about their operation; therefore, a relaxed period of instruction just before discharge is helpful, and a **written** set of instructions is essential. The patient must have a 24-hour phone contact provided in case of problems or concerns, and the anesthesia team should contact them directly at least once each day following discharge. Most patients are willing and capable of removing their catheters at home, but frequently require some support by phone at this time. A useful tool is to instruct the patient to watch the PACU nurse remove the intravenous line before discharge, and plan to expect the same sensation and experience, without any bleeding.
4. **Common problems.** Phone calls from patients are surprisingly rare, especially outside of regular hospital hours (43). The most common challenges are not frequent, and usually easily resolved.
   a. **Inadequate analgesia.** In this event, the patient is instructed to administer a bolus and to reprogram the pump (if possible) to deliver a higher rate. If these techniques do not work, there is some suspicion that the catheter may have **migrated** or become **disconnected,** and the patient may need to return to the hospital for further evaluation and potential replacement or treatment with a long-acting single injection. Another possible explanation is unrecognized opioid dependency, which might require oral opioid therapy despite adequate sensory analgesia (see Chapter 23).
   b. **Dislodgment** is another common event. It can happen by the simple constant migration of tubing with movement, but is more frequently associated with inadvertent tension on the catheter by dropping the pump or stepping or pulling on the catheter line. Replacement of the catheter is often a challenging prospect, and simple reversion to oral analgesia may be preferred, especially if substantial time has already passed since surgery.
   c. **Fluid** under the dressing is common, due to leakage back along the catheter track. This can usually be managed by reassurance.
   d. True **infection** is rare, but any signs of redness or tenderness should prompt a return to the hospital for inspection of the site.
   e. Local anesthetic **toxicity** is also primarily a theoretic concern and has not been reported with the volumes and concentrations used in peripheral catheters.
   f. Difficult **removal** is also rare, but if pain, or especially paresthesias occur on attempted removal, the patient should return to the hospital for assessment and assistance.
   g. Many minor issues can be resolved by simple **education,** such as the patient's concern about the sense of tingling or heaviness associated with the block. Patients also need to be counseled that they can use small doses of oral opioids to control pain outside the blocked area (back of the

knee for femoral, top of the foot for popliteal block). Patients also need to be educated that analgesia will persist a few hours after discontinuation of the catheter, but that they need to start taking oral analgesics in that time frame to maintain their pain relief.

VI. Summary

Regional techniques, particularly continuous catheters after painful procedures, offer significant advantages to outpatients. Better analgesia, less nausea and vomiting, and faster discharge are well documented with peripheral nerve blockade of the arm, leg, and trunk. Neuraxial techniques require careful choices of drugs and doses if prolonged discharge is to be avoided. For all techniques, use of fast-acting local anesthetics and an induction or block room will help overcome the perceived time delay of using regional. Every effort should be made to overcome these challenges because the benefits are impressive.

REFERENCES

1 **Liu SS, Strodtbeck WM, Richman JM, et al. A comparison of regional versus general anesthesia for ambulatory anesthesia: a meta-analysis of randomized controlled trials. *Anesth Analg* 2005;101:1634–1642.**

2 **Armstrong KP, Cherry RA. Brachial plexus anesthesia compared to general anesthesia when a block room is available. *Can J Anaesth* 2004;51:41–44.**

3 Chan VW, Peng PW, Kaszas Z, et al. A comparative study of general anesthesia, intravenous regional anesthesia, and axillary block for outpatient hand surgery: clinical outcome and cost analysis. *Anesth Analg* 2001;93:1181–1184.

4 D'Alessio JG, Rosenblum M, Shea KP, et al. A retrospective comparison of interscalene block and general anesthesia for ambulatory surgery shoulder arthroscopy. *Reg Anesth* 1995;20:62–68.

5 Williams BA, Kentor ML, Williams JP, et al. Process analysis in outpatient knee surgery: effects of regional and general anesthesia on anesthesia-controlled time. *Anesthesiology* 2000;93:529–538.

6 Vaghadia H, McLeod DH, Mitchell GW, et al. Small-dose hypobaric lidocaine-fentanyl spinal anesthesia for short duration outpatient laparoscopy. I. A randomized comparison with conventional dose hyperbaric lidocaine. *Anesth Analg* 1997;84:59–64.

7 Bodily MN, Carpenter RL, Owens BD. Lidocaine 0.5% spinal anaesthesia: a hypobaric solution for short-stay perirectal surgery. *Can J Anaesth* 1992;39:770–773.

8 Ben-David B, Levin H, Solomon E, et al. Spinal bupivacaine in ambulatory surgery: the effect of saline dilution. *Anesth Analg* 1996;83:716–720.

9 **Liu SS, Ware PD, Allen HW, et al. Dose-response characteristics of spinal bupivacaine in volunteers. Clinical implications for ambulatory anesthesia. *Anesthesiology* 1996;85:729–736.**

10 Kouri ME, Kopacz DJ. Spinal 2-chloroprocaine: a comparison with lidocaine in volunteers. *Anesth Analg* 2004;98:75–80.

11 **Casati A, Danelli G, Berti M, et al. Intrathecal 2-chloroprocaine for lower limb outpatient surgery: a prospective, randomized, double-blind, clinical evaluation. *Anesth Analg* 2006;103:234–238.**

12 Drasner K. Chloroprocaine spinal anesthesia: back to the future? *Anesth Analg* 2005;100:549–552.

13 Korhonen AM, Valanne JV, Jokela RM, et al. A comparison of selective spinal anesthesia with hyperbaric bupivacaine and general anesthesia with desflurane for outpatient knee arthroscopy. *Anesth Analg* 2004;99:1668–1673.

14 Valanne JV, Korhonen AM, Jokela RM, et al. Selective spinal anesthesia: a comparison of hyperbaric bupivacaine 4 mg versus 6 mg for outpatient knee arthroscopy. *Anesth Analg* 2001;93:1377–1379.

15 **Mulroy MF, Salinas FV, Larkin KL, et al. Ambulatory surgery patients may be discharged before voiding after short-acting spinal and epidural anesthesia. *Anesthesiology* 2002;97:315–319.**

16 Mulroy MF, Larkin KL, Hodgson PS, et al. A comparison of spinal, epidural, and general anesthesia for outpatient knee arthroscopy. *Anesth Analg* 2000;91:860–864.

17 Kopacz DJ, Mulroy MF. Chloroprocaine and lidocaine decrease hospital stay and admission rate after outpatient epidural anesthesia. *Reg Anesth* 1990;15:19–25.

18 Reuben SS, Sklar J, El-Mansouri M. The preemptive analgesic effect of intraarticular bupivacaine and morphine after ambulatory arthroscopic knee surgery. *Anesth Analg* 2001;92:923–926.

19 Ritchie ED, Tong D, Chung F, et al. Suprascapular nerve block for postoperative pain relief in arthroscopic shoulder surgery: a new modality? *Anesth Analg* 1997;84:1306–1312.
20 Reuben SS, Bhopatkar S, Maciolek H, et al. The preemptive analgesic effect of rofecoxib after ambulatory arthroscopic knee surgery. *Anesth Analg* 2002;94:55–59.
21 Reuben SS, Connelly NR, Maciolek H. Postoperative analgesia with controlled-release oxycodone for outpatient anterior cruciate ligament surgery. *Anesth Analg* 1999;88:1286–1291.
22 Urmey WF, Stanton J, Peterson M, et al. Combined spinal-epidural anesthesia for outpatient surgery. Dose-response characteristics of intrathecal isobaric lidocaine using a 27-gauge Whitacre spinal needle. *Anesthesiology* 1995;83:528–534.
23 Klein SM, Buckenmaier CC III. Ambulatory surgery with long acting regional anesthesia. *Minerva Anestesiol* 2002;68:833–847.
24 Brown AR, Weiss R, Greenberg C, et al. Interscalene block for shoulder arthroscopy: comparison with general anesthesia. *Arthroscopy* 1993;9:295–300.
25 Hadzic A, Williams BA, Karaca PE, et al. For outpatient rotator cuff surgery, nerve block anesthesia provides superior same-day recovery over general anesthesia. *Anesthesiology* 2005;102:1001–1007.
26 Al-Kaisy A, McGuire G, Chan VW, et al. Analgesic effect of interscalene block using low-dose bupivacaine for outpatient arthroscopic shoulder surgery. *Reg Anesth Pain Med* 1998;23:469–473.
27 Chelly JE, Greger J, Al Samsam T, et al. Reduction of operating and recovery room times and overnight hospital stays with interscalene blocks as sole anesthetic technique for rotator cuff surgery. *Minerva Anestesiol* 2001;67:613–619.
28 Krone SC, Chan VW, Regan J, et al. Analgesic effects of low-dose ropivacaine for interscalene brachial plexus block for outpatient shoulder surgery-a dose-finding study. *Reg Anesth Pain Med* 2001;26:439–443.
29 Neal JM, McDonald SB, Larkin KL, et al. Suprascapular nerve block prolongs analgesia after nonarthroscopic shoulder surgery but does not improve outcome. *Anesth Analg* 2003;96:982–986.
30 Chilvers CR, Kinahan A, Vaghadia H, et al. Pharmacoeconomics of intravenous regional anaesthesia vs general anaesthesia for outpatient hand surgery. *Can J Anaesth* 1997;44:1152–1156.
31 Hadzic A, Arliss J, Kerimoglu B, et al. A comparison of infraclavicular nerve block versus general anesthesia for hand and wrist day-case surgeries. *Anesthesiology* 2004;101:127–132.
32 Koscielniak-Nielsen ZJ, Rasmussen H, Hesselbjerg L, et al. Infraclavicular block causes less discomfort than axillary block in ambulatory patients. *Acta Anaesthesiol Scand* 2005;49:1030–1034.
33 McCartney CJ, Brull R, Chan VW, et al. Early but no long-term benefit of regional compared with general anesthesia for ambulatory hand surgery. *Anesthesiology* 2004;101:461–467.
34 Hadzic A, Karaca PE, Hobeika P, et al. Peripheral nerve blocks result in superior recovery profile compared with general anesthesia in outpatient knee arthroscopy. *Anesth Analg* 2005;100:976–981.
35 Mulroy MF, Larkin KL, Batra MS, et al. Femoral nerve block with 0.25% or 0.5% bupivacaine improves postoperative analgesia following outpatient arthroscopic anterior cruciate ligament repair. *Reg Anesth Pain Med* 2001;26:24–29.
36 Hansen E, Eshelman MR, Cracchiolo A III. Popliteal fossa neural blockade as the sole anesthetic technique for outpatient foot and ankle surgery. *Foot Ankle Int* 2000;21:38–44.
37 Terheggen MA, Wille F, Borel Rinkes IH, et al. Paravertebral blockade for minor breast surgery. *Anesth Analg* 2002;94:355–359.
38 Toivonen J, Permi J, Rosenberg PH. Analgesia and discharge following preincisional ilioinguinal and iliohypogastric nerve block combined with general or spinal anaesthesia for inguinal herniorrhaphy. *Acta Anaesthesiol Scand* 2004;48:480–485.
39 Hadzic A, Kerimoglu B, Loreio D, et al. Paravertebral blocks provide superior same-day recovery over general anesthesia for patients undergoing inguinal hernia repair. *Anesth Analg* 2006;102:1076–1081.
40 Klein SM, Greengrass RA, Weltz C, et al. Paravertebral somatic nerve block for outpatient inguinal herniorrhaphy: an expanded case report of 22 patients. *Reg Anesth Pain Med* 1998;23:306–310.
41 Carroll NV, Miederhoff P, Cox FM, et al. Postoperative nausea and vomiting after discharge from outpatient surgery centers. *Anesth Analg* 1995;80:903–909.
42 Ilfeld BM, Enneking FK. Continuous peripheral nerve blocks at home: a review. *Anesth Analg* 2005; 100:1822–1833.
43 Swenson JD, Bay N, Loose E, et al. Outpatient management of continuous peripheral nerve catheters placed using ultrasound guidance: an experience in 620 patients. *Anesth Analg* 2006;103:1436–1443.
44 Ilfeld BM, Esener DE, Morey TE, et al. Ambulatory perineural infusion: the patients' perspective. *Reg Anesth Pain Med* 2003;28:418–423.
45 Capdevila X, Dadure C, Bringuier S, et al. Effect of patient-controlled perineural analgesia on rehabilitation and pain after ambulatory orthopedic surgery: a multicenter randomized trial. *Anesthesiology* 2006;105:566–573.

46 Ilfeld BM, Morey TE, Enneking FK. Continuous infraclavicular perineural infusion with clonidine and ropivacaine compared with ropivacaine alone: a randomized, double-blinded, controlled study. *Anesth Analg* 2003;97:706–712.

47 Ilfeld BM, Morey TE, Wright TW, et al. Continuous interscalene brachial plexus block for postoperative pain control at home: a randomized, double-blinded, placebo-controlled study. *Anesth Analg* 2003;96:1089–1095.

48 Klein SM, Grant SA, Greengrass RA, et al. Interscalene brachial plexus block with a continuous catheter insertion system and a disposable infusion pump. *Anesth Analg* 2000;91:1473–1478.

49 Ilfeld BM, Morey TE, Enneking FK. Continuous infraclavicular brachial plexus block for postoperative pain control at home: a randomized, double-blinded, placebo-controlled study. *Anesthesiology* 2002;96:1297–1304.

50 Williams BA, Kentor ML, Vogt MT, et al. Reduction of verbal pain scores after anterior cruciate ligament reconstruction with 2-day continuous femoral nerve block: a randomized clinical trial. *Anesthesiology* 2006;104:315–327.

51 Borgeat A, Blumenthal S, Lambert M, et al. The feasibility and complications of the continuous popliteal nerve block: a 1001-case survey. *Anesth Analg* 2006;103:229–233.

52 Ilfeld BM, Morey TE, Wang RD, et al. Continuous popliteal sciatic nerve block for postoperative pain control at home: a randomized, double-blinded, placebo-controlled study. *Anesthesiology* 2002;97:959–965.

53 White PF, Issioui T, Skrivanek GD, et al. The use of a continuous popliteal sciatic nerve block after surgery involving the foot and ankle: does it improve the quality of recovery? *Anesth Analg* 2003;97:1303–1309.

54 Zaric D, Boysen K, Christiansen J, et al. Continuous popliteal sciatic nerve block for outpatient foot surgery—a randomized, controlled trial. *Acta Anaesthesiol Scand* 2004;48:337–341.

55 Ilfeld BM, Morey TE, Enneking FK. The delivery rate accuracy of portable infusion pumps used for continuous regional analgesia. *Anesth Analg* 2002;95:1331–1336.

56 Ilfeld BM, Morey TE, Enneking FK. Portable infusion pumps used for continuous regional analgesia: delivery rate accuracy and consistency. *Reg Anesth Pain Med* 2003;28:424–432.

23 Postoperative Pain Management

Susan B. McDonald

I. INTRODUCTION

A. Over the last few decades there has been a rapidly **growing appreciation** for how important a role adequate postoperative analgesia plays in patient recovery.

1. The traditional method of nurse-administered intramuscular (IM) opioid analgesia has been replaced by modern reliance on a combination of drugs and delivery approaches. Although opioids remain the principal analgesics, the variable effectiveness and side effects have led to the development of alternative delivery systems, such as **patient-controlled analgesia (PCA)** and routes (epidural, subarachnoid, and peripheral). The desire to avoid opioid side effects has also led to a greater reliance on local anesthetics and other analgesics.
2. The **risks and benefits** of the various approaches have been comparatively studied, and several complete textbooks describe in extensive detail the application of these techniques (1–4).
3. The need to deliver complex and multimodal care has led to the development of **"acute pain services,"** with anesthesia caregivers as an integral part of the development (5).

B. The **importance of appropriate pain management** has received national attention in the United States. **The Joint Commission has implemented their own standards requiring organizations to address pain control,** making it a requirement for patients to have appropriate pain assessment and management. It has mandated that pain be considered **"the fifth vital sign"** and that its management is a **"patient's right"** (6).

C. Anesthesiologists have joined discussion of the **ethical and medicolegal implications** of assessing and addressing pain control. Some authors have recognized it as a "fundamental human right" with the failure to treat such pain as "negligent" and "professional misconduct" (7). Others have asserted that using opioid analgesics alone in the treatment of postoperative (and chronic) pain adds unnecessary risk of sedation, respiratory depression, nausea, and pruritus (6). **Therefore, opioid-sparing techniques, such as regional blocks, can be an important factor in acute postoperative pain management.**

II. PCA

A. The first major improvement in postoperative analgesia was the development of a more appropriate delivery system, specifically, the introduction of intravenous (IV) **PCA**.

1. **PCA is superior to the traditional IM route** because effective blood levels are produced immediately with little overshoot. The on-demand patient control allows each patient to titrate the exact level that is needed for his or her analgesic requirement and to adjust that dosage to varying levels of activity.
2. There are a multitude of pumps in the market that allow the patient to inject a small bolus of an IV opioid drug whenever he or she feels pain, and thereby

maintain the analgesic blood level in the range that is appropriate. Each of the machines has a "lockout" system, which provides an adequate delay time for the patient to achieve analgesia from each injected dose. **Excessive dosing is avoided by the patient's own titration** and, if inappropriate dosing occurs, the sedation that it produces during the lockout period usually prevents the patient from giving an overdose that would lead to respiratory depression. Because this delivery system only maintains a blood level, the initial production of adequate analgesia requires a bolus injection of an opioid, usually provided by a loading dose programmed for each patient.

3. One problem with this method is the **need for constant reinjection to maintain adequate blood levels**, most frequently resulting in interrupted sleep. Most machines will allow a continuous infusion mode that provides a constant background infusion of drug, which may alleviate this problem. The constant infusion mode does not reduce the total quantity delivered; it does increase the potential for respiratory depression by removing the patient control (8). Nevertheless, it may be useful for overnight setting, particularly on the first postoperative night.
4. All standard PCA orders should include alternatives that allow the nursing staff to increase the incremental doses or decrease the lockout interval to meet the patient's needs.
5. Virtually all of the available opioids have been administered by this route (Table 23.1) (9).
   a. **Morphine** is the least expensive and often the drug of first choice. The development of side effects (pruritus, nausea, dysphoria) may require switching to an alternative.
   b. **Meperidine** is equally effective, but with a slightly shorter duration of action. Meperidine is less commonly used because of toxicity from its primary metabolite, normeperidine, especially with prolonged use or high doses (9).
   c. Hydromorphone is a potent analgesic, and can be considered an acceptable alternative to other opioids.
   d. Fentanyl is more expensive, but it has been used in patients with sensitivity to other opioids. The PCA delivery mode overcomes the usual disadvantage of the short duration of this drug, but the patient will need to inject more frequently.
6. As mentioned, the delivery systems appear to be safe. Mechanical problems are rare (9). Although central depression does occur (8), it is no more common than with any other delivery technique. **The use of continuous**

Table 23.1 Intravenous patient-controlled administration: drugs and doses

Drug	Loading dose (mg)	Increments
Morphine	5–20	0.5–2.5
Meperidine	50–250	10–25
Hydromorphone	1–2	0.05–0.25
Fentanyl	0.075–0.1	0.010–0.050

infusions or the presence of advanced age increases the risk of respiratory depression. The major problem with this modality has been when control of the device is shifted to a family member rather than the patient, which risks unintentional overdose and respiratory depression.

7. Overall, this delivery system has been highly effective in providing appropriate analgesia for postoperative patients.
   a. PCA, when compared to nurse-administered opioids, whether IV or IM, provides better analgesia and patient satisfaction (10).
   b. It **is very effective for peripheral and lower abdominal surgery, but neuraxial opioids appear superior for upper abdominal and thoracic procedures** (see Section IV).

B. The **PCA modality has been adapted** to subcutaneous, perineural, and epidural catheters, and has been highly effective with the targeted delivery systems discussed in the subsequent text.

III. **Local and peripheral nerve analgesic techniques.** Several local and peripheral regional techniques are used to provide ongoing analgesia. The advantages of **specifically targeting analgesia to one area** include minimal limitations of mobility and reduction of systemic side effects such as sedation and nausea. Peripheral infusions usually employ low concentrations of local anesthetics, but opioids and α_2-agonists are also useful in some situations. The efficacy and popularity of continuous peripheral techniques have been enhanced by the introduction of new continuous catheter delivery systems and smaller portable pumps.

A. **Surgical wound infiltration**

1. Simple infiltration of the wound with dilute local anesthetic **can provide 4 to 8 hours of analgesia,** depending on the location.
   a. This technique is **particularly useful in the pediatric patient**, especially with penile or groin blocks following urologic surgery.
   b. Local infiltration is also effective for **adult outpatients,** allowing them to be discharged without the side effects of systemic opioids.
2. For inpatients, the analgesia in smaller wounds can be extended by the insertion of a multiorifice catheter and provision of a continuous infusion of solutions such as 0.1% bupivacaine or ropivacaine at 6 to 12 mL/h. Orthopaedic surgeons have used this technology with disposable pumps to provide 24 hours of analgesia after shoulder surgery for outpatients.
3. Another variation of this is injection of the knee joint following arthroscopic surgery. Bupivacaine will provide several hours of analgesia, and there is a suggestion that the addition of opioids such as morphine may prolong the analgesia considerably (11), although this remains controversial.

B. **Intrapleural Catheters**

1. Injection of local anesthetics through intrapleural catheters has been used to relieve postoperative pain. The technique is described in Chapter 10.
2. For postoperative analgesia, 20 mL 0.5% bupivacaine can be injected every 6 to 12 hours, or a continuous infusion can be instituted. Satisfactory results have been reported in some patients with subcostal incisions for cholecystectomy as well as with thoracotomy patients. Other authors have found **variable analgesia and a significant potential for systemic toxicity** with the doses required.
3. This technique is **not as effective as epidural opiates for thoracotomy procedures** (12).

C. **Repeated intercostal blockade**

1. Injection of the 6th to the 11th intercostal nerves with 3 to 5 mL 0.25% bupivacaine with 1:200,000 epinephrine at 12-hour intervals will provide excellent continuous analgesia (12). It is **utilized infrequently because of the personnel and time required to provide reinjections every 12 hours,** compared to the ease and efficacy of epidural infusions.
2. Insertion of a continuous catheter will reduce some of the technical and time problems. Its use is usually limited to the occasional frail patient requiring special attention, or the trauma patient suffering from multiple rib fractures in whom respiratory depression from systemic opioids is undesirable and epidural analgesia is contraindicated.

D. **Peripheral nerve catheters.** Peripheral nerve blocks provide excellent postoperative analgesia for both inpatients and outpatients, which can be prolonged with continuous catheters (13,14). Interest in this technique has rapidly increased over the last decade as a result of **new technology** that aids in the placement (stimulating catheters, ultrasound guidance) and management (reliable, portable, and disposable pumps) of these blocks.

1. See previous chapters for an in-depth discussion of the placement of peripheral nerve catheters (Chapters 15 and 16 for lower extremity and Chapter 12 for upper extremity).
2. **Delivery systems**
   a. Pumps designed for PCA, such as inpatient epidural analgesia, can be used to deliver local anesthetic (with or without adjuncts) to the peripheral nerve catheter.
   b. **Portable pumps** are available that can allow patients to be discharged home with the catheter in place (see Chapter 5).
      (1) Early generation included elastomeric spheres that delivered solutions at a specific continuous rate, without bolus capabilities, until empty or discontinued.
      (2) Newer models are disposable battery-operated pumps with light emitting diode (LED) display/controls that allow a set continuous rate and intermittent patient-controlled boluses. These pumps are filled with 2 to 3 days of local anesthetic solution and **once empty are discarded.** Patients can **remove their own catheters at home,** under their anesthesia provider's direction.
3. **Drugs**
   a. **Dilute local anesthetic solutions** are the most commonly used, especially long-acting amides. Ropivacaine 0.2% offers similar analgesic profile as 0.15% bupivacaine with potentially less motor blockade and lower cardiotoxicity risk.
   b. Adjuncts such as clonidine and opioids have been advocated by some (15), whereas others have failed to show a clinically relevant benefit.
4. **Outcomes**
   a. Interscalene catheters, used for 2 days postoperatively, can **decrease pain and opioid use** (along with such adverse effects as nausea and sleep disturbance) in patients undergoing moderately painful ambulatory shoulder surgery (14).
   b. Femoral nerve catheters provide **better pain relief, improve the recovery time, and shorten the rehabilitation time** following total knee

replacement after inpatient surgery, compared to conventional opioids or epidural infusions (16). However, long-term functional outcomes, such as mobility, are likely no different between continuous and single-shot femoral nerve blocks in these patients (16).

c. Feasibility studies have demonstrated that with the use of portable delivery systems, total **joint replacements** (including knees, hips, and shoulders) can be done in a subset of patients **as overnight-stay or outpatient procedures** (17,18).

5. Complications **and adverse effects are rare.** Local inflammation and infection rates are less than 1% even when catheters remain in place for 4 to 7 days (19). Even outpatient use of continuous techniques has been associated with few major complications (20). Knotting of catheters around anatomic structures, including nerves, has been reported (21).

IV. Neuraxial opioid analgesia

A. The use **of neuraxial administration of opioids** has been the major advancement in acute analgesic therapy (22,23).

1. Opioids applied to the spinal cord are effective in blocking pain perception **at the dorsal root entry zone** in doses that are substantially smaller than those required to produce systemic analgesia.
2. The direct application of opioids to the specific receptor site **reduces the systemic side effects** of respiratory depression and sedation usually associated with IM and IV injection.
3. This effect is seen with **both subarachnoid and epidural injection,** although **epidural application requires higher doses (by a factor of 10)** to produce penetration of the membranes.
4. This route has been demonstrated to produce **superior analgesia for thoracotomy and abdominal procedures** (12,24–26).

B. **Choice of opioids.** Virtually all of the opioids have been employed in both the subarachnoid and epidural space (Table 23.2).

1. **Epidural delivery**

a. **Morphine.** Because of its poor lipid solubility, morphine has a **relatively slow penetration into the lipid layers of the spinal column** (22). Although early investigators found that they could overcome this by using higher doses, it was quickly discovered that these doses were also associated with a higher incidence of side effects, specifically the production of central sedation and respiratory depression as the

Table 23.2 Epidural opioid infusions

Drug	Loading dose (mg)[a]	Maintenance
Morphine	1–3	0.04 mg/mL, 4–8 mL/h
Meperidine	20–100	1 mg/mL, 8–12 mL/h
Hydromorphone	1–2	0.02 mg/mL, 4–10 mL/h
Fentanyl	75–100	4 mg/mL, 8–16 mL/h
Sufentanil	50	2 mg/mL, 8–12 mL/h

[a]Lower rates effective if local anesthetic added.

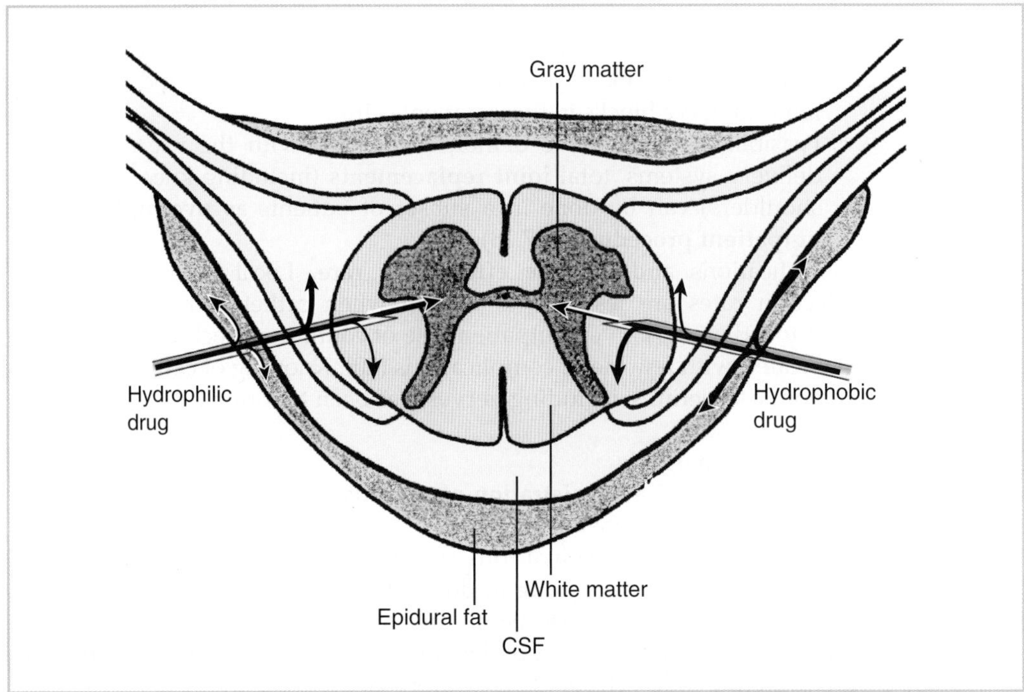

Figure 23.1. Any drug placed in the epidural space will distribute among local tissues based on its physicochemical properties. For example, relative to hydrophilic drugs, hydrophobic drugs will be taken up into epidural fat to a greater degree, cleared into plasma to a greater extent as they diffuse through the rich capillary network in the dura mater, reside in cerebrospinal fluid (CSF) for a much shorter period of time and be sequestered in the rich lipid environment of the spinal cord white matter to a greater degree. As a result, relative to hydrophilic drugs, a much smaller percentage of the administered dose of a hydrophobic drug reaches the spinal cord dorsal horn. If the drug is a local anesthetic this is not a significant problem because the site of action is the relatively hydrophobic environment (i.e., myelinated axons) of the nerve rootlets suspended in CSF. However, for drugs that target receptors in the spinal cord dorsal horn (e.g., opioids, α_2-agonists, etc.), a significant amount of the drug administered epidurally is taken up into other tissues, thereby reducing the bioavailability of the drug in the dorsal horn.

water-soluble morphine diffused cephalad in the cerebrospinal fluid (CSF) (Figure 23.1).

(1) Appropriate low bolus doses [1–5 mg for most patients, based primarily on patient age (27)] will produce adequate pain relief with minimal side effects if a single dose is administered early enough to allow 60 minutes for the onset of action.

(2) Use of a continuous infusion of morphine avoids the peak and valley phenomenon of intermittent injections, and also appears to be associated with a lower incidence of side effects (28).

b. Fentanyl. Because this drug has higher lipid solubility, it **diffuses less readily in the CSF** (Figure 23.2). Historically, it was thought that fentanyl (as the prototypical highly lipid-soluble opioid) would produce a more localized segmental band of analgesia with less likelihood of centrally mediated respiratory depression and other side effects. Currently, **many disagree on whether epidural fentanyl provides a significant effect at**

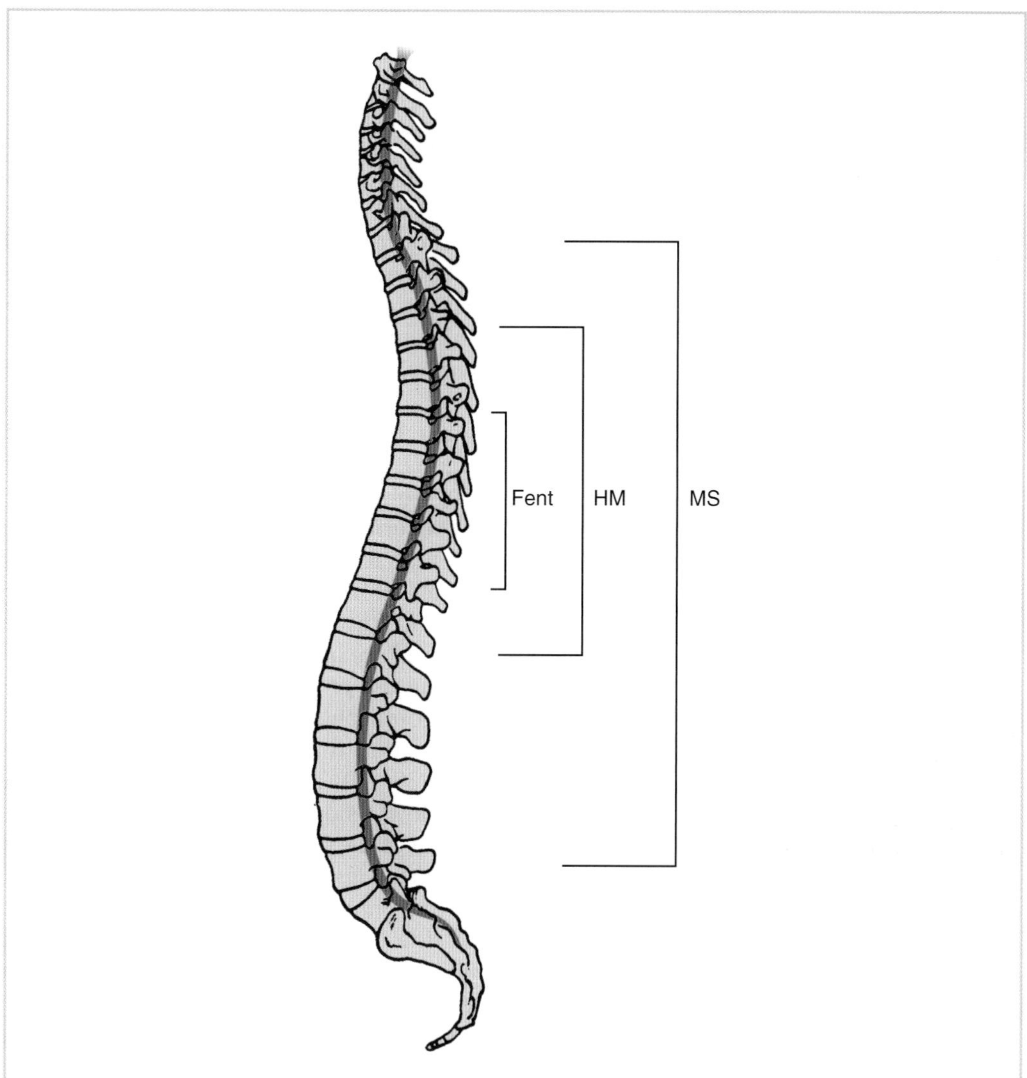

Figure 23.2. The extent of spread of epidurally administered opioids is related to the degree of water solubility. Less water-soluble drugs such as fentanyl (Fent) will produce a narrow band of segmental analgesia surrounding the insertion site, while hydromorphone (HM) and morphine(MS) will produce wider bands of analgesia.

the spinal cord versus largely systemic effect from plasma absorption (see Chapter 7).

(1) Epidural fentanyl has been shown to produce localized segmental anesthesia as required for post-thoracotomy pain (12,23), with some suggestion of a lower side effect profile (29).

(2) There is significant uptake into the blood stream (30), and in several studies the blood levels attained with epidural infusion have equaled the blood levels with IV administration. Some have questioned whether there is really a direct spinal action at all, and whether these drugs have any use in neuraxial analgesia (31,32).

(3) Other data suggest that with bolus doses, rather than by infusion, there is a local effect in the spinal cord, but only near the immediate area of injection (33).

(4) Despite the laboratory studies suggesting only systemic effects, there are large clinical studies demonstrating a high degree of effectiveness with epidural fentanyl infusions (29,34). These series demonstrate that the location of the catheter tip is critical; it must be located near the dermatomal source of pain. They also demonstrate that the combination with a local anesthetic is important for adequate analgesia with this opioid. If a large number of spinal segments are to be provided analgesia, higher doses (and systemic effects) may be required, and alternative opioids with a wider spread may be more desirable.

c. **Sufentanil.** Because of its higher lipid solubility, even larger doses are required. For effective analgesia, doses of sufentanil equivalent to the fentanyl dose are required. Although sufentanil may be an effective analgesic, there is nevertheless **concern that its effects are also simply due to systemic blood levels.** As with fentanyl, this has been confirmed when higher doses are used. The use of higher volumes of a more dilute solution for sufentanil infusions will improve its analgesic effects, but advantages of this drug over fentanyl are unclear.

d. **Meperidine, hydromorphone.** The use of intermediate-solubility opioids such as meperidine or hydromorphone provides a spinal cord action with wider spread and duration than seen with fentanyl, and perhaps less frequent side effects (35–37). This class may represent an ideal balance of good spread with lower side effects.

e. **Optimizing epidural opioid delivery.** Generally, there appears to be a relationship that suggests that drugs producing sufficient spread to provide excellent analgesia (morphine) do so at the price of side effects. The lower frequency of side effects of the lipid-soluble drugs is associated with lower efficacy, unless such high infusion rates are used that systemic levels are attained. This has led many to believe that the use of the **lipid-soluble drugs should be limited to cases where the catheter is at or near the "epicenter" of a narrow band of painful dermatomes,** such as thoracotomy incisions (and therefore pain can be relieved with small doses). The more water-soluble opioids appear to be more appropriate for distant catheters (lumbar placement for thoracotomy pain) or wider incisions (abdominal cases). Unfortunately, there are **insufficient comparative studies** between the various opioids to support the personal choice of drug.

2. **Intrathecal delivery**

a. All of the opioids have also been administered as subarachnoid injections. The **doses required are significantly less than the epidural route,** but the efficacy of this route is limited by the (usually) single injection. (Table 23.3)

b. After administration, intrathecal opioids not only bind to receptors in the dorsal horn of the spinal cord but also traverse the dura mater into the epidural space, travel in the CSF to more cephalad binding sites, and enter the plasma. As with epidural opioids, the **degree of binding is related to the drug's lipophilicity** (38).

Table 23.3 Spinal opioid doses for postoperative analgesia

Drug	Dose (mg)	Duration (h)
Morphine	0.1–0.3	8–24
Meperidine	10–30	10–24
Fentanyl	5–25	2–6

(1) Lipophilic opioids like **fentanyl and sufentanil** rapidly cross the dura into the epidural space and rapidly bind to spinal cord receptors and are cleared into the plasma. Such pharmacodynamics limits the analgesic duration but also the degree of side effects, including respiratory depression (Figure 23.3).

(2) **Morphine,** as a hydrophilic compound, remains in the CSF for a longer duration. While this prolongs the analgesia (24 hours or more), it also significantly increases the risk of cephalad spread of the drug, which may lead to respiratory depression. There is a narrow dose–response relationship, and a relatively high incidence

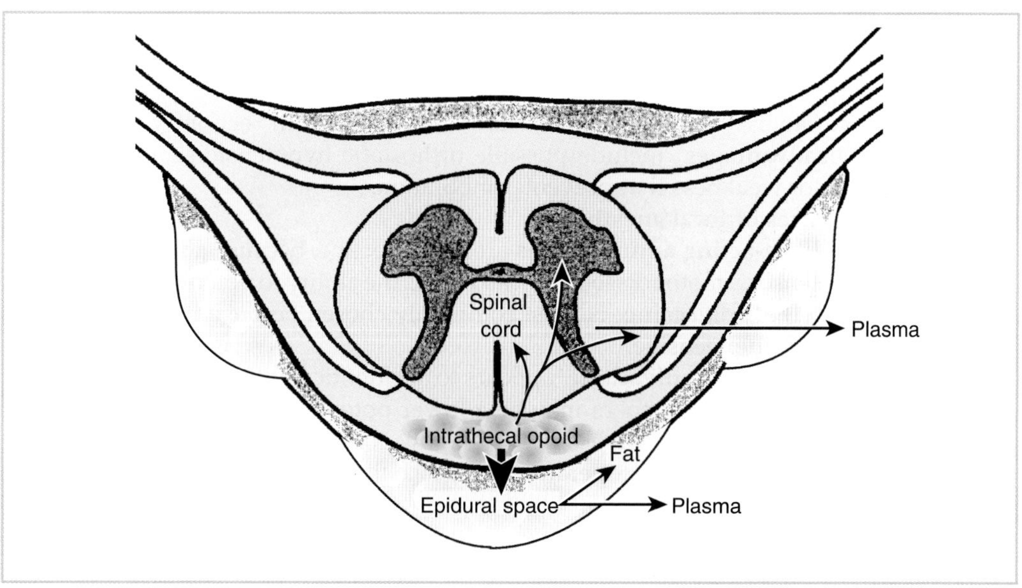

Figure 23.3. Disposition of opioid after intrathecal administration. After intrathecal administration, the disposition of opioids is complex and multicompartmental. Simultaneously, intrathecal opioids (i) travel cephalad within the cerebrospinal fluid (CSF), (ii) enter the spinal cord, and (iii) traverse the dura mater to enter the epidural space. The clinical properties of each opioid (speed of onset, duration of action) and degree of rostral spread result from the sum of effects for each route. Lipophilic opioids (fentanyl/sufentanil) display rapid onset, limited and brief rostral spread and a narrow band of analgesia surrounding the site of injection, and a relatively short duration of action. In contrast, the hydrophilic opioid morphine traverses the dura slowly to the epidural space, demonstrating slow onset, extensive and prolonged rostral spread and a broad band of analgesia surrounding the site of injection, and a relatively long duration of action. (Adapted from Rathmell JP, Lair TR, Nauman B. The role of intrathecal drugs in the treatment of acute pain. *Anesth Analg* 2005;101(Suppl 5):S30–S43.)

of side effects (39). **Although respiratory depression is the greatest concern, it is fortunately rare (less than 0.5%).** Decreased level of consciousness is a more reliable indicator of respiratory depression than pulse oximetry or respiratory rates. Nausea and urinary retention can also occur, each with an incidence of approximately 30%. **Most common is pruritus,** disturbing more than half of the patients.

C. **Addition of local anesthetics**
   1. **The efficacy of epidural opioids is improved** by the addition of a dilute concentration of local anesthetics, such as 0.05% bupivacaine.
   2. Although higher concentrations of bupivacaine (0.1%) may occasionally be required, the maximum potentiation seems to occur in the 0.05% range. Higher concentrations may provide enhanced analgesia by providing some sensory analgesia, but the higher doses increase the potential for motor block and hypotension due to sympathetic blockade (29).
   3. **Advantages of adding local anesthetic** to the epidural infusion
      a. The **potency of epidural opioids is significantly increased.**
         (1) Worthwhile adjunct therapy for both lipid-soluble and water-soluble (29,34,40) opioids.
         (2) Provides a significant **synergistic improvement in analgesia,** especially with movement or coughing, which is particularly evident with the lipid-soluble opioids (23,41).
      b. Local anesthetics **speed the return of normal bowel function** after abdominal surgery (42,43).
      c. Other outcome-based measures are discussed in Section IV.
   4. **Disadvantages** include possible orthostatic hypotension and sensory or motor weakness that prevents ambulation.
   5. **Choices of local anesthetic**
      a. Long-**acting aminoamides** are also effective, because all possess a good sensory-motor dissociation as well as the ability to potentiate the opioids.
         (1) **Bupivacaine** is most commonly chosen because it is effective and inexpensive.
         (2) **Levobupivacaine** appears to act identically to the racemic mixture. Although there may be a lower potential for cardiac toxicity than racemic bupivacaine, at the low concentrations and infusion rates used for postoperative analgesia, this advantage may not justify the additional cost.
         (3) **Ropivacaine** has been studied as a potential analgesic infusion without opioid. It produces less motor blockade than bupivacaine in the same concentrations, but still has a significant potential for motor blockade in the concentrations needed to produce analgesia without opioids. When combined with fentanyl in low concentrations, there does not appear to be a significant difference compared to equipotent mixtures with bupivacaine (23,44,45). Again, there is less potential for cardiotoxicity, although this is not as significant a risk with these low doses of drug.
      b. Despite a plethora of published studies of almost every conceivable combination of opioid and local anesthetic for almost every type of surgery, there are **no clear guidelines for the ideal proportion for combination therapy.**

(1) Because of the synergism, any reduction in one component requires an increase of the other. Using a complex "direct search" method, Curatolo demonstrated this interdependence between bupivacaine, fentanyl, and clonidine dose (46).

(2) A useful approach is to choose an opioid, and start with a combination with 0.05% bupivacaine. If analgesia is inadequate with patient-controlled epidural anesthesia (PCEA), the basal infusion rate can be increased a few times as a first step, and then concentration of bupivacaine increased to 0.1% as the next alternative. If a lipid-soluble opioid was the initial choice, conversion to a more water-soluble (wider spreading) drug is another alternative.

D. Other adjuvants

1. Several other adjuvants show promise in potentiating epidural opioids or in having analgesic properties themselves.
   a. **α_2-Agonists (clonidine, dexmedetomidine).** Clonidine appears to be the most effective, but at the price of a higher frequency of hypotension and sedation (23), which may limit the use of this drug to peripheral nerve infusions. Currently, dexmedetomidine is not approved for epidural infusion in humans in the United States.
   b. ***N*-methyl-D-aspartate (NMDA) antagonists (ketamine).** Ketamine has been shown to be effective, but its safety in the epidural space has not been confirmed.
   c. Epinephrine has been shown to intensify analgesia with bupivacaine–fentanyl mixtures.
2. At this time, most postoperative analgesia services appear to be interested in using the simplest combination of ingredients until there is more evidence of enhanced analgesia or reduced side effects with adjuvants.

E. Delivery system. As with the drug combinations, there are a number of reports, but a dearth of good comparisons. However, there have been some evidence-based conclusions:

1. The use of a thoracic epidural catheter for thoracic and upper abdominal procedures provides ideal analgesia with the lowest dose and lowest frequency of motor blockade (23,29), especially with the more lipid-soluble opioids.
2. Although continuous infusions appear to have replaced bolus injection methods, the addition of a PCA component also improves analgesia and allows better titration to varying patient needs. PCEA does not appear to be effective without a background infusion, but that combination appears to provide the best analgesia with lowest side effect profile.

F. Multimodal analgesia

1. **No ideal single drug infusion exists to provide total analgesia without side effects or interference with ambulation or recovery of bowel function.**
2. Combinations of several modalities are more effective than a single-analgesic regimen (47).
   a. The **synergism** of local anesthetics plus opioids in the epidural space provides better analgesia than either alone and is also more effective in promoting return of normal bowel function than the use of opioids (either PCA or epidural) alone.
   b. The use of supplemental systemic analgesics that act by a separate mechanism provides additional synergism (48).

(1) Specifically, administration of nonsteroidal anti-inflammatory drugs (**NSAIDs**) on a regular basis has been shown to improve analgesia while reducing opioid requirements in many procedures, and therefore the potential for the side effects of respiratory depression or ileus is reduced. Most pain services now add NSAIDs to almost all regimens.

(2) The use of acetaminophen on a regular basis has similar benefits, and is also included as a baseline in many pain services.

(3) Centrally acting antidepressants and anticonvulsive drugs such as gabapentin and pregabalin have recently been shown to augment analgesia (49), and may be useful when given preoperatively.

3. There are **other factors** that determine final recovery in addition to adequate analgesia. The return of bowel function appears to be especially important, and accelerated recovery has been shown in patients who are treated with an analgesic regimen that reduces ileus combined with early feeding of low-fat diets. Nonpharmacologic treatment including early feeding and aggressive ambulation appears to be beneficial and is clearly an area for further study.

G. Preemptive application

1. Animal data suggest that the presurgical application of neuraxial opioids will significantly blunt the phenomenon of spinal cord excitation usually associated with painful stimuli, and will reduce analgesic requirements for postinjury pain therapy (50). At this point, the human data are still unclear (51).
2. Although epidural opioids do not provide adequate analgesia for surgery itself, they may reduce anesthetic requirements by 30% to 40%.
3. A definite preemptive effect cannot be documented at this point. A recent meta-analysis demonstrated that preemptive epidural analgesia resulted in lower postoperative pain scores, less consumption of overall analgesic medication, and longer time until first rescue analgesia (51). It appears to be worthwhile to initiate epidural analgesia early in the surgical course, perhaps by placing the epidural catheter before surgery and administering the anesthetic with a combined technique that includes local anesthetic and opioids during surgery. This allows a smooth transition to an epidural infusion for postoperative analgesia.

H. Treatment of side effects

1. **Respiratory depression is the greatest concern.**
   a. It is no greater risk than with IM opioids or IV PCA if appropriate doses are employed (8,23).
   b. All patients receiving neuraxial opioids should be **monitored** for signs of respiratory depression.
      (1) Respiratory depression may occur 6 to 18 hours after initial injection or start of an infusion.
      (2) For intrathecal morphine, most agree that such monitoring should continue for at least 24 hours after injection.
      (3) For intrathecal fentanyl, there has been no reported case of respiratory depression after 2 hours, and is therefore considered safe in the ambulatory setting.
   c. Patients **at greatest risk** are the elderly, especially those who have received other systemic opioids or sedatives. Upper abdominal and

Table 23.4 Risk factors for respiratory depression

Intravenous PCA	Epidural opioids	Both
Continuous infusion mode	Thoracic, abdominal incisions	Advanced age
Family interference	Dural puncture	Overdosage
Respiratory disease	Intrathecal vs. epidural Thoracic catheter ASA status >3 Surgery >4 h	Other narcotics/sedatives

PCA, patient-controlled administration; ASA, American Society of Anesthesiologists.

thoracic surgeries also increase risk. Patients receiving chronic opioid administration are more resistant (Table 23.4).

d. Mechanical monitoring devices have not proved useful (52). With appropriate education of nursing staff and patient monitoring, neuraxial opioids have been used successfully on patients in general hospital wards, and need not be limited to application in intensive care units (23,29,34,40,52).

(1) **Decreased level of consciousness is the best indicator** of impending respiratory failure, especially when coupled with a decreasing respiratory rate (less than 10 breaths/min), and should be treated with an opioid antagonist.

(2) **A single IV dose of naloxone is not adequate**; depression will recur within 20 minutes as the naloxone effect dissipates. A continuous infusion of naloxone (5 μg/kg/h) will reverse the respiratory depression without antagonizing the analgesia, and may even be an advisable prophylactic measure in high-risk patients.

2. **Pruritus** is the most common complaint with neuraxial opioids. (Table 23.5)

a. **Antihistamines** are effective treatment, but histamine release is not the mechanism of the symptom. This treatment frequently produces sedation and somnolence.

b. A more effective treatment is with an **opioid antagonist**. A small dose of an antagonist will relieve the side effect without reversing the analgesia. This is true with pure antagonists, such as naloxone, or with

Table 23.5 Epidural opioid side effects

Side effects	Frequency	Treatment
Respiratory depression	Rare: <0.2%	Naloxone bolus followed by infusion
Pruritus	20%–60%	Mild: antihistamines Moderate: systemic nalbuphine, 1–3 mg Severe: naloxone infusion Reduced with infusions, lipid-soluble drugs
Nausea	6%–50%	Mild: antiemetics Moderate: opioid antagonist
Urinary retention	4%–40%	Indwelling catheter

agonist-antagonists, such as nalbuphine, which has been used in doses of 1 to 3 mg intravenously or 10 mg subcutaneously to relieve these symptoms.

3. **Nausea** is less common, but also disturbing to the patient.
   a. Symptomatic treatment with any of the common antiemetic drugs is useful
   b. A low-dose antagonist or agonist-antagonist is also appropriate.
4. **Urinary retention** is the other troublesome side effect and, unfortunately, is not readily reversed with antagonist therapy. Without good justification, many postsurgical patients treated with epidural opioids are simultaneously treated with an indwelling bladder catheter until the opioid infusion is halted.
5. **Infection** at the site of catheter placement is not a common problem. Epidural analgesia can be continued for several days or weeks, as long as the original dressing was placed in an aseptic manner and is monitored daily.
6. **Epidural hematoma** is a rare but major complication. The performance of epidural injections (or removal of catheters) should be considered carefully in the presence of coagulation abnormalities. If there is any concern about the possibility of hematoma formation, it is best to remove any local anesthetic from the epidural infusion (to remove any ambiguity about motor weakness) and to institute evaluations of motor function every 2 hours (see Chapter 7).
7. **Inadequate analgesia** is an occasional problem, especially when low doses are chosen for the elderly or ''standard'' doses are used for young vigorous patients. When using epidural analgesic infusions:
   a. A bolus injection of fentanyl (50–100 μg) or of the infusion solution itself will usually improve the analgesia for a few hours, but the basic infusion rate must be increased if a continued improvement in analgesia is desired.
   b. If repeated boluses and rate increases do not improve analgesia, the efficacy of the epidural catheter should be tested by injection of 5 to 10 mL 1.5% lidocaine or 2% chloroprocaine. This will usually produce analgesia for 2 hours and confirm that the catheter is in the appropriate location.
   c. The most difficult patients to treat in this regard are those who have been habituated to opioid drugs preoperatively, and therefore have a higher tolerance and perhaps even dependence. In this situation, increasing the opioid dose or the use of a more potent opioid in the epidural space may be helpful (53). Another alternative is to use an epidural infusion of local anesthetic alone and provide the patient with an IV PCA of opioid to provide them with the ''reassuring'' signs of systemic effects, while allowing them to titrate to a level that meets their needs.

V. Outcome

All of the methods described, especially epidural opioid infusions, require some increased effort and imply some assumption of additional risks. It is important to place the use of regional techniques for postoperative analgesia in an **appropriate risk–benefit perspective**.

A. Despite the risks of side effects and the effort involved, the use of epidural infusions of local anesthetics and opioids for postoperative analgesia has been shown to improve patient outcome in several significant areas.

1. **Superior pain relief**, especially dynamic pain after thoracotomy and upper abdominal procedures (12,24–26).
2. **Postoperative respiratory complications** are less frequent (55).
3. **Return of bowel function** is more rapid (42).
4. The usual hypercoaguable state of the perioperative period is reversed, leading to fewer complications with vascular grafts (56) and a reduction in **thromboembolic complications** (57).
5. There is a trend toward reduction in the hormonal stress response to surgery (54) including a reduction in catecholamine release (58), which may be related to a trend to reduced **cardiac complications** (54).
6. In high-risk groups prone to cardiac ischemia, data also confirms that optimal pain relief provided by epidural analgesia leads to a reduction in **cardiac morbidity** (59).
7. Some evidence that use of optimal epidural analgesic regimens may reduce the potential for the development of **chronic postoperative pain states** (60).

B. Peripheral nerve blockade also confers advantages in pain relief and in **rehabilitation**. With this growing body of data, it appears that the benefits of the analgesic regimens discussed here are significant, and merit use of these techniques.

VI. Acute pain service

A. The use of these modalities is obviously complex and usually requires the creation of a **dedicated anesthesia pain service** (5). Overall, the institutions that have instituted the pain service have found that it offers significant advantages to the patients in their postoperative coverage.

B. **Major challenges** of acute pain service include:

1. **Education of nursing personnel and surgeons** about the limitations and complications of the therapies described is vital.
2. **Expert coverage is also required** to modify the dosages with these techniques and handle the unusual complications and, especially, the technical problems when epidural or peripheral nerve catheters appear to malfunction. These problems require that an experienced team of anesthesiologists be available on a 24-hour basis. This service requires the commitment by the anesthesia staff and, in larger hospitals, often requires a continuous in-house presence. It has been possible to provide coverage for pain services by at-home call in smaller community hospitals, but this requires intensive education of all the nursing staff and a thorough set of standing orders to cover eventualities. Ideally, this team will round at least twice a day on the pain patients and be readily available for consultation.
3. An essential component of the service is the **development of standing orders** that provide clear guidelines to ward staff about recognition and initial management of the complications and side effects discussed earlier. The use of standard protocols for administration of continuous analgesics is also helpful, as well as a set of standing orders for management of complications. The standing orders should specifically include the appropriate respiratory monitoring and the authorization for the nursing staff on the floor to initiate treatment (usually with naloxone) before the arrival of the pain team for evaluation.

C. The work of a pain service is greatly enhanced if a **nurse specialist** is included. This person is helpful in educating and supporting ward nurses, as well as in providing a more constant and consistent level of patient care.

REFERENCES

1 Ferrante FM, VadeBoncouer TR. *Postoperative pain management.* Philadelphia: WB Saunders, 1993.
2 Macintyre PE, Schug S. *Acute pain management.* Philadelphia: WB Saunders, 2007.
3 Rawal N, Jones RM, Aitkenhead AR. *Management of acute and chronic pain.* London: BMJ Publishing, 1998.
4 Hadzic A. *Textbook of regional anesthesia and acute pain management.* McGraw-Hill, 2007.
5 Ready LB, Oden R, Chadwick HS, et al. Development of an anesthesiology-based postoperative pain management service. *Anesthesiology* 1988;68:100.
6 White PF, Kehlet H. Improving pain management: are we jumping from the frying pan into the fire? *Anesth Analg* 2007;105(1):10–12.
7 Brennan F, Carr DB, Cousins M. Pain management: a fundamental human right. *Anesth Analg* 2007;105: 205–221.
8 Etches RC. Respiratory depression associated with patient-controlled analgesia: a review of eight cases. *Can J Anaesth* 1994;41:125.
9 Macintyre PE. Safety and efficacy of patient-controlled analgesia. *Br J Anaesth* 2001;87:36.
10 Hudcova J, McNicol E, Quah C, et al. Patient controlled opioid analgesia versus conventional opioid analgesia for postoperative pain. *Cochrane Database Syst Rev* 2006;(4):CD003348.
11 Stein C, Comisel K, Haimerl E, et al. Analgesic effect of intraarticular morphine after arthroscopic knee surgery. *N Engl J Med* 1991;325:1123.
12 Kavanagh BP, Katz J, Sandler AN. Pain control after thoracic surgery. A review of current techniques. *Anesthesiology* 1994;81:737.
13 Richman JM, Liu SS, Courpas G, et al. Does continuous peripheral nerve block provide superior pain control to opioids? A meta-analysis. *Anesth Analg* 2006;102:248–257.
14 Ilfeld BM, Enneking FK. Continuous peripheral nerve blocks at home: a review. *Anesth Analg* 2005;100: 1822–1833.
15 McCartney CJ, Duggan E, Apatu E. Should we add clonidine to local anesthetic for peripheral nerve blockade? A qualitative systematic review of the literature. *Reg Anesth Pain Med* 2007;32(4):330–338.
16 Salinas FV, Liu SS, Mulroy MF. The effect of single-injection femoral nerve block versus continuous femoral nerve block after total knee arthroplasty on hospital length of stay and long-term functional recovery within an established clinical pathway. *Anesth Analg* 2006;102(4):1234–1239.
17 Ilfeld BM, Gearen PF, Enneking FK, et al. Total hip arthroplasty as an overnight-stay procedure using an ambulatory continuous psoas compartment nerve block: a prospective feasibility study. *Reg Anesth Pain Med* 2006;31(2):113–118.
18 Ilfeld BM, Gearen PF, Enneking FK, et al. Total knee arthroplasty as an overnight-stay procedure using continuous femoral nerve blocks at home: a prospective feasibility study. *Anesth Analg* 2006;102(1): 87–90.
19 Wiegel M, Gottschaldt U, Hennebach R, et al. Complications and adverse effects associated with continuous peripheral nerve blocks in orthopedic patients. *Anesth Analg* 2007;104(6):1578–1582.
20 Swenson JD, Bay N, Loose E, et al. Outpatient management of continuous peripheral nerve catheters placed using ultrasound guidance: an experience in 620 patients. *Anesth Analg* 2006;103:1436–1443.
21 Offerdahl MR, Lennon RL, Horlocker TT. Successful removal of a knotted fascia iliaca catheter: principles of patient positioning for peripheral nerve catheter extraction. *Anesth Analg* 2004;99(5):1550–1552.
22 Cousins MJ, Mather LE. Intrathecal and epidural administration of opioids. *Anesthesiology* 1984;61:276.
23 Wheatley RG, Schug SA, Watson D. Safety and efficacy of postoperative epidural analgesia. *Br J Anaesth* 2001;87:47.
24 Liu S, Carpenter RL, Neal JM. Epidural anesthesia and analgesia. Their role in postoperative outcome. *Anesthesiology* 1995;82:1474.
25 Wu CL, Cohen SR, Richman JM, et al. Efficacy of postoperative patient-controlled and continuous infusion epidural analgesia versus intravenous patient-controlled analgesia with opioids: a meta-analysis. *Anesthesiology* 2005;103(5):1079–1088.
26 Block BM, Liu SS, Rowlingson AJ, et al. Efficacy of postoperative epidural analgesia: a meta-analysis. *J Am Med Assoc* 2003;290(18):2455–2463.
27 Ready LB, Chadwick HS, Ross B. Age predicts effective epidural morphine dose after abdominal hysterectomy. *Anesth Analg* 1987;66:1215.
28 Dahl JB, Rosenberg J, Hansen BL, et al. Differential analgesic effects of low-dose epidural morphine and morphine-bupivacaine at rest and during mobilization after major abdominal surgery. *Anesth Analg* 1992;74(3):362–365.

29 Liu SS, Allen HW, Olsson GL. Patient-controlled epidural analgesia with bupivacaine and fentanyl on hospital wards: prospective experience with 1,030 surgical patients. *Anesthesiology* 1998;88:688.
30 Ummenhofer WC, Arends RH, Shen DD, et al. Comparative spinal distribution and clearance kinetics of intrathecally administered morphine, fentanyl, alfentanil, and sufentanil. *Anesthesiology* 2000;92:739.
31 de Leon-Casasola OA, Lema MJ. Postoperative epidural opioid analgesia: what are the choices? *Anesth Analg* 1996;83:867.
32 Peng PW, Sandler AN. A review of the use of fentanyl analgesia in the management of acute pain in adults. *Anesthesiology* 1999;90:576.
33 Ginosar Y, Riley ET, Angst MS. The site of action of epidural fentanyl in humans: the difference between infusion and bolus administration. *Anesth Analg* 2003;97(5):1428–1438.
34 Scott DA, Beilby DS, McClymont C. Postoperative analgesia using epidural infusions of fentanyl with bupivacaine. A prospective analysis of 1,014 patients. *Anesthesiology* 1995;83:727.
35 Chaplan SR, Duncan SR, Brodsky JB, et al. Morphine and hydromorphone epidural analgesia. A prospective, randomized comparison. *Anesthesiology* 1992;77:1090.
36 Liu S, Carpenter RL, Mulroy MF, et al. Intravenous versus epidural administration of hydromorphone. Effects on analgesia and recovery after radical retropubic prostatectomy. *Anesthesiology* 1995;82:682.
37 Paech MJ, Moore JS, Evans SF. Meperidine for patient-controlled analgesia after cesarean section. Intravenous versus epidural administration. *Anesthesiology* 1994;80:1268.
38 Rathmell JP, Lair TR, Nauman B. The role of intrathecal drugs in the treatment of acute pain. *Anesth Analg* 2005;101(Suppl 5):S30–S43.
39 Murphy PM, Stack D, Kinirons B, et al. Optimizing the dose of intrathecal morphine in older patients undergoing hip arthroplasty. *Anesth Analg* 2003;97:1709–1715.
40 de Leon-Casasola OA, Parker B, Lema MJ, et al. Postoperative epidural bupivacaine-morphine therapy. Experience with 4,227 surgical cancer patients. *Anesthesiology* 1994;81:368.
41 Solomon RE, Gebhart GF. Synergistic antinociceptive interactions among drugs administered to the spinal cord. *Anesth Analg* 1994;78:1164.
42 Steinbrook RA. Epidural anesthesia and gastrointestinal motility. *Anesth Analg* 1998;86:837.
43 Jorgensen H, Wetterslev J, Moiniche S, et al. Epidural local anaesthetics versus opioid-based analgesic regimens on postoperative gastrointestinal paralysis, PONV and pain after abdominal surgery. *Cochrane Database Syst Rev* 2000;(4):CD001893.
44 Hodgson PS, Liu SS. A comparison of ropivacaine with fentanyl to bupivacaine with fentanyl for postoperative patient-controlled epidural analgesia. *Anesth Analg* 2001;92:1024.
45 Senard M, Joris JL, Ledoux D, et al. A comparison of 0.1% and 0.2% ropivacaine and bupivacaine combined with morphine for postoperative patient-controlled epidural analgesia after major abdominal surgery. *Anesth Analg* 2002;95(2):444–449.
46 Curatolo M, Schnider TW, Petersen-Felix S, et al. A direct search procedure to optimize combinations of epidural bupivacaine, fentanyl, and clonidine for postoperative analgesia. *Anesthesiology* 2000;92:325.
47 Brodner G, Van Aken H, Hertle L, et al. Multimodal perioperative management combining thoracic epidural analgesia, forced mobilization, and oral nutrition reduces hormonal and metabolic stress and improves convalescence after major urologic surgery. *Anesth Analg* 2001;92:1594.
48 Dahl V, Raeder JC. Non-opioid postoperative analgesia. *Acta Anaesthesiol Scand* 2000;44:1191.
49 Tiippana EM, Hamunen K, Kontinen VK, et al. Do surgical patients benefit from perioperative gabapentin/pregabalin? A systematic review of efficacy and safety. *Anesth Analg* 2007;104(6):1545–1556.
50 Woolf CJ, Chong MS. Preemptive analgesia treating postoperative pain by preventing the establishment of central sensitization. *Anesth Analg* 1993;77:362.
51 Ong CK, Lirk P, Seymour RA, et al. The efficacy of preemptive analgesia for acute postoperative pain management: a meta-analysis. *Anesth Analg* 2005;100(3):757–773.
52 Ready LB, Loper KA, Nessly M, et al. Postoperative epidural morphine is safe on surgical wards. *Anesthesiology* 1991;75:452.
53 de Leon-Casasola OA. Postoperative pain management in opioid-tolerant patients. *Reg Anesth* 1996;21:114.
54 Kehlet H, Holte K. Effect of postoperative analgesia on surgical outcome. *Br J Anaesth* 2001;87:62.
55 Ballantyne JC, Carr DB, deFerranti S, et al. The comparative effects of postoperative analgesic therapies on pulmonary outcome: cumulative meta-analyses of randomized, controlled trials. *Anesth Analg* 1998;86:598.
56 Christopherson R, Beattie C, Frank SM, et al. Perioperative Ischemia Randomized Anesthesia Trial Study Group. Perioperative morbidity in patients randomized to epidural or general anesthesia for lower extremity vascular surgery. *Anesthesiology* 1993;79:422.
57 Rodgers A, Walker N, Schug S, et al. Reduction of postoperative mortality and morbidity with epidural or spinal anaesthesia: results from overview of randomised trials. *Br Med J* 2000;321:1493.

58 Breslow MJ, Parker SD, Frank SM, et al. The PIRAT Study Group. Determinants of catecholamine and cortisol responses to lower extremity revascularization. *Anesthesiology* 1993;79:1202.
59 Beattie WS, Badner NH, Choi P. Epidural analgesia reduces postoperative myocardial infarction: a meta-analysis. *Anesth Analg* 2001;93:853–858.
60 Perkins FM, Kehlet H. Chronic pain as an outcome of surgery. A review of predictive factors. *Anesthesiology* 2000;93:1123.

Index

Note: Page numbers followed by f indicate figures; those followed by t indicate tables.